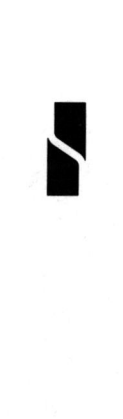

How to Divide

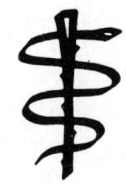

Over
Twenty-five
Thousand Words
in Common Usage
Showing
Their Spellings
and
Combinations into
Syllables

Medical Words

By RICHARD V. LEE, M.D.

And DORIS J. HOFER

SOUTHERN ILLINOIS UNIVERSITY PRESS
Carbondale and Edwardsville

Feffer & Simons, Inc.
London and Amsterdam

Contents

Apologia

WITHIN the last few years we have been somewhat peripherally involved in a very fine educational and training program of S.I.U.'s Vocational and Technical Institute, designed to produce medical secretaries. During a portion of this training program, students have been assigned a work experience within one of the medical departments of the university. In this supervisory capacity we constantly encountered the pragmatic usefulness of such secretarial aids as *20,000 Words* (Louis A. Leslie [New York: McGraw-Hill, 1965]) and *Word Division* (Supplement to Government Printing Office Style Manual, 1962) as they relate to secretarial work generally, and deplored the absence of such an aid more specifically related to the kind of transcription and dictation expected of those in the many fields of medicine. We sincerely hope this aid answers to what we perceived as a need.

In designing the format, we felt generic, chemical, and trade names of drugs and medications could be usefully combined, and they in turn kept separate from the main text of words. Trade names are identified beginning with capital letters, and like other proper names, are not to be divided.

We wish to express our deep and sincere appreciation to Misses Janet Gibson, Priscilla Beard, and Simin Bahmanyar, students themselves, without whose assistance with the manuscript this effort would yet be incomplete.

It is to you, however, who have use of this aid—you who regularly toil amidst the frustrations of incoherent dictation, compound words and descriptive terminology stemming from the Greek, Latin, Arabic, French, Anglo-Saxon, and other cultures, ancient and modern—that this work is most affectionately dedicated.

THE AUTHORS

Southern Illinois University
October 1971

Drugs and Medications

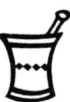

A

A-Caps
A-C Troches
A-C-D Solution
A.C.N.
ACTH
A and D Cream
A and D Hemorrhoidal
    Suppositories
A and D Ointment
A D C Drops
A-D-R Capsules
A.E.A. Tablets
AMO Sulfa Tablets
AMO Tabs
A-M-T
A.N.R.
A. P. Forte
A.P.L.
A.R.D. Anoperineal
    Pads
A.S.A.
A.S.A. Compounds
A.S.A. & Codeine
AVC Cream
AVC Cream w/Dien-
    estrol
AVC Suppositories
Aasquel
Abdec Drops
Abdol w/Minerals
Accelerase
Accelerase-PB
Acedoval Tablets
Acedyne Tablets
acenocoumarin
Acetabar
acetaminophen

Acetated Ringer's
acetazolamide
acetic acid
Aceto-Cort
acetohexamide
acetone
acetophenazine maleate
acetphenolisatin
Acetycol
acetylcarbromal
acetylcholine
acetylcysteine
acetyldigitoxin
Achrocidin Tablets
Achromycin
Achromycin V
Achrostatin V
Acid Mantle Creme
Acidolate
Acidol-Pepsin
Acidulin
Aci-Jel
Acitamin
Acna-Flage
Acnaveen
Acne-Aid Cream
Acne-Aid Detergent
    Soap
Acne-Cort-Dome Creme
Acnederm
Acne-Dome
Acnestrol
Acnomel Cream
Acogesic
Acon Capsules
acrisorcin
Acrobolic Tablets
Actasal Pediatric
    Drops
Actest Gel
Acthar
Actidil

Actifed
Actifed-C
Activol Liquid Soap
Actol Solution
Acutuss
Acylanid
Adabee
Adacal w/Fluoride
Adalan Lanatabs
Ad-Cebrin Drops
Ade Tablets
Adeflor B Drops
Adeflor Chewable
Adeflor Drops
Adeflor M Tablets
Adeno Twelve
Adenocrest
Adenolin Forte
adenosine
    5-monophosphate
Adenotinate
Ade-Vet
Adhesivease
Adipex Ty-Med
adiphenine hydro-
    chloride
Adipo Tablets
Adjudets
Ad-Nil #2
Adrenalin
Adrenalin in Oil
Adrenalin Solution
Adrenatrate
adrenocorticotropic
    hormone
Adrenosem Salicylate
Adrestat
Adrocaine Solution
Adroyd Tablets
Advicin Cream
Aeroderm Lotion
Aerohalor

Aerolate Sr. & Jr.
Aerolone Compound
Aeroplast Dressing
Aeroseb-HC
Aerosept
Aerosporin
A-Fil
Aflus Suspension & Tablets
Aflus-P Tablets
Afrin
Afrodex
Agoral
Akalon-T '5'
Akineton
Akrinol Cream
Alacta
Aladrine Tablets
Alamine
Alamine-C
Alamine Expectorant
Alased
Ala-Trist
Al-ay Tablets
Albamycin
Albasulphidi Lotion
albumin
Albuspan
Alcopara Dispersible Granules
Aldactazide
Aldactone
Aldiazol-M
Aldoclor
Aldomet
Aldonnal
Aldoril
Alepsal
Alertonic
Alevaire
Algic
Algoson

Alidase
Alkagestabs
Alkaline Cordial
Alkaopectin
Alka-Phen
Alkarau
Alka-Seltzer
Alkatabs
alkavervir
Alkeran
Alkets
allantoin
Allbee-T
Allbee w/C Capsules
Allercaf
Allercreme
Allerdon
Allerest
allergenic extracts
Allergex
Allergyl Tablets
Allernix
Allersone
Allerspan
allobarbital
allopurinol
Allpyral
Allylgesic
Allylgesic w/Ergotamine
Alma-Tar Bath
Almay Hypo-Allergenic
Almebex Plus
Almediol
Almeret '1000'
Almetropin
Almetussin
Almezyme
Almocarpine
Almora
Alophen
Alo-Tuss
Aloxed

Alpen
Alpha Chymar
Alphadrol
Alpha-Keri
Alphalin Gelseals
Alphamin
Alphamul
alphaprodine hydrochloride
Alpha-Ruvite
Alpha-T
Alphosyl Lotion
Alprine BiTabs
alseroxylon
Alsical Powder
Alteryn Injection
Alucen
Aludrox
Alumadrine
alumina (fused)
aluminum acetate
aluminum hydroxide
aluminum hydroxide gel
aluminum nicotinate
aluminum potassium sulfate
aluminum sulfate
Alupec
Alurate
Aluscop
alverine citrate
Alvinine Shampoo
Al Vite
Alvodine
Alysine Elixir
Alzem Spray
Alzinox
Amalgin
amantadine hydrochloride
Amaril "D" Spancap

4

Amaril Spancap
Amatrol
Ambar
Ambenyl
Ambodryl
Ambot Vials
ambutonium bromide
Amcill
Amcill Chewables
Amcill-S
Amephytal
Americaine
Amerital
Amerotol Ear Drops
Amertan Jelly
Amesec
Amex
Amfrecin Douche
Amgesic
Amicar
Amid-Sal
Amilixir
Aminabel
aminacrine
Aminet Suppositories
amino acid
9-amino acridine
Amino Hep Injectable
aminoacetic acid
aminobenzoic acid
aminocaproic acid
Amino-Cerv
Aminodrox
Aminodrox-Forte
Aminodur Dura-Tabs
Aminoform-Sr.
    Suppositories
Aminophyllin
    Supposicones
aminophylline
Aminophylline &
    Amytal

aminosalicylate sodium
aminosalicylic acid
Aminosol 5% Solution
Aminyl Liquid
amitriptyline
    hydrochloride
Amlax Tablets
Ammens Medicated
    Powder
Ammonia Aromatic
ammonium chloride
ammonium-quaternary
Amnestrogen
amobarbital
amobarbital sodium
Amobile
Amocillin
Amocine
Amo-Derm
Amodex Junior
Amodex Tablets
Amodex Timed Capsules
Amo-Dextrosule Sr.
Amodin
Amodin-A
Amodin-Plus
Amodril Spancap
Amodril Tablets
Amodrine
Amoebicon
Amogel
Amogel P.G.
Amogel Plus
Amohist
Amolate
Amonidrin
AmORdex
Amosan
Amosene Tablets
Amostat T.D.
Amozar
Ampelose

Ampha-Caps
Amphaplex
Amphedase
Amphene
Amphenol
amphetamine
amphetamine sulfate
Amphicol
Amphojel
Amphone
Amphor
amphotericin B
ampicillin
ampicillin trihydrate
Amplex
Ampyrox
Amril
Amsed
Amsed Spancap
Amsed T.D.
Amsodyne
Amsustain
Amtet
Amurex
Amvicel
Amvicel-X
Am-Vite
Amyl Nitrite
a-Amylase
amylolytic enzyme
Amyospasmol
Amytal
Amytal Sodium
Am-Zyme
Anabolin
Anachloric A
Analbalm
Analeptone
Analgesine
Analgesine-MN
Analgestine
Analsedine

Analucin
Analval
Anamine
Anamine T.D.
Ananase
Anaphen
Anasorb
Anatola
Anatuss
Anavac
Anavar
And-Est
Andesterone
Andoin
Andrestraq
Andriol
Andro L.A. Injectable
Andro Medicone
Andro "50"
Andro "100"
androgens
Androgyn
Androgyn L. A.
Android
Android E
Android-H.B.
Android Plus
Android X
Androlin
Andronaq-25
Andronaq-50
Anectine
Anergex
Anestacon
Anesthone
Anexsia-D
Anexsia w/Codeine
Angio-CONRAY
angiotensin amide
Anhydron
Anhydron K
Anhydron KR

anisotropine
   methylbromide
Anizol
Anodynos
Anodynos-DHC
Anodynos Forte
Anovo
Ansemco
Ansolysen
Antabuse
antazoline phosphate
Antepar
anterior pituitary
Anthra-Derm
anthralin
anthraquinone
Anthryl
Anthryl 5X
Anti-Hemophilus
anti-hemophilus
   influenzae
antihistamine
Antime
Anti-Nausea Supprettes
Antirabies Serum
Anti-Rust Tablets
Antistine phosphate
Anti-Tussive
antivenin (crotalidae)
   polyvalent
Antivenin Lyovac
Antivenin Polyvalent
Antivert
Antora
Antora-B
Antora-H
Antrenyl
Antrin
Antrocol
Antuitrin-S
Anturane
Antussal Syrup

Anucaine
Anugesic
Anusol
Anusol-HC
Apac
Apamide
Apatate
ApORvite
Appetrol
Appetrol-S.R.
Apresoline
Apresoline-Esidrix
Aprisac
aprobarbital
AP-Sub Tablets
Apyrexin
Aquabarb Supprettes
Aquachloral
Aquacort
Aquadiol
Aqua-Ivy
Aqualin
Aqualin-Plus
Aquamin
Aquamul HC
Aquasol A
Aquasol E
Aquatag
Aralen
Aralen Hydrochloride
Aralen Phosphate
Aramine
Aranthol
Arazem
Arbon
Arcofac
Arco-Lase
Arcoret
Arcotinic
Arcylate
Arda Timed Capsules
Ar-Ex Hypo-Allergenic

6

Argyrol
Aridose
Aristocort
Aristogesic
Aristomin
Aristospan
Arithmin
Arlidin
Armour Thyroid
Arovite LF
Artane
Arteril
Arthralgen
Arthralgen-PR
Arthripred
Arthrolate
Arthropan
artificial tears
Arvette
Asbron
As-Ca-Phen
Asco Solu Caps
Asco Tablets
Ascodeen-30
Ascoramide
ascorbic acid
Ascorbicap
Ascorbo-Thiamine
    Compound
Ascorbuf
Ascriptin
A-Sec Supprettes
Asmabar
Asmacol
Asmadil Unicelles
Asmakets
Asmerol
Asminorel
Asminyl
Asmolin
Asphac-G
Asphamal-D

Asphates
Aspir-B
aspirin
Aspirin Aluminum
Aspirin Supprettes
Aspirocal
Aspodyne
Aspred-C Kotinated
Asthmacon
Asthma Meter Mist
Astrafer
Astrovite
Astrovite-F
Atabrine
Atarax
Ataraxoid
Athemol
Athemol-N
A-3 Foot Powder
Athrombin-K
Atoka
Atrobarbital
Atrobar-M
Atrobyl
Atrocholin
Atromid-S
atropine
Atropisol
attapulgite
Attenuvax Lyovac
Atussin-D.M.
Atussin Expectorant
Aura-Bell Liquid
Aural Acute
Auralgan
Aural-O1 Improved
Aureomycin
Auristil Dropules
Aurol Otic
aurothioglucose
Autoplex
Autozyme

Avazyme
Avcen Vaginal Cleanser
Aveeno-Bar
Aveeno Colloidal
    Oatmeal
Aveeno Lotion
Aveeno Oilated
Aveeno Ointment
Avenol Bath
Aventyl
Avlosulfon
Axotal
Ayrcap S.R.
Azironal
Azlidon
Azlimed
Azlytal
Azmadrine
Azo-Aflus-P
Azo Gantanol
Azo Gantrisin
Azolate
Azo-Mandelamine
Azomer
Azo Methalate
Azosul
Azo Sulfisoxazole
Azo-Sulfstat
Azo-Sulfurine
Azotrex
Azulfidine
azuresin

B

BAL in Oil
BCG Vaccine
B & O Supprettes
B_{12} Plus
Bacid Capsules

Baciguent
Bacimycin
bacitracin
Bacitracin Ointment
Bactine
Baculin Vaginal Tablets
B.A.-Graduals
Baker's Infant Formula
Baker's Ready-4
Balamin Gel
Balamin 1000
Balancel Forte
Balatrin
Balmex
Balneol
Balnetar
balsam Peru
Bamadex Sequels
Bamadex Tablets
Banalg
Banausea Tablets
Bancaps
Bancaps-C
Banesin Forte
Banthine
Barbatrin-Hexett
Barbatro
Barbel Graduals
Barbella
Barbeloid
Barbidonna
Barbipil
barbiturate
Barbtheo
Bar-Cy-A
Bar-Cy-Amine
Bardase
Bar-Don
Barhoma
Barnes-Hind
Barnes-Hind-Wetting
    Solution

Baroflave
Barosperse
Barotrast
Barphyllin
Barseb HC
Barseb Scalp Lotion
Bartime T. D.
Bartone
Bar-Tropin
Barval
Basaljel
Baselan
Basigets
Basigets Ultima
Bassoran
Baumodyne
Bayer Aspirin
BC-Vite
Beclysyl 5%
Becomco
Becoplex
Becotin
Becotin c̄ Vitamin C
Becotin-T
Becyte
Bedoce
Beesix Injectable
Bejectal
Bejex
Belakoids TT
Belap
Belap Ty-Med
Belbarb
Belbarbzyme
Belexal
Belfac
Belfer
Belkatal
Belladenal
belladonna
Belladonna Ergotamine
Bellafedrol AH

Bellafoline
Bellagrant
Bellaphen
Bellastal
Bellergal
Bellkatal
Bellophene
Beltiver
Belvedrox
Belvetin
Beminal-500
Beminal Forte
Bemotinic
benactyzine hydro-
    chloride
Benadex
Benadryl
Bena-Fedrin
Benasept
Benat w/B_{12}
Ben-Caine B-B
Bendectin
bendroflumethiazide
Benecap
Benemid
Benizol
Benizol Plus
Benoquin
Benoxyl
Bensulfoid
Bentyl Hydrochloride
Benylin Expectorant
benzalkonium chloride
Benzapas
Benzedrex
Benzedrine Sulfate
benzethonium chloride
benzocaine
benzoic acid
benzonatate
benzophenones
benzoyl peroxide

8

n' benzoylsulfanilamide
benzphetamine hydro-
    chloride
benzthiazide
benztropine mesylate
benzyl alcohol
Bēplete
Bēpron
Berocca
Berocca-C
Berubigen
Bescorbic
Besertal
Besta
Beta-Chlor
Betacrest
Betadine
Betadine Douche
Betadine Mouthwash
Betadine Ointment
betahistine hydro-
    chloride
betaine hydrochloride
Betaine-Inositol-
    Choline B_{12}
Betalin
Betalin Complex
Betalin Complex F.C.
Betalin S Ampoules
Betalin 12
betamethasone
betamethasone valerate
Betaprone
Betathiolin
Beta-Vite
bethanechol chloride
Bethiamin
Bevidox
Bewon
Bexar
Bexibee

Bexo-C
Bexomal
Bextral B_{12}
B-G-Phos
Biamin
Bicalpho In-A-Tab
Bicholate
Bicholax
Bicillin
Bicillin All-Purpose
Bicillin C-R
Bicillin P·A·B
Bidrox
Bidtinic
Bifacton
Biferone
Bifran
Bihistol
Bilamide
Bilate
Bilezyme
Bilezyme-Plus
Bilogen
Bilron
Binestro
Bintron
Biocalate
Bio-Crest
bioflavonoids
Bi-O-Kal
Biokets
Biomydrin
Biomydrin F Nasal Spray
Biomydrin Otic
Biosulfa
Biosynephrine
Biothesin
Biotran
Biotres
Biotres-HC
Bioxatphen
Biozyme

Biozyme-HC
biperiden
Bi-Phene
Biphetacel
Biphetamine
Biphetamine-T
bisacodyl
Bisceral
bishydroxycoumarin
Bisilad
Bismakaolin
Bismapec
Bismosalicate
Bismuth
bismuth (anti-syphilitic)
Bismuth Cevitamate
bismuth crystal violet
Bismuth & Paregoric
bismuth subcarbonate
bismuth subgallate
bismuth subnitrate
Bismuth Violet
Bistrimate
Bitrate
Bitrinsic-E
Bivalent Botulism
    Antitoxin
B-K-P Mixture
B-K-Z Tablets
black widow spider
    antivenin (equine)
Blandlube
blastomycin
Blemak Lotion
Blexcon
Blinx
Blockain Hydrochloride
    Injection
Bluboro
B-Nutron
Bonacal Plus
Bonadoxin

Bonatabs
Bonazin
Bon-Du Powder
Bonine
Bonmiotin
Bontril
boric acid
Bornate
Borofax
borotannic complex
botulism antitoxin
Boules Quies Ear Plugs
B-Plex
Brāsivol
Bremil
Brevital
Bristacycline I.V.
Bro-B, B-Complex
Bro-Bexin 6/50
Brohembione
Bro-Lac Sterile
bromelains
bromide
Bromide & Chloral
    Hydrate
bromisovalum
Bromo Quinine
brompheniramine
    maleate
Bromsulphalein
Bromul
Bromural
Bronchobid Duracap
Bronchohist
Broncholin
Brondecon
Brondilate
Bronesina
Bronkephrine
Bronkolixir
Bronkometer
Bronkosol

Bronkotabs
Bronkotabs-Hafs
Bron-Sed
Bro-Parin
Brucellergen
Brucellin
B-Scorbic
B-Tropic
Bubarbital
Buchu-Methenamine
Bucladin
Buclamase
buclizine hydrochloride
Budon
Bufazo Solu Caps
Buff-A
Buff-A Comp
Buff-A #2
Buffadyne
Buffagesic Tablets
Buffer Solution
Buffered Parasal
Buffered Parasal-INH
Bufferin
Buffonamide
Bufosal
Bufosal-K
Buren Tablets
Buro-Sol
Burowets
Burow's solution
Burrizem
Bur-Veen Wet Dressing
busulfan
butabarbital
Butabell HMB
Butacalm
Butadeine
Butagem
Butagesic
butalbital
Butalix

Butamin
Butapap
butperazine maleate
Butasaron
Butatran
Butatrax
Butatrope
Butazem
Butazolidin
Butesin Picrate
Butibel
Butibel R-A
Butibel-Zyme
Buticaps
Butigetic Repeat Action
Butiserpazide
Butiserpine
Butiserpine R-A
Butisol Sodium
Butisol Sodium R-A
Butizide
Butseco
Butyn Metaphen
Butyn Sulfate
Butyn Sulfate &
    Metaphen
butyrophenone

C

C.G. Chorionic
    Gonadotropin
C M
C M w/Paregoric
C.M.R. Tablets
C.P.H.
C.R.C.
C Speridin
C & T
C.V.P.

C.V.P. w/Vitamin K
C Z O
Cafaryl
CaFe w/Folic Acid
Cafergot
Cafergot P-B
caffeine
Cafrose
Caladryl
calamine
Calathesin
Calcabex
Calcicaps
Calcid Tablets
Calcide Tablets
Calcidin
Calcidrine
calciferol
Calcinatal
Calcisalin
Calcitinic Tablets
calcium acetate
calcium aminosalicylate
calcium ascorbate
calcium bis-(dioctyl
    sulfosuccinate)
calcium carbaspirin
calcium carbonate
Calcium Carbonate,
    Aromatic
Calcium Disodium
    Versenate
calcium gluconate
calcium gluconogalac-
    togluconate
calcium glycerophos-
    phate
calcium iodide
calcium lactate
Calcium Leucovorin
calcium pantothenate

calcium phosphate, di-
    basic
calcium-protein
calcium thiosulfate
Calciwafers
Caldecort
Caldesene
Caldin
Caleate Z/M
Calferbee
Calferbee Lactate
Calfer-Vite
Calfos-D
Calidro
Calinate
Calinate FA
Calmaphine
Calmative-Analgesic
Cal-O-B
Calodex
Caloxide
Calphosan
Calphosan B_{12}
Cal-Prenal
Cal-Ron O.B.
Calsamate
Calsarbain
Calscorbate
Caltase
Calurin
Calverol
Cal-Zo Ointment
Camirol
Camoform Hydro-
    chloride
Camollient
Camoquin
Campho-Phenique
camphor
Camphor & Soap Lini-
    ment
Camusol

Candeptin Vaginal
candicidin
cantharidin
Cantharone
Cantil
Capa
Capas
Capiloid
Capla
Caplaril
Ca-PLUS
Capré
Capré FLOR
Caprylium Vaginal
Capsebon
Capsolin
15-90 Capsules
Caquin
caramiphen edisylate
carbamazepine
carbamide
Carbamiotin
Carbanesin
Carbarsone
Carbased
carbazochrome salicylate
carbetapentane tannate
carbinoxamine maleate
Carbocaine
Carbo-Cort Creme
carbohydrates
carboxymethylcellulose
    sodium
carboxyphen
Carbrital
carbromal
Carbropent
Carcholin
Cardalin
Cardalin-Phen
Cardamom Compound
Cardenz

11

Cardilate
Cardilate-P
Cardiografin
Cardio-Green
Cardioquin
Cardrase
Carfusin
Carica-Bile
Caripeptic
carisoprodol
Cari-Tab Softab
Caroid & Bile Salts
Carrhist
Carrhist Forte T.D.
Carrtime
Carrtinic
Carrvite
Cartussin
Cartussin-NN Syrup
Cartrax
Casafru
Casakol
Casa-Laud
casanthranol
casanthrol
cascara sagrada
Casec
Cas-Evac
Castaderm
castor oil
Casyllium
Causalin
C-B Time Capsules
C-B Time Liquid
C-Bex Tablets
Cebefortis
Cebenase
Cebetinic
Cebo-Caps
Cebro Tablets
Cebrogen
Cebromone

Cebrovas
Cebum Shampoo
Cecon Dulcet
Cecon Solution
Ce-De-Flor
Cedilanid
Cedilanid-D
Ceebec
Celestone
Cell-O-Dex
cellulase
cellulolytic enzyme
cellulose, oxidized
Celmol
Celontin
Cenac for Her
Cenac for Him
Cenagesic
Cenalene
Cenalene-M
Cenamal
Cenasert
Cendex
Cendexal
Cenolate
Ceo-Two Suppositories
Cepacol
Cephalgesic
cephaloridine
cephalothin
Cerebro-Nicin
Ceremia Tablets
Cerespan
Cer-O-Cillin
Cerose
Cerose Compound
Cerose-DM
Cer-O-Strep
Cerumenex Drops
cervical caps
Cesul
Cetacort

Cetaphil
Cetazine
Cetazo
Cetro-Cirose
Cetyben
cetylpyridinium
   chloride
Cevalin
Cevatol
Cevipak
Cevirate
Ce-Vi-Sol
Chamo-Powder Packets
Charcoal w/Phenabel
Chardonna
Chemovag "Supps"
Chenatal
Chera Sulfa
Cheracol
Cheracol D
Cherri-B
Chew-Tinic
Chexit Tablets
Child-ron
Child's Drikof
Child's Ongestol
Child's Rhi-Lief
Chlo-Amine
chlophedianol hydro-
   chloride
chloral betaine
chloral hydrate
Chloral-Methylol
Chloramate
chlorambucil
chloramphenicol
chloramphenicol pal-
   mitate
chloramphenicol sodium
   succinate
Chlor-Anodyne
Chloraseptic

Chloraseptine
chlorcyclizine hydrochloride
chlordantoin
chlordiazepoxide
chlordiazepoxide hydrochloride
Chloresium
Chloretone
chlorhydroxyquinoline
chlormadinone acetate
chlormerodrin
chlormezanone
chloroform
Chlorohist
Chloromycetin
chlorophyll
chloroprocaine hydrochloride
chloroquine hydrochloride
chloroquine phosphate
Chloro-Salicylate
chlorothiazide
chlorotrianisene
Chlorotron
Chlorotron Spancap
chlorphenesin carbonate
chlorpheniramine
chlorpheniramine gluconate
chlorpheniramine maleate
chlorpheniramine resin
chlorpheniramine tannate
chlorphenoxamine
chlorphentermine hydrochloride
Chlorpred
chlorpromazine

chlorpromazine hydrochloride
chlorpropamide
chlorprothixene
chlorquinaldol
chlortetracycline
chlorthalidone
Chlor-Trimeton
Chlor-X
chlorzoxazone
Chobile
Chobile-Pan
Chocks
Cho-Free Formula Base
Cholan-DH
Cholan-HMB
Cholan-V
Cholarace
Chola-Zem
Choledyl
Cholelith
Choleo-Caps
cholera vaccine
choleretics
cholestyramine
Cholimeth
Cholinaz
choline bitartrate
choline dihydrogen citrate
choline theophyllinate
Chol* Cholografin
Cholorebic
Choloxin
Chorex
chorionic gonadotropin
Choritrope
Choron
Chromagen
Chronodial
Chymar

Chymolase
Chymoral
Chymotest
chymotrypsin
Chytryp
Cidicol
Cimadrox
Cinagill
Cinatabs
Cinbisal
cinnamates
Cinnasil Graduals
Cinnasil Tablets
cinoxate
Ciramine
Circavite T
Cirin
Citanest
Cithal
Citra
Citra Forte
Citralka
Citrasulfas
citric acid
Citrin
Citrocarbonate
Clara Ointment
Claratrate
Clarets
Clarnatal
Cledonal
clidinium bromide
Clistanal
Clistin
Clistin-D
Clistin R-A
Clocream
clofibrate
Clomid
clomiphene citrate
Clopane Hydrochloride
Clorpactin

13

Clusivets
Clusivol
Coagustat Injection
Cobalamed 100
Cobaldrox-12
Cobalin
Cobetaron
Cobroxin
Cocaine
coccidioidin
Coco-Diazine
Coco-Quinine
cod liver oil
Codalan
Codalex
codeine phosphate
codeine sulfate
Codel
Codempiral
Codenate A.H.
Codexin
Codexin-T
Codimal DH
Codimal PH
Codinets
Codistan
Coditrate
Co-Elorine 25
Co-Ferrin Hy-B
Cofron
Co-Gel
Cogentin
Cohema
Co-Iron
Colabee
Colace
cola syrup
ColBENEMID
colchicine
Colcylate
Coldate
Colicell

Colicon
colistimethate sodium
colistin sulfate
Colitussin
colloidal oatmeal
Collosul
Collyrium, Eye Lotion
Colo-Bar
Cologel
Colrex
Colsalide
Co-Lu-Gel
Co-Lu-Gel M-T
Columag
Col-Vi-Nol
Coly-Mycin M
Coly-Mycin S
Combahist
Combex
Combichole
Combid
Combi-Tuss
Combogenic
Combrion
Comēdad
Comfortine
Compazine
Compocillin-V
Compocillin-VK
Compren
Comycin
Conar
Conar-A
Conestron
Conex
Congespirin
Conjutabs
Conray
Conray-400
Consotuss
Contactisol
Contrablem

Contra-Creme
Contramal
Controlyte
Convertin
Convertin-H
Converzyme
Cool-Vapor Humidifers
Copavin
Cope
Coplexin
copper sulfate
Co-Pyronil
Coradyl
Coralsone
Coramine
Coraval
Cordex
Cordex-Forte
Cordran
Cordran-N
Coricidin
Coriforte
Corilin
Corobid
coronary vasodilators
Coro-nol
Corovas
Corovas Tymcaps
Corparex Meta-Kaps
Corparid Solu Caps
Cort-Acne Lotion
Cortalex
Cor-Tar-Quin Creme
Cor-Tar-Quin Forte
Cortate Pellets
Cort-Dome Creme
Cortef
Cortenema
cortex rhamni frangulae
Corticaine Cream
Corticloron
Cortigel-40

14

Cortigel-80
Cortinaq Injectable
Cortiprel
Cortisone
cortisone acetate
Cortisporin
Cortomixin
Cortone
Cort-Quin Creme
Cortril
Cortrophin Gel
Cortrophin-Zinc
Coryban-D
Coryza
Coryzaid
Coryzoil
Coryztime
Cosadein
Co-Salt
Cosanyl
Cosanyl-DM
Cosmegen
Cotazym
Cotazym-B
Cothera Compound
Co-Tinic
Cotton Syrup
cottonseed oil
Cotussis Syrup
CO-Tylenol
Coumadin
coumarin
Covanamine
Covangesic
Covap
Covermark
Covicone Cream
Covisten
Covite
Co-Xan
C-Quens
Cradol

Cremesone
Cremo-Carbonates
Cremomycin
Cremosuxidine
Cremothalidine
Creodol
Cresatin
Crestabolic Injection
Crestef
Cresterra
Crestinic
Cresylone
C-Ron
crotamiton
cryptenamine
cryptenamine tannate
Crysticillin A.S.
Crystifor 400
Crystivite
Crystodigin
Crystoids Anthelmintic
C-Tabs
Cube Pessaries
Cuemid Powder
Cuprimine
Curban-P
Curbetite
Cyadesine
Cyamine
Cyanest
cyanocobalamin
Cyanover
Cyclaine
cyclamate
Cyclamycin
cyclandelate
Cyclex
cyclizine
Cyclogesterin
Cyclogyl
cyclomethycaine
Cyclomydril

cyclopentamine hydro-
   chloride
cyclopentolate hydro-
   chloride
cyclophosphamide
cycloserine
Cyclospasmol
cyclothiazide
Cydril
Cynal
cyproheptadine hydro-
   chloride
cysteine
Cystitabs
Cystizem
Cystokon
Cystospaz
Cytal
Cyte
Cytellin
Cytobolin
Cytoferin
Cytomel
Cytora
Cytoxan
Cytran

D

D-11 T.D.
DBI
D.C.P. Tablets
D.C.P. 340
D.H.E. 45
D. P. T.
D V B-15
Daca
Dacriose
Dactil
Dactilase

Dainite Tablets
Dainite-KI
DaL Sinus Tablets
Dalex
Dalibour
Dalicote
Dalicreme
Daliderm
Dalidome
Dalidyne
Dalifort
Daligesic
Dalihist
Da-Li-Kaps
Dalimycin
Dalisept
Dalitabs
Dalivim
Dallergy
Danilone
Danivac
Danthro-Lax
danthron
Daprisal
Dapta
Dara Soapless Shampoos
Daranide
Daraprim
Darbid
Darcil
Daricon
Daricon PB
Daro Jr.
Daro Tablets
Dartal
Darvon
Darvon Compound
Darvon w/A.S.A.
Darvo-Tran
Dasikon
Dasin
Dasin-CS

Davoxin
Daxalan
Dayalets
Daylets-M
Dayamin
Dayteens
Day-Vite
DBI-TD
Deaner
Deanol
Debrox
Decadron
Deca-Durabolin
Decagesic
Decalbion
Decapryn
Deca-Vi-Flor
Deca-Vi-Sol
Decholin
Decholin w/Belladonna
Decholin-BB
Declofen
Declomycin
Declostatin
Declostatin 300
Deco-Disc
Decodult
Decogest
Decolate
Deconamine
Decostat
Decotussin
Dee-Caps
deferoxamine mesylate
Definate
Degest
Dehist
dehydrocholic acid
Deladumone
Deladumone OB
Delalutin
Delatestryl

Delavan Hand Creme
Delenar
Delestrogen
Delfen
Delkadon
Delomets
Delphicol
Delta-Cortef
Delta-Dome
Deltalin
Deltasmyl
Deltasone
Deltolate
Delta
Deluteval 2X
Delvinal
Demazin
Demerol
Demerol-APAP
demethylchlortetra-
 cycline
Denamone
Denol M/R
Dentafluor
Dentalgia
Dentalone
Dentavite
Depancol
Dep-Androle
Dep-Estrole
Depinar
Dep-Neutrole
Depo-ACTH
Depo-Cer-O-Cillin
Depo-Duomed
Depo-Estradiol
Depo-Estromed
Depogen
Depo-Heparin
Depo-Medrol
Depo-Penicillin
Depo-Provera

Depo-Testadiol
Depo-Testosterone
Depo-Testromed
Deprol
Derfule
Dergong
Dergong Forte
Derifil
Dermacid
Dermadram
Dermalac
Dermalotion HC
Dermal Rub
Derma Medicone
Derma Pack
Dermarex
Dermasulf
Derma 10
Dermatophytin
Dermatophytin "O"
Dermaval
Dermogen
Dermolate
Dermoplast
Dermovan
Deronil
Desabam
Desacholine
Desa Hist
Desamycin
Desarex
Desatrate
Desatric H
Desbutal
Descillin
Desenex
deserpidine
Desferal
Desicol
desipramine hydro-
    chloride
Desitin

deslanoside
Des-Oxa-d
desoxycholic acid
desoxycorticosterone
    acetate
desoxycorticosterone
    pivalate
desoxyephedrine
    hydrochloride
Desoxyn
desoxyribonuclease
desPlex
Detachol
Detoxogen
Detrex
Dexacortin
Dexadon
Dexalme-S
Dexameth
dexamethasone
Dexamine
Dexamyl
Dexaspan
dexbrompheniramine
    maleate
Dex-Cell-Ate
dexchlorpheniramine ma-
    leate
Dex-Cobar
Dexedrine
Dexobee
Dex-O-Curb
Dex-O-Tuss
Dexoval
dexpanthenol
Dex-Sed
Dexstim
Dex-Tend
Dextran 6%
dextran-40
Dextran-70
dextrans

dextriferron
Dextri-Maltose
dextro-amphetamine
    hydrochloride
dextro-amphetamine
    phosphate
dextro-amphetamine
    sulfate
dextro-amphetamine
    tannate
Dextrolate
dextromethorphan
    hydrobromide
Dextrosule 15.
dextrothyroxine
Dextro-Tussin
Diabinese
Diacryst
Diafen
Diagnex Blue
Dial-A-Gesic
Dialix
Dialixir
Dialog
Dialose
Dialose Plus
Diamerco
Diamond Antiseptics
Diamox
Diamox, Sequels
Dianabol
Diaparene
Diaparene Peri-Anal
    Creme
Diaprene Ointment
DIA-quel
Diasal
Diasone
Diasporal
Diasporal-Tar
diatase
Diastyl

17

Diatraegus
Diatric
diatrizoate
diatrizoate sodium
diazepam
Dibenzyline
dibucaine hydro-
    chloride
Dibuline Sulfate
Dicalcium Phosphate
Dical-D
Dicaldimin
Dicarbosil
dichloralphenazone
Dicodid
Di-Cold Tablets
Dicorvin
Dicumarol
Dicurin Procaine
dicyclomine hydro-
    chloride
Didrex
dienestrol
Dienestrol Cream
Di-Est
Dietene
diethylcarbomazine
    citrate
diethylpropion
diethylpropion
    hydrochloride
diethylstilbestrol
Diettes
Di-Factor Tablets
Di-Ferrin
digalloyl trioleate
Di-Genik
Digestamic
Digestant
Digifortis
Digiglusin
Digitaline Nativelle

digitalis
digitalis glycoside
Digitora
digitoxin
Digolase
digoxin
Dihycon
Di-Hydrin
dihydrocodeine bi-
    tartrate
dihydroergotamine
    mesylate
dihydroergotamine
    methanesulfonate
dihydromorphinone
    hydrochloride
dihydrostreptomycin
    sulfate
dihydrotachysterol
Di-Isopacin
dihydroxy aluminum
    aminoacetate
dihydroxyacetone
dihydroxyanthra-
    quinone
diiodohydroxyquinoline
Dilabid
Dilac
Dila-min
Dilantin
Dilantin D.A.
Dilaudid
Dilaves
Dilocol
Dilone
Dilor
DilORbron
Dilor-G
Dilyn
dimercaprol
dimenhydrinate
Di-Met

Dimetane
Dimetapp
Dimetapp Extentabs
Dimethacol
dimethindene maleate
dimethisoquin hydro-
    chloride
dimethisterone
dimethoxanate hydro-
    chloride
Dimindol
Diminic
dioctyl potassium
    sulfosuccinate
Di-Odine
Diodoquin
Diodrast
Diofed
DioMedicone
Diostate D
Diosuccin
Dio-Sul
Diothane
Diothron
Dioviburnia
dioxybenzone
dioxyline
Dipaxin
diperodon
diphenhydramine
diphenidol
diphenoxylate hydro-
    chloride
diphenylhydantoin
diphenylhydantoin
    sodium
diphenylpyraline
    hydrochloride
Diphtheria & Tetanus
    Toxoids
diphtheria & tetanus
    toxoids combined

18

Diphtheria & Tetanus
  Toxoids & Pertussis
  Vaccine
diphtheria toxin
Diphtheria Toxin for
  Schick Test
Diphylets
dipyridamole
dipyrone
Direct Sky Blue
Direx
Disipal
d-Isoephedrine Sulfate
Disolan
Disomer
Disonate
Disophrol Chronotab
Di-Sosul
Disotuss
Dispatabs
Dissol Ophthalmic
Di-Steroid
disulfiram
Diupres
Diurbital
Diuril
Diurnal-Penicillin
Diutensen
Diutensen-R
Divarine
Diviron
Doak Oil
Doak's Liquor Carbonis
  Detergents
Dobrolic Injection
Doca Acetate
Doctate
Doctate-P
dodecaethyleneglycol
Dodex
Dolagraine
Dolate

Dolonil
Dolophine
Dolor
Dolar Plus
Domeboro
Domeform-HC
Dome-Paste
Domerine
Domogyn
Domol Bath
Domolene-HC
Donabarb
Donabarb-SR
Donapas
Donatussin
Doncillin-G
Doncillin-V
Doncycline
Donna Extentabs
Donnagel
Donnagel-PG
Donnagesic
Donnalate
Donna Sed
Donnasep
Donnasep-MP
Donnatal
Donnatal Extentabs
Donnatal No. 2
Donnatal Plus
Donnazyme
Donphen
Donphyllin
Donquil
Donsolone
Donzyd
Donzyd + B-6
Dophenco
Dopram
Dorana
Dorbane

Dorbantyl
Dor-C Pediatric
Dorcol
Doriden
Dormal
Dornavac
Dorsacaine
Dosarbital
Dosoxy
Doss
Doss-300
Doveram
Doveret
Doverin
Doxan
doxapram
Doxegest
doxepin hydrochloride
Doxidan
Doxinate
Doxinate w/Danthron
Doxol
Doxychol-AS
Doxychol-K
doxycycline
doxylamine succinate
Dralserp
Dramamine
Dramamine-D
Drest
Drilitol
Drinus
Drisdol
Dri-Toxen
Drixoral
Drize
Drize M
Drocogesic No. 3
Drolban
dromostanolone
Dronactin
droperidol

Drotic No. 2
Droxomin
Drusilate
Drydoxin
Dry-Hist Meta-Kaps
Dryvax
d-Sorbitol
Duad
Duadacin
Ducobee Depot
Ducobee-HY
Ducobee "1000"
Dularin
Dularin TH
Dulcolax
Dumogran
Dumone
DUO-C.V.P.
Dougen
Duo-Gesic
Duo-Kestrin
Duolate-Q
Duo-Med
Duo-Medihaler
Du-Oria
DuoSpan
Duosterone
Duotrate
DuoTuss
Duoval P.A.
Duovent
Duphaston
Duphrene
Durabolin
Dura-C 500
Duracillin
Duracillin F.A. One
    Million
Duracillin Fortified
Duracton
Duradyne
Duragesic

Duramid
Duratrad
Duribex
Dyazide
Dyclone
dydrogesterone
Dykatuss
Dylephrin
Dymelor
Dynapen
Dynosal
Dynovas T.D.
Dynsed
Dy-O-Derm
dyphylline
Dyrenium
Dynsne-Inhal
Dysonil

E

Ear Drops-Presco
Ear Ease
Earobex
Ear-O1 Liquid
echothiophate iodide
Eclabron
Ecliserp
Eclispan
Ecotrin
Ectasule Sr.
Edecrin
Edrisal
Edrisal w/Codeine
edrophonium chloride
Efacin
Efedron-Hart Nasal Jelly
E-Ferol Capsules
E Ferol Ointment
E-Ferol Succinate

Effergel
Effersyl
Effersyllium
Effervescent Parasal
Efricon
Efroxine
E-Graph
Eisenzucker Tablets
Ekko Sr.
Ekomine
Ekrised
El
Elase
Elase Ointment
Elavil
El-Da-Mint
Eldec Kapseals
Eldecon
Eldecort
Elder's Cold-Tabs
Eldertonic
Eldezol
Eldiatric
Eldo-B & C
Eldofe
Eldonal
Eldopaque
Eldoquin
Eldovite
Elixir Hep-Iron
Elixophyllin
Elixophyllin-KI
Elkosin
Elmaloin
El-Ped-Ron
El-Petn
Elprecal
Elserpine
Elzyme
Embron
Emeracol
Emesert

Emetrol
Emfaseem
Emivan
Emko Vaginal Foam
Emo-Spasms
Emphysal
Empiral
Empirin Compound
Empirin Compound
    w/Codeine
Emprazil
Emprazil-C
Emulave
Emul-O-Balm
E-Mycin
Enarax
En-Cebrin
En-Cebrin F
En-Chlor
Endallergy
endocrine
Endoglobin Forte
Endotussin
Endrate
Enduron
Enduronyl
Enfamil
Enfamil Nursette
Enfamil w/Iron
Engran
Engran-HP
Ennade
Enovid-E
Enovid 5 mg.
Enterex
Enterodon
Enterosulfon
Entero-Vioform
Entozyme
entsufon
Enuretrol
Enzactin

Enziflur
Enzobile
Enzo-Cal Cream
Enzyle
Enzymet
Enzypan
ephedrine
ephedrine hydro-
    chloride
ephedrine sulfate
ephedrine tannate
Ephoxamine
Epicort
E-Pilo Ophthalmic
Epinephricaine
epinephrine
epinephrine bitartrate
epinephrine hydro-
    chloride
epinephryl-borate
Epi-pHil Cream
Eiptrate
Eplus
epoxymethamine bro-
    mide
Eppy
Epragen
Eprolin
Epsilan-M
Equagesic
Equalysen
Equanil
Equanitrate
Equgen
Equihemin
Equilet
Equinex
Equi-Plex
Ercal Sublingual
Ergkatal
Ergomar
ergonovine maleate

Ergophene
ergot
ergotamine tartrate
Ergotatropin
Ergotrate
Erucyte
erythrityl tetranitrate
Erythrocin
erythromycin
erythromycin estolate
erythromycin ethyl
    succinate
erythromycin lactobi-
    onate
erythromycin stearate
Es-A Creme
Es-A-Cort
Esangen
Eschatin
Esdone
Esdone D-Lay
Esgic
Esidolene
Esidrex-K
Esidrix
Esimil
Eskabarb
Eskadiazine
Eskaphen B
Eskaserp
Eskatrol
Eskay's Neuro Phos-
    phates
Eskay's Theranates
Esophotrast Oratrast
Esromiotin
Essential-8
Estan
Estate
Estinyl
Estivin
Estomul

Estopherol
estradiol
estradiol benzoate
estradiol cypionate
estradiol dipropionate
estradiol valerate
Estradurin
Estralate
Estra-Plex
Estratab
Estratest
Estraval-P.A.
estriol
Estrocon
estrogens, conjugated
Estro-Med
estrone
Estronol
Estrosed
EstroSpan
Estrovag "Supps"
Estrovarin S.S.
Estro-V Supprettes
Estrugenone
Estrusol
Etamon
ethacrynic acid
ethambutol hydro-
    chloride
ethamivan
Ethanacol
ethaverine hydro-
    chloride
ethchlorvynol
Ethicort
ethinamate
ethinyl estradiol
Ethiodol
ethisterone
Ethobral
ethohoptazine citrate
ethosuximide

ethotoin
ethyl alcohol
ethyl aminobenzoate
ethylnorepinephrine
    hydrochloride
ethylpapaverine hydro-
    chloride
ethynodiol diacetate
Etnabolate
Etnaclor
Etnacyclin
Etnapa
Etnasclerin
Etnatol
Etnorcon
Etnotin
Etrafon
eucalyptol
Eudicaine
Euphenex
euprocin hydrochloride
Eurax
Euresol
Euthroid
Eutonyl
Eutron
Evac-U-8
Evac-U-Gen
Evac-U-Lax
Evac-U-Mint
Evagen
Everone
Evex
E-Vital
Exabese
Excedrin
Exna
Exna-R
Expansatol
Expectrosed
Extendryl
Extralin

Extralin B
Extralin F
Eye-Mo

F

F-B-C Tabs
F.M.-200
F.M.-400
factor ix complex
Falvin
fatty acids
F-Cortef
Febridol
Fedahist
Fed-Mycin
Fednal
Fedrazil
Fedrex
Feglumin
Fello-Sed
Felsules
Femogen
Fenbane
Fendol
fentanyl
Fentropine
Feosol
Feosol Plus
Feosol Spansule
Feostat
Feostim
Fe-PLUS
Feramel
Ferancee
Ferate-C
Feratin
Ferbetrin
Fer-Bid
Fergon

Fergon c C
Fergon Plus
Fer-In-Sol
Ferisorb
Ferlon
Fermalox
Fermatin
Fernacid
Fernisolone
Fernisone
Fero-Folic-500
Fero-Grad-500
Fero-Gradumet
Ferretts
ferric ammonium citrate
ferric pyrophosphate
Ferritrinsic
Ferro-Betalin
Ferro-Chews
Ferrocol
Ferro-Desicol
Ferro Drops
Ferro-Gent
ferroglycine sulfate
    complex
Ferrolac
Ferrolip
Ferro-Mandets
Ferro Nemia
Ferronese
Ferronord
Ferronord-DLA
Ferro-Sequels
ferrous fumarate
ferrous gluconate
ferrous sulfate
Ferrovite
Ferro-win
Fertilo-Paks
Feryl-C
Feryl-Vita Ovalets
Festal

Festalan
Fetabarb-Plus
Fetamin
FevOR Elixir
fibrinogen
fibrinolysin
Fibro-AHF
Filibon
Filibon F.A.
Filibon Forte
Filibon OT
Fiorinal
Flagyl Tablets
Flagyl Vaginal Inserts
Flanithin
Flavo-Hist
Fleet
Fleet Enema
Fletcher's Castoria
Flights Chewable
Floracream
Floraquin
Florinef
Florinef-S
Florisobarb
Flornal
Floropryl
Florotic
Floxamine
Fluax
fludrocortisone acetate
flumethasone pivalate
fluocinolone acetonide
Fluogen Influenza Virus
Fluonid
Fluonid-n
Fluoravite
fluoride
fluorine
Fluor-I-Strip
Fluoritab
fluorometholone

fluorouracil
fluoxymesterone
fluphenazine dihydro-
    chloride
fluphenazine enanthate
fluphenazine hydro-
    chloride
flurandrenolide
Fluress
Flutussin
Foille Antiseptic
Foille Liquid
Foille Ointment
Fola Bee
Folavite
Folbesyn
folic acid
Folidozin-R
Follestrol
Follutein
Folvite
Folvron
Fomac
Forhistal
Formalin
Formatone
Formatrix
Formtone-HC
Formula #81
Forosteo
Fortespan
Forthane
Forticon-c
Fortiferplex
Fortizyme
Fosfree
Fostex
Fostril
Fostril-HC
Four S's
Four-Sulfazem
4-Way Cold Tablets

Fragicap
Fragicap-K
Franol
Frenquel
Freon
Fre-Tense
Fructose
Fuadin
Ful-Glo
Fuller Shield
Fulvicin
Fulvicin-U/F
Fuma-Drops
Fumaral
Fumasorb
Fumatinic
Fumatrin-Forte
Fumex
Funda-Vite
Fungizone
Furacin
Furacin-E
Furacin-HC
Furacin Urethral Inserts
Furacin Vaginal
    Suppositories
Furacort
Furadantin
furazolidone
Fu-Ron
Furonatal
furosemide
Furoxone

G

G-1 Tablets
G-2
G-3
G.B.-Prep

G. B. S.
G.G.I. Expectorant
G. I. 8
GVS
GVS Vaginal
Gadoment
Gallogen
Gamastan
Gamatet
Gamatran
Gamimune
gamma benzene hexa-
    chloride
Gammacorten
Gammagee
gamma globulin
Gamulin
Gamulin T
Ganatrex
Gantanol
Gantrisin
Garamycin
Gargaline
Gasterone
Gastralme-M
Gastrical
Gastroenterase
Gastrografin
Gastrolic
Gastromycin
Gaysal
Gel-A-Neutrin
gelatin
Gelazine
Gelfilm
Gelfoam
Gel-Kote
Gelsodyne
Geltabs Vitamin D
Gelusil
Gelusil-M
Gemonil

Genapax
gentamicin sulfate
gentian violet
Gentia-Jel
Gentlax
Gentle Shampoo
Gentz Rectal
Geralin
Geramine
Gerandrest
Gera Pet
Gerets
Geri-Ace
Geriamic
Geri-Bath
Gericaps
Gericrest
Geridalin
Geri-Lam
Gerilets
Gerilid
Geriliquid
Gerinats-H
Gerinats-T
Geriplex
Geriplex-FS
Geristone
Geritag
Geritinic
Geritonic
Gerix
Gerizyme
Germicin
Ger-O-Foam
Geroid
Geroniazol
Gest Tablets
Gesterol
Gestest
Gevizol
Gevrabon
Gevral

Gevramet
Gevrestin
Gevrine
Gevrite
Giasol
Ginsopan
Ginsopen
Gitaligin
gitalin
Givalex
Glaucon
G-Lixir
Globin Zinc Insulin
Globotrin
globulin, immune serum
globulin, poliomyelitis
    immune
Glucagon
Gluco-Calcium
Gluco-Fedrin
Glucoron w/B₁₂
Glucose
Gluco-Tinic
Glucotropin
Glucovite
Glukor
Glu-Sal
Glutalam
glutamic acid
glutamic acid hydro-
    chloride
Glutan H-C-L
Glutasyn
Glutavene
Glutazyme
Glutest
glutethimide
glycerin
glycerin dehydrated
glycerophosphate
Glycero-Saline
glyceryl guaiacolate

glyceryl trinitrate
glycine
glycobiarsol
Glycogel
glycopyrrolate
Glycotuss
Glycyrrhiza
Gly-Oxide
Glyrol
Glysennid
Glytinic
Godoform
Gonadoplex
Gotas Ce
Gourmase
GPC-Expectorant
Gradumet
Gramicidin
Gravidox
Gray's Compound
G-Recillin
Grecort
Grifulvin
Grifulvin V
Grillodyne
Grisactin
griseofulvin
gris Owen
Guaiacodyl
guaiacol
Guaiafage
Guaiamine
guanethidine mono-
    sulfate
guanethidine sulfate
guar gum
Guia-Camph
Gui-Acua
Guiaform
Guiamine
Guiosan
Guistrey

gum karaya
GU-70
Gustalac
Gustase
G-V Vaginal
Gynben
Gynergen
Gyne-Sec
Gynetone
Gynogen Injectable
Gynogen L. A.
Gynogen R. P.
Gynorest
Gyn Tablets

H

HBP 100
HC Creme
HCV Creme
H.I.L.-20
HL-5
HP Acthar Gel
HVC
H Y V A Gentian Violet
Halabar
Halazone
Haldol
Haldrone
Halercol
Haley's M-O
Haliver Oil
Halodrin
haloperidol
Halotestin
Hapamine
Harmonyl
Harmonyl-N
Hasacode
Hasamal

Hasanone
Hasp Elixir
Haugase
Hautosone
Haxsen
Hazel-Balm
Head & Shoulders
HEB-Cort
Hedco Drops
Hedulin
Heliobrom
Hemafolate
Hemalgen
Hemaliquid
Hematinic
Hematone C
Hematovals New
Hematrinsic
Hemethica
Hemicin
Hemobon
Hemocrine
Hemocyte
Hemo-Forte
Hemogen "100" LF
Hemonex
Hemo-Vite
Hemo Vitol
Hep Nine-B
Hepa-Desicol
Hepaferron
Hepamine
Hepaphytol B$_{12}$
Heparam
heparin
Heparplex
Hepathrom
Hep-Forte
Hepicebrin
Hepp-Iron
Hepron
heptabarbital

Hepteryl-12
Heptuna Plus
Hescor
Hesper-C
hesperidin
Hetrazan
Hexa-Betalin
hexachlorophene
Hexacrest
Hexaderm
Hexadrol
Hexalet
Hexalol
Hexathricin
Hexatropine
Hexavibex
hexocyclium methyl-
    sulfate
Hi-Bee w/C
Hiprex
Hiscaspray
Hiscatabs
Hisdrin
Hiserpia
Hispril
Histabid
Histabs
Histacalma
Hista-Cap
Hista-Clopane
Hista Compound
Hist-A-Cort-E
Hista-Derfule
Histadur
Histadyl
Histadyl & A.S.A.
Histadyne
Histalet Forte T.D.
Histalog
Histam
Histamic-SR
Hista-Sed 25

Histaspan
Histene
histoplasmin
HistOR-D
Hist-Oxa-Mine
Histrey Syrup
Hi-Temp phials
Hiwolfia
Hollandex Silicone
    Ointment
Homagenets
Homapin
Homaspan
Homatrophen
homatropine methyl-
    bromide
Homicebrin
Homo-Tet
Homvite
Hormale
Hormestrin
Hormogen
Hormonin
Hormoplete
Hormo-Provimine
Hormovite
Hospi-Lotion
Hovizyme
H-R Electrode Contact
H-R Sterile Lubricating
    Jelly
H-R Steri-Wipe
Humacort
Humatin
Humorsol Ophthalmic
Hurricaine Oral
Hyadrine
Hyalex
Hy-Ampha-Barb
Hy-Asmatabs
Hyasorb Penicillin
Hyatro

Hyazyme
Hybalamin
Hybephen
Hybolin
Hycodan
Hycoff
Hycomine
Hy-Cort Cream
Hydantal
hydantoin derivative
Hy-Decon
Hydeltrasol Injection
Hydeltrasol-Ophthalmic
Hydeltra-T.B.A.
Hydergine
Hydocaine
Hydoxin
Hydra-Kit
hydralazine hydro-
   chloride
Hydra-Mag
Hydra-Mat
Hydra Nasal Spray
Hydraserp
Hydrea
Hydrelt
Hydrelt-AC
Hydriodic Acid
Hydro-Bilein
hydrochloric acid
hydrochlorothiazide
Hydrochol
hydrocholeretics
Hydrocil
hydrocodone bitartrate
hydrocodone resin
hydrocortisone
hydrocortisone acetate
Hydrocortone
Hydrocortone Acetate
Hydrocortone Phos-
   phate

HydroDIURIL
HydroDIURIL-Ka
hydroflumethiazide
Hydrolose
hydromorphone
hydromorphone hydro-
   chloride
hydromorphone sulfate
Hydromox
Hydrone
Hydrophen
Hydrophilic Ointment
Hydropres
Hydropres-Ka
hydroquinone
Hydrosone
Hydrospray
Hydro-Tar
Hydro-Tet
Hydro-12
Hy-Drox
Hydroxal Gel
Hydroxy B-12
hydroxyamphetamine
   hydrobromide
hydroxychloroquine
   sulfate
hydroxyprogesterone
   caproate
8-hydroxyquinoline
   sulfate
hydroxyurea
hydroxyzine hydro-
   chloride
hydroxyzine pamoate
Hydryllin
Hygefem
Hygroton
Hykinone
Hylugel Plus
Hymenol
Hyonatol

hyoscine hydrobromide
1-hyoscyamine
hyoscyamine hydro-
   bromide
hyoscyamine sulfate
hyoscyamus
Hypan
Hy-Panthron
Hypaque
Hypaque Meglumine 60%
Hypaque-M, 75% .
Hypaque-M, 90%
Hyparotin
Hyper-Cholate
Hyperloid
Hypertensin
Hyper-Tet
Hypertussis
Hypnaldyne
Hypnette
Hypnos Solution
Hypobeta-20
Hy-Po-Tone
Hyptran
Hy-Quad-Phed
Hyquin Cream 50
Hyrye Injectable
Hyp-Sen
Hy-Scopamine
Hysobel
Hysone
Hytakerol
Hytinic
Hytone
Hytrona
Hytuss
Hyvanol
Hy-Zorbis
Hyzyd

I

I.L.X. Elixir
IMF
Iatric
Iberet
Iberol Filmtab
Ichloroquin
ichthammol
Ichtho-Cort
Ichthyol
Idotein
idoxuridine
Iletin, Regular
Iletin, Semilente
Iletin, Ultralente
Iletin Lente
Iletin U-500
Ilocalm
Ilomel
Ilopan
Ilopan-Choline
Ilosone
Ilotycin
Imbicoll
Imenol
Imferon
imipramine hydro-
    chloride
Immolin
Immu-G
Immuglobin
Immune Serum Globulin
Immunovac Oral
Immunovac (Parenteral)
IMMU-Tetanus
Impregon Concentrate
Imuran
Incorpohist
Incorposol
Incremin

Inderal
Indocin
indocyanine green
indomethacin
Indorex
Infa-Digin Tablets
Infadorm
Infagen
Infantovit
Infantussis
Inflamase
influenza virus vaccine
Influenza Virus Vaccine
    Bivalent
Initia Drops
Innovar
inositol
Inoton
Inpersol
Insect Antigen
Inserfem
Insta-Perm
insulin
insulin, delayed
insulin, globin zinc
insulin NPH
insulin, protamine zinc
intasedol
Inthol
intra-uterine devices
Intribex
Intrin
Intrinase
intrinsic factor
Intri-Vite
Intromycin
Intron
Inversine HCL
Iocort
Iocortar
iodine
Iodized Lime

iodochlorhydroxyquin
Iodomax
Iodo-Niacin
Ioklon
ionamin
Ionax
Ionil
Ionosol B
Ionosol D
Ionosol D-CM
Ionosol G
Ionosol K
Ionosol MB
Ionosol PSL
Ionosol T
Ion-o-trate Potassium
    Chloride
Ion-o-trate Sodium
    Chloride
Ion-o-trate Sodium
    Lactate
Iotein
iopanoic acid
iothiouracil sodium
Ipaterp
ipecac
ipodate
Ipral Calcium
Ipsatol
Ircon Tablet
irish moss
Iromin-G
iron
Ironate
iron choline citrate
Ironco-B
iron dextran injection
Ironized Yeast Tablets
iron, peptonized
iron sorbitex
Irosorb-59
Irradol-A

Isalax
I-sedrin
Ismelin
Iso-Asminyl
Iso-Brovite
isocarboxazid
Isoclor
Isodine
isoetharine
Isofedrol
Isogesic
Isogram
Isohalant
Isohist
Isoject
Isomel
isometheptene hydro-
  chloride
isometheptene mucate
isoniazid
Isopacin
Isophrin Nasal
isopropamide
isopropyl alcohol
Isopropyl Alcohol
isopropyl myristate
isopropyl sebacate
isoproterenol
isosorbide dinitrate
Isordil
Isordil Tembids
Iso-Tabs 60
Isotogen
Isotonic Sodium
  Chloride
Isovex-60
Isovex-100
isoxsuprine hydro-
  chloride
Isufranol
Isuprel
Isuprel Mistometer

Isuprel 1:5000
Itrumil
Ivarest Poison Ivy Cream
Ivax
Ivy-Eze
Ivyoak
Ivyol
Ivy-Rid

J

JV Vitamins
Jacobson's Solution
Jayne's P-W Vermifuge
Jayne's R-W Vermifuge
Jayron Tablets
Jectofer

K

KIE
KMC Electrolyte
KNL (Darrow's
  Solution)
K O L Capsules
K.P.G.-400 Powder
Kalpec
Kamadrox
kanamycin sulfate
Kantrex
Kanulase
Kanumodic
Kaochlor
Kao-Con
kaolin
Kaomagma
Kaomin
Kaomuth

Kaomycin
Kaon
Kaopectate
Kappadione
Karidium
Karigel
Kato Powder
Kavacaps
Kay Ciel
Kayexalate
K-Cillin
Keflin
Kelatrate
Kelex
Kemadrin
Kenacort
Kenalog
Kenalog-S
Kenpectin
Kenpectin-P
Ken Span
Keoparic
Keotin
Kerid Drops
Keri Lotion
Kerodex
Kesso-Bamate
Kessodanten
Kessodrate
Kessolana
Kesso-Pen
Kesso-Tetra
Kestrin
Ketochol
Ketosox
Key-Gesic
Key-Pred
Key-Pyrone
Key-Sed
Key-Serpine
Keysone
Kiddi-Vites

Kin Protective Cream
Kiophyllin
Kisol Syrup
Klaron
Kler-Ro
Kloride
Klorlyptus
K-Lyte
Knollide
Koglucoid
Kolantyl
Koloyd
Komal
Komed Acne Lotion
Konakion
Kondremul
Konsyl
Kontrol
Konyne
Konzyme
Koro-Flex Diaphragm
Koromex Coil Spring
  Diaphragm
Koromex Douche
  Powder
Koromex Introducer
Koromex Jelly
Koromex Matrisalus
  Diaphragm
Koromex Mensinga Flat
  Spring Diaphragm
Koromex-A Vaginal Jelly
Kortrate
Koryza
Kosate 100
Kos-House Otic
K-PEN
K-Phos
K-Predne-Dome
Kremplex
Kreso Dip No. 1
Kronohist

Kryl
Kryzen
K-20
Kudrox
Kused
Kutapressin
Kutrase
Ku-Zyme
Kwell Cream
  Lotion
  Shampoo
Kynex

L

L. A. Formula
L A Testosterone
L. C. D. Cream
L. F. B. 12
L. F. B. 12-100
LMD 10%
L. O. L. Lotion
Lacticaps-M
Lactinex
lactobacillus acidophilus
lactobacillus bulgaricus
Lactocal
Lambase
Lam-B-Doce
Lam-B-Tol
Lanacillin "400"
Lanahex
Lanamin
lanatoside C
Lanatuss
lanolin
Lanoline
Lanoxin
Lanvisone
Largon

Larylgan
Laryngene
Lasix
Lastomone
Lastrogen
Laudacin
Laud-Iron
Lavacol
Lavatar
Lavema Compound
  Solution
Laxaid
Laxinate 100
Lax-O-Cat
Laxogen
Laxsil
Layered Lific B_{12}
Lecipure
lecithin
Ledercillin VK
Lederplex
Lembrose
Lemiserp Ty-Med
Lenic HP
Leptagesic
Leptinol
Leritine
Les-Cav
Lestemp
Lethopherol
Letter
Leucovorin
leucovorin, calcium
Leukeran
levallorphan tartrate
levamfetamine succinate
Levamine
Levanil
levarterenol bitartrate
Levatrol
Levo-Dromoran

levo-epinephrine
  hydrochloride
Levoid
Levophed
Levoprome
levorphanol tartrate
Levsin
Levsin-C
Levsinex
Lexavite
Lextron
L-Glutavite
Liafon
Libco-12
Li-Betaron
Libigen
Librax
Libritabs
Librium
Lidaform-HC Creme
Lida-Mantle Creme
lidocaine
Lidosporin
Lific B_{12} "100"
Lifolbex
Lincocin
lincomycin
Lini-Balm
liothyronine
Lipiodol
Lipiodol Ascendant
Lipo-Adrenal Cortex
Lipo-Anasal
Lipo-Art
Lipocaps
Lipoflavonoid
Lipo Gantrisin
Lipo-Hepin
lipoiodine
Lipoliquid
Lipo-Lutin
lipolytic

Lipomechol
Lipomul-Oral
Lipo Nicin
Lipo-Sinahist
Lipo-Tol
Lipotosse
Lipotriad
Lipotron
Lipotropic
Liprotein
Liquaemin
Liquamar
Liquibarine
Liqui-Cee
Liquid Kler-ro
Liqui-Doss
Liquimat
Lirugen
Lisacort
Listica
Litwelfo
Liva Injection
liver concentrate
liver, desiccated
Liv-Fer-B
Livibron
Livitamin
Livitol
Liv-O-Rex
Livroben
Lixaminol
Lixophen
Lobana
lobeline sulfate
Locorten
Lofenalac
Lomotil
Lonalac
Lorex Dermal
Lorfan
Loridine
Lorophyn

Loroxide
Lorvic Decalcifier
Lorvic Rinse
Lorvic Vapor Phase Rust
  Inhibitor
Loryl
Lotio Alsulfa
Lotioblanc
Lotocreme
Lotusate
Lowila
Lowila Cake
Lozets
Lozilles
Luasmin
Lubafax
Lubasporin
Lubath
Lubricort Cream
Lubriderm
Lubritine
Lucidon
Lufyllin
Lufyllin-EPG
Lufyllin-GG
Luminal
Lunaspas
Luride
Lusyn
Luton
Lutrexin
lututrin
Lycinate
Lycolan
Lycoral
Lyforcin
Lygranum S. T.
lymphogranuloma venerum
  antigen
Lynoral
Lyo B-C w/B_{12}
Lypho-Bex-C

1-lysine
Lysmins
Lyteers
Lytren

M

MCT Oil
MG Capsules
M.I. 30%
MSC Triaminic
M-T Suppository
M.V.I.
Maalox
Macrodantin
Macrodex
Madribon
mafenide acetate
mafenide hydrochloride
magaldrate
Magcyl
Magcylax
Maginal-HM
Magmalin
Magnagel
Magnatril
magnesium carbonate
magnesium hydroxide
magnesium nicotinate
magnesium oxide
magnesium para
    aminobenzoate
magnesium phosphate
magnesium sulfate
magnesium trisilicate
Magoleum
Maizette
Makrogen
Malanesin
Malatonic

Malcogel
Malcotabs
Malcotran
Maleen
Mallagesic
Mallenzyme
Mallo-B
Mallo-Plex
Mal-O-Fem
Malogen
malt extract
Maltsupex
Malumel
Mammol Ointment
Manacid
Mandacon
Mandalay
Mandelamine
Mandex
Manibee
Manniphen
Manophyllin
Mantadil
Manvertin
Maolate 400 mg.
Mapharsen
Marax
Marbec
Marblen
Marezine
Marfonyl
Marinex
Marlyn Formula 50
Marmine
Marpex T.D.
Marplan
Marsone
Marsulfas
Maseda Foot Powder
Masse Breast Care
    Cream
Massengill Powder

Matulane
Maturon
Maxibolin
Maxipen Tablets
Maxitate w/Rauwolfia
Maytrex
Maywolfia
measles vaccines
Measles Virus Vaccine
Mebaral
Meb-Byl
Mebroin
meclizine preparations
Medache
Medadent
Medaline
Medaprin
Meda Tex
Medcohist Tablets
Mediatric
Medicone
Mediconet
Medigesic
Medihaler
Medi-Ject
Mediplex
Medi-Skreen
Meditussin
medium chain trigly-
    cerides
Medomin
Medotopes
Medrol
Medrol Medules
medroxyprogesterone
    acetate
mefenamic acid
meglumine diatrizoate
meglumine iodipamide
Melan Tablets
Melfiat Unicelles
Mellaril

Meloxine
melphalan
Melynor
menadiol sodium
  diphosphate
Menagen
Menest
Menformon (A)
Menic
Menotab-M
Menrium
Menseze
Menta-Bal
Menthalgesic
menthol
Mentholaire Vaporizer
  Fluid
Mentholine
menthyl anthranilate
Mentran-H
Meonine
mepenzolate bromide
Mepergan
meperidine
  hydrochloride
mephenesin
mephenytoin
mephobarbital
Mepho-d
Mephosal
Mephyton
mepivacaine
  hydrochloride
Meprane
meprobamate
Meprospan
Meprotabs
meralluride
Meratran
mercaptomerin, sodium
mercaptopurine
Mercodol

Mercresin
Mercuhydrin
Meribam
Mericillin
Mericycline
Meride
Merigesic
Meritene
Merlenate Ointment
Merpectogel
Merphene
Merithiolate
Meruvax Lyovac
Mesantoin
Mesopin
Mestinon
mestranol
Mestrone
Mesulfin
Metachlor
Metahydrin
Metalex
Metamine
Metamucil
Metandren
Metaphen
Metatensin
Metatone
metaxalone
Meted Shampoo
methacycline hydro-
  chloride
methadone hydro-
  chloride
Methajade
Methakote
Methalate
Methaloid
Metham
methamphetamine
methandrostenolone
Methaphor

methapyrilene
methapyrilene fumarate
methapyrilene hydro-
  chloride
methaqualone
metharbital
Methatar
Meth-Averin
Methazem
methdilazine
Methedrine
methenamine
methenamine hippurate
methenamine mandelate
methenamine-
  sulfosalicylate
Methendelate
Methergine
methicillin sodium
methimazole
Methine
methiodal sodium
methionine
Methioplex
Methischol
methixene hydro-
  chloride
methocarbamol
methohexital sodium
Methotrexate
methotrimeprazine
methoxamine hydro-
  chloride
methoxyflurane
Methoxyphyllin
methscopolamine bro-
  mide
methscopolamine ni-
  trate
methsuximide
methyclothiazide
methyl salicylate

33

methylbenzethonium chloride
methylcellulose
Methyldiol
methyldopa
methylene blue
methylergonovine maleate
methylisooctenylamine hydrochloride
methylisooctenylamine mucate
methylphenidate hydrochloride
methylphenylsuccini-mide
methylprednisolone
methylrosaniline chloride
methyltestosterone
methyprylon
methysergide maleate
Meticortelone
Meticorten
Meti-Derm
Metimyd Ophthalmic
Metopirone
Metranil
Metrazol
Metreton
Metrogesic
metronidazole
Metropectin
Metropine
Metubine Iodide
Metycaine
metyrapone
Mevanin-C
Mevatinic-C
Mevitonic
Mezo Ointment

Mg-PLUS
Mg-+"C"
Mi-Cebrin
Mi-Cebrin T
Microsyn
Microzyme
Midicel
Midol
Midrin
Migral
Migralam
Migrinil
Mikedimide
Milestro
Milex Creme
Milex Folding Pessaries
Milibis
Milibis w/Aralen
Milkinol
Milontin
Milpath
Miprem
Miltown
Miltrate
Minacap
mineral oil
Minit Rub
Minnehaha Soap
Minoplex
Minro-Plex
Mintezol
Mio-Carpine
Miochol
Mio-Pressin
miotics
Mi-Pilo
Miradon
Mity-Mycin
Mity-Quin
Mixiro
MMP Mold Allergens
Mobisyl

Modane
Moderil
Modilac
Modumate
Modutrol
Moebiquin
Mol-Iron
Mol-Iron Panhemic
Mol-Iron w/Vitamin C
Monacet
monamine-oxidase inhibitors
Monichol
monobenzone
Monodral
Monomeb
Monotheamin
Mono-Vacc
8-MOP
Morestin
Moruguent
Morumide & Phenacaine
Morusan
Movicol
Moxine
Mucamide
Mucilloid
Mucilose
Mucomyst
Mucoplex
Mucotin
Mucusol
Mudrane
Mudrane GG
Mull-Soy
Mul-Sed
Multi-B-K
Multi-B-Plex
Multical
Multicebrin
Multidex Injection
Multifluor

Multifuge
Multihist
Multi-Vi-Rex
Multivitalin
Multivitamins
Multron
Mulvidren
Mulvitab
Mulvitol
mumps immune
    globulin
mumps vaccine
Mumpsvax
Murel
Muripsin
Murocoll Atropine
        Eucatropine
        Fluorescein
        Homatropine
        Isoflurophate
        Methyl Cel-
            lulose
        Physostigmine
        Pilocarpine
        Scopolamine
        Tetracaine
Muro's Contact Lens
    Irrigating Solution
    Wetting & Cleaning
        Solution
Mus-L-Tone
Mustargen
Muvica
M-Vac Measles Virus
Myadec
Myambutol
My-B-Den
Mychel
Mycifradin
Myciguent
Mycinol
Mycitracin

Mycofan
Mycolog
Myconef
Mycostatin
Mycozol
Mykocert
Mylanta
Mylaxen
Myleran
Mylicon
Myo-B
Myocholine
Myochrysine
Myodigin
Myoflex Creme
Myomephetane
Myospaz
Myotrate
Mypron
Myringacaine
Mysoline
Mysteclin-F
Mytelase
M-Z Solution

N

NCP-500
ND-8
NPH Iletin
nTz
Na Pent
Na-Co-A1
Nactisol
Nacton
nafcillin, sodium
Nadol
Naldecon
Naldetuss
Nalertan

nalidixic acid
Nalline HCl Injection
nandrolone decanoate
nandrolone phen-
    propionate
naphazoline hydro-
    chloride
Napril
Napsed
Naptrate
Naqua
Naquival
Nardil
Narine Gyrocaps
Narone
Nascobarb
Nasprin
Natabec
Natabec-F. A.
Natacrest
Natalac
Nata-Lam
Natalets-F
Natalins
Natalins Plus
Natatabs
Natola
Natri-Pas
Naturetin
Naturetin c̄ K
Nautrol Suppositories
Navane
ND-Gesic
ND-Stat
Nebair
Nebralin
nebulizers
Negatan
NegGram
Neko Soap
Nembudeine
Nembu-donna

Nembu-Gesic
Nembu-Serpin
Nembutal
Neo-Amniotin
Neobase Greaseless
    Ointment Base
Neo-Beta
Neo-Betalin 12
Neobile
Neobiotic
Neo-Calglucon
Neocarbon
Neocet
Neocholan
Neo-Corovas
Neo-Corovas Tymcaps
Neo-Cort-Dome
Neo-Cortef
Neocurtasal
Neo-Cutone
Neocylate
Neocylone
Neocyten
NeoDecadron
NeoDECASPRAY
Neo-Delta-Cortef
Neodex
Neo-Domeform-HC
Neo Fernisone Cream
Neo Gel w/Sulfa
Neogen
Neogesic
Neo-Grecort
Neo-Heprin
Neo-Hombreol
Neo-Hydeltrasol
Neohydrin
Neo-Hydrosone
Neo-Hytone
Neo-Iopax
Neo-Kondremul
Neolax

Neoloid
Neo-Lopax
Neo-Medrol
Neomersyl
Neo-Mull-Soy
neomycin
neomycin palmitate
neomycin sulfate
Neonic
Neo-Nysta-Cort
Neo-Oxylone
Neopap
Neoparbel
Neoparbrom
Neopasalate
Neopavrin
Neopectin
Neo-Polycin
Neo Prescel
Neo-Propisol
Neoquess
Neo-Rhiban
Neo-Sedaphen
Neo-Silvol
Neo-Slowten
Neosone
Neosorb
Neosporin
neostigmine bromide
neostigmine methyl-
    sulfate
Neo-Synalar
Neo-Synephrine
Neo-Tab
Neotep
Neo-Tet
Neothalidine
Neothylline
Neotinic
Neotrizine
Neotuss
Neo Vitwel

Neoxyn
Neozyl w/Codeine
Nepritin
Neptazane
Nepto Lotion
Nepytol
Nergestic
Nesacaine
Nethaphyl
Nethaprin
Neurinase
Neuro B$_{12}$
Neurogyn
Neuronidia
Neurophytol
Neurosine
Neutracomp
Neutralox
Neutrapen
Neutra-Phos
Nevrotose
Nexorin
niacin
niacinamide
Niadox
Nialex
Nialift
Niamid
Niapent
Niatinic
Niazole
Nibesol-M
Nicalex
Nickerson's Medium
Nicocap
Nicolexin
Nico-Metrozol
Niconyl
Nicoscorbine
Nico-Span
Nicotal
Nicotinex

nicotinic acid
nicotinyl alcohol
Nicotron
Nicozol
Nidar
Niferex
nifuroxime
Niglycon
nikethamide
Nikorin
Nilatus
Nilevar
Nimo-Tex
Ninhydrin
Nio-A-Let
Niodolin
Nionate
Niondox
Nioric
Nipirin
Nisaval
Nisentil
Nisept
Nisine
Nisolone
Nisulfazole
Nitora
Nitralox
Nitranitol
nitrate
Nitrazine Paper
Nitrin
nitrite
Nitro-Bid
nitrofurantoin
nitrofurazone
nitroglycerin
Nitroglyn
nitromersol
Nitroglyn-Sublingual
Nitrol
Nitronet

Nitrong
Nitrospan
Nitro- T.D.
Nitrovas
No Doz
Nobese
Noctec
Noctel 500
Nodalin
Nolamine
Noludar
nonoxynol-9
Noracee T
Noracin
Noradrin
Noradryl
Noralac
Noramide
Noraminic
Noraphen-Plus
Noratuss
Norbrin
NORchrome
Nor Drops
Nordryl
Norel
norethindrone
norethynodrel
Norflex
Norgesic
norgestrel
Norimex
Norinyl 1 + 80 21-Day
Norinyl 1 + 80 28-Day
Norisodrine
Norlestrin Fe 1 mg.
Norlestrin 2.5 mg.
Norlestrin 21 1 mg.
Nor Lief
Norlutate
Norlutin
Normacid

Normaderm
Norma-Skreen
Normatar
Normosol-M & Surbex T
  in D5-W
Normosol-M 900 Cal
Normosol-M in D5-W
  Solutions
Normosol-R
Normosol-R pH 7.4
Normosol-R in D5-W
Normosol-R/K + in
  D5-W
Norocaine
Norocol w/Codeine
Norodin
Norophylline
Norotons
Noroxine
Norozol
Norpramin
Norquen
Norstrone
nortriptyline hydro-
  chloride
Nortussin
noscapine
Noscaps
Noscoline
Novacebrin
Novahistine
Novalene
Novatrin
Noviplex
Novisyn
novobiocin
Novocain
Novogran
Novrad
Nuclomin
Nucodan
Nudox

Nugestoral
NúLeven
Numa Dura-Tabs
Numorphan
Nupercaine
Nurosal
Nursmatic Nursers
Nutra-500
Nutracort
Nutraderm
Nutramigen
Nutraspa
Nutricol
Nutricon
Nutritive Capsules
nux vomica
Nuxaphen
Nydrazid
nylidrin
Nylmerate
Nyloxin
Nymore
Nyomin
Nyral Lozenges
Nysta-Cort Lotion
Nysta-Dome Lotion
Nystaform-HC Ointment
Nystaform Ointment
nystatin

Obalan
Obedrin
Obegyn
Obesa-Mead
Obesavit
Obestat
Obetrol
Obeval

Obex
Obid
Obnatal
Obocell
Obolip
Obotan
Obrical
Obron-6
OB-Tabs
Octin
Octinum Mucate
Oc-U-Zin Solution
Oenethyl
Ogen
Oilatum Cream
Oilatum Soap
ointment
Olac Powder
Olbese No. 1
oleandomycin
O1-Vitum
Omega-P.A.
Ominal
Omnipen
Omni-Tuss
Oncovin
One-A-Day Multiple
    Vitamins
One-Iron
Onycho-Phytex
Opacedrin
Opasal
OpH Eye Drops
Ophthaine
Ophthalgan
Ophthel
Op-Hydrin
Opidice
Op-Isophrin
opium
opium (tincture of)
Op-Sulfa-10

Op-Sulfa-30 Sterile
    Ophthalmic
Optef Drops
Optho-Derm-A
Optihist
Optilets
Optilets-M-500
Optimyd Ophthalmic
Optiphyllin
Optival Ophthalmic
Orabase Emollient
Orabiotic
Oracon
Oradash
Oragrafin Calcium
Oragrafin Sodium
Orahema
Orahesive Intraoral
    Bandage
Oral Calscorbate
Oral Pentacresol
Oralphyllin
Oraminic
Orasoxol
Oraspan
Orbedec
Orbiferrous
Orbigesic
Orbipec w/Neomycin
Orbisulfas AD
Ordway's Solution
Orenzyme
Oretic
Oreticyl
Oreton
Oreton Aqueous
    Suspension
Oreton Methyl
Orexin
Organidin
Orgaphen
Orifer

Orimune Poliovirus
  Vaccine
Orinase
Orinase Diagnostic
Oriodide-131 Oral
  Solution
Ornade Spansule
Orovite
orphenadrine citrate
orphenardine hydro-
  chloride
Orprine
Ortho-Creme
Ortho Diaphragm
Ortho-Gynol
Ortho-Novum SQ
  Tablets
Ortho-Novum 1 mg.
Ortho-Novum 2 mg.
Ortho-Novum 10 mg.
Ortho-Novum 1/80 ☐ 21
Orthoxicol
Orthoxine
Os-Cal
Os-Cal-Gesic
Os-Cal-Mone
Osmōglyn
Osmopak
Ostone
Os-Vim
Otalgine
Otall
Otic Domeboro Solution
Otic Lidaform-HC
Otic Neo-Cort-Dome
Otobione
Otobiotic
Otocort
Otodyne
Otolgesic
Otomide
Otomyxin

Otoreid-HC
Otos-Mosan
Otosone-F
Otrivin
Ovlin
Ovocylin
Ovofen
Ovogyn
Ovral
Ovulen
Ovulen-21
Ovulen-28
Oxabar
Oxabil
oxacillin, sodium
Oxadron
Oxaine
oxazepam
ox bile extract
oxethazaine
Oxiphen
Oxolax
Oxsoralen
Oxsorbil
oxybenzone
Oxycel
Oxychinol
Oxycodone
Oxydess
Oxy-Kesso-Tetra
Oxylone
oxymetazoline hydro-
  chloride
Oxymetholone
oxymorphone
Oxynitral w/Veratrum
  Viride
oxyphenbutazone
oxyphencyclimine
  hydrochloride
oxyphenisatin acetate
oxyphenonium bromide

oxyquinoline sulfate
oxytetracycline
oxytocin
Oxyvatine

P

P.A.C. Compound
P.A.C. w/Cyclopal
P.A.D. Tablets
PE Ophthalmics
PETN Plus
PETN 30
PMB-200
PNS Rectal
P.R. Syrup
PTZ Tablets
Paadon
Pabafilm
Pabalate
Pabalate-HC
Pabalate-SF
Pabanol
Pabirin
Pabirin AC
Pabirin AC Buffered
Pabizol
Pagitane
Paisoxine
Paladac
Palaflor
Palatol
Palbar
Palgesic
Palminate
Palmiron
Palmiron-C
Palocarp
Palocillin-5
Palocillin-S

Palodyne
Palohist
Palonad
Palonyl
Palsorb
Paltet
Paludrine
Pama
Pam B$_{12}$' 1000
Pamcillin
Pamine
Pamine PB
Pamisyl
Panabarb
Panafil Ointment
Panafil-White Ointment
Panalgesic
Panazyme
Pan B Plex
Panbutal
Pancard
Pancard 30 TPA
Pancebrin
Pancidin
Pancobile
Pancof
Pancohemin Improved
Pan-Concemin
Pancort
Pancreatic Hormone
pancreatin
Pancreatin, Triple
    Strength
Pancrobilin
Pan D Plex
Pan-Estra MT
Pan-Estra 20 mg. L.A.
Pan-Estra 40 mg. L.A.
Panfem Powder
Panheprin
Panitol
Panitol H.M.B.

Panitone
Panjet
Pan K
Panmycin
Pannaz
Pan Nutron M
Pan OB
Panoral
Panosate
Panpaba
PanPav TP
Panpyro
Panquil
Panrau
Panrexin TP
Panritis
Pantabeeroid No. 2
Pantemic
Panteric Capsules
Pan-Test 100 L.S.
Pan-Test 200 L.A.
panthenol
Panthoderm
Pantho-F Cream
Pantholin
Pantopaque
Pantopon
pantothenate, calcium
Pantrin
Panverm
Pan-Vi
Panvitex
Panwarfin
Panzalone
Panzol
Panzyme
Paocin
Paoguan
papain
Papase
Papavatral
Papavatral L.V.

papaverine hydro-
    chloride
para-aminobenzoate
para-aminobenzoic acid
parachlorometaxylenol
Paradione
Paradol
Paraflex
Parafon Forte
Parafon w/Codeine
Parafon w/Prednisolone
Paral
paraldehyde
parmethadione
paramethasone
Parasal
Paraspan T.D.
Parba-K
Parba-KP
Parbexin
Parbocyl
Parcatol
paregoric
Paredrine
Paredrine Sulfathiazole
    Suspension
Parelixir
Parenogen
Parenteral B Vials
Parenzyme
Parepectolin
Parest
Par-F
Pargel
pargyline hydrochloride
Parkodene Syrup
Parlite Vitamins B w/C
Parnate
Paroidin
Parsidol
Pasara
PAS-C

Pasca Pack Granules
Pasca Tablets
Paskalium
Pasna Pack Granules
Pasna Powder
Pasna Tri-Pack
Passi-Barb
Passiphen
Pathibamate
Pathilon
Pathocil
P-A-V
Pavabid Plateau CAPS
Pavadel
Pavalets
Pava-Span
Paveril
Paveril Phosphate & Amytal Tablets
Paverolan
Pavricol
Paxarel
Pazo Formula
P-B-Sal-C
peanut oil
Peaton
pectin
Pectocel
Pectoguanidine
Ped O Sul
Pedameth
Pediacof
Pediaflor
Pedialyte
Pediamycin
Pediatric Isophrin Nose Drops
Pediatric Phenergan Expectorant
Pediatric Piptal w/Phenobarbital
Pedimin

Pedituss
Pedric
Peganone
Pektamalt
Penalate
Penbritin
Penbritin-S
Penicillin G
penicillin g, benzathine
penicillin g potassium
pencillin g procaine
penicillin g sodium
penicillin (oral)
penicillin, phenoxy-methyl
penicillin (repository)
penicillin v
penicillinase
Pentacine
Pentacresol
pentaerythritol tetra-nitrate
Pentafort-T
Pentagesic
Pentagill
pentapiperide methyl-sulfate
Pentarcort
pentazocine hydro-chloride
pentazocine lactate
Pentazyme
penthienate bromide
Penthrane
Pentids
pentobarbital
Pento-Del
Pentothal Sodium
Pentraline
Pentritol
Pentryate

Pentryate Timed Capsules
Pen.Vee Drops
Pen.Vee K
Pen.Vee Oral
Pen.Vee Sulfas
pentylenetetrazol
Pep-O-Wafers
pepsin
peroxide
perphenazine
pertussis immune globulin
pertussis vaccine
Peptenzyme
Pepto-Ferrin
Peptolin
Peptron
Pepulcin
Perandren propionate
Perborate Compound
Perbuzem
Percobarb
Percodan
Percogesic
Percorten
Perfolin
Periactin
Peri-Colace
Peridial
Peridin-C
Perifoam Aerosol
Perihemin
Perin Syrup
Perithiazide S A
Peritinic
Peritrate
Peritrate c̄ Pb.
Peritrate Sustained Action
PERKé
Permapen

Permitil
Pernaemon
Pernavit
Pernox
Persadox
Persantine
Persistin
Personamine
Personaphen
Personatinic
Pertofrane
Petabolic
Petacal D
Peta Gel
Pet A Vite
Petrocel
Petrogalar
Petro-Phylic Soap
Pfizerpen
Pfizerpen-AS
Phallos Capsules
Phantos
Pharycidin
Phasphorone
Phazyme
Phedoxe 4B
Phedral
Phelantin
Phe-Mer-Nite Ointment
Phe-Mer-Nite Throat
    Tablets
Phemerol Chloride
    Solution
Phemerol Topical, 3%
phenacemide
phenacetin
Phenaderm
Phenagesic
phenaglycodol
Phenahist
Phenaphen
Phenaphen Plus

Phenaphen w/Codeine
Phenapirin
Phenate
Phenatuss
Phenazem
Phenazo
phenazopyridine
phenazopyridine hydro-
    chloride
Phencasal
Phencaset
phendimetrazine
    bitartrate
Pheneen Sanitizer
Pheneen Solution N.R.I.
Phenergan
Phenergan Cream
Phenergan Expectorant
Phenergan VC
    Expectorant
phenethicillin potassium
phenformin
phenindamine tartrate
phenindione
Phen-Iodine #2
pheniramine maleate
phenmetrazine hydro-
    chloride
phenobarbital
Phenodrox
Phenodyne
phenol
Phenolax
Phenoleum Antiseptic
    Sponges
phenolphthalein
phenolsulfonphthalein
Phenolsulfonphthalein
    Injection
phenothiazine
Phenoxene

phenoxybenzamine
    hydrochloride
Phensal
phensuximide
phentermine resin
phentolamine
Phenurone
phenylalanine
phenylbutazone
phenylephrine
phenylephrine bitartrate
phenylephrine hydro-
    chloride
phenylephrine tannate
Phenylin
phenylmercuric acetate
phenylmercuric nitrate
phenylpropanolamine
phenylpropanolamine
    hydrochloride
phenyl salicylate
phenyltoloxamine
phenyltoloxamine
    dihydrogen citrate
phenyltoloxamine resin
    complex
Pheny-Pas-Tebamin
Phetabarb
pHil-Acne-Cort
Phillips' Milk of
    Magnesia
pHisoAc
pHisoDan
pHisoderm
pHisoHex
Phoam Cleanse Pac
pHorsix
Phos-Flur
pHos-pHaid
Phosphaljel
Phospholine

phosphorated carbohydrate solution
phosphorus
Phospho-Soda
Phyatromine-H
Phylacogen
Phyldrox
Phyllicin
physostigmine salicylate
Physotropin
Phytex
phytonadione
Picro-Benzyl Ointment
Pil-Digis
Pilo B
Pilocar Ophthalmic Ointment
pilocarpine hydrochloride
Pilomiotin
Pima
P-I-N Forte
Pinkette Lotion
Pinrou
Pipanol
pipenzolate bromide
piperazine
piperidolate hydrochloride
Pipizan Citrate
pipobroman
pipradrol hydrochloride
Piptal
Piptal-PHB
Piptelate
Piromen
Pirseal
piSEC
Pitocin
Pitressin
pitressin tannate
Pituitrin

Pituitrin (S)
Placidyl
plague vaccine
plantago seed
Plantamucin
Plaquenil
plasma fractions
Plasmanate
Plax Lotion
Plebex
Plegine
Plenozyme
Plestran
Plexon
Plexonal
Plexovims
Plimasin
Pluravit
Plus Factor Tablets
Pneumocolon
p-nitrosulfathiazole
Piodiaspray
podophyllin
Poisonivi-Oral
Poisonok-Oral
Polanil
Polaramine
Poldine Methylsulfate
poliovirus vaccine
Poliovirus Vaccine, Live, Oral
Polybrade
polycarbophil
Polycillin
Polycillin-N For Injection
Polycin
Polycitra
Polyectin
polyestradiol phosphate
polyethyleneglycol
Polygesic

Poly-Guentum
Polykol
Polymagma
polymyxin
polymyxin b sulfate
Polyonic M-56 in 5% Dextrose
Polyonic M-900
Polyonic R-148 in 5% Dextrose in Water
Polyonic R-148 in Water
polyoxyethylene lauryl ether
Polysal in water w/5% Dextrose
Polysal-M w/2 1/2, 5%, 10%
Polysept
Polysorb
Polysorbin
Polysporin
Polytar Bath
Polytar Soap
polythiazide
polythionate
Poly-Vi-Flor
polyvinylpyrrolidone
Poly-Vi-Sol
Pomalin
Ponodyne
Ponstel
Pontocaine
Portagen
Postacne Lotion
Postopack No. 2
Potaba
potassium acetate
potassium acetylsalicylate
potassium acid phosphate

potassium bicarbonate
potassium chloride
potassium citrate
potassium gluconate
potassium guaiacol-
   sulfonate
potassium iodide
potassium oxyquinoline
   sulfate
potassium phosphate,
   dibasic
potassium phosphate,
   monobasic
potassium salicylate
potassium salts
Potassium Sulfocyanate
Potassium Thiocyanate
Potassium Triplex
Pot. Iod. Theocalcin
Povan
povidone-iodine
Poyaliver
Poyamin
Poyaplex
Pradase
Pragmatar
Pramet
Pramilets
Pramilets FA
Pramosone Lotion
pramoxine hydro-
   chloride
Pranone
Prantal
Prantal Repetabs
Precalcin
Precalcin-D
Preceptin Contraceptive
Predalone
Pred-5
Pre-Diluted Cytal

Predisal
Prednaman Tablets
Predne-Dome
Prednigesic
Prednilan
prednisolone
prednisone
Predoxine
Predsem
Pre-Enthus
Pregent
Pregnyl
Prelamin
Prelaron
Preltron
Preludin Endurets
Preludin Tablets
Premarin Cream
Premarin Intravenous
Premarin Lotion
Premarin Tablets
Pre-Mens
Premtal
Prenabex
Prenalac
Prenatal Dri-Kaps
Prenatal-Federal
Prequest
Pre-Sate
Preseptic
Prestets
Prestogen
Presulin Cleanser
Pre-Test Tablets
Priatest
Pricortin
Priferon
Pri-Gera
prilocaine hydro-
   chloride
Primabalt
Primacel

Primafolin
Primafort
Primaphos
Primaplex
primaquine phosphate
Primatone
Primenol
Primestrin
primidone
Primogen
Primone
Principen
Principen/N
PriORbarb
Priscoline
Privine
Probana
Pro-Banthīne
Pro-Banthīne P.A.
Pro-Banthīne w/Dartal
Pro-Banthīne
   w/Phenobarbital
Probec
Probec-T
probenecid
Probilagol
Probital
Pro-Blem
Probutylin
procainamide hydro-
   chloride
procaine
procaine hydrochloride
procarbazine hydro-
   chloride
Pro-Ception
prochlorperazine
Proctalme Ointment
Proctocaine
Proctocort
Proctodon
Proctofoam-HC

Proctoform Suppositories
Pro Cute Lotion
procyclidine hydrochloride
Pro-Duosterone
Profenil
progesterone
Pro-Gestive
Progestoral
Pro-Gest-Roid
Progiatric
Proglobin
Progynon
Proketazine
Proklar
Prolaire
Proliculin
Prolixin
Proloid
Proluton
Promacetin
promazine hydrochloride
Promenstrin
promethazine hydrochloride
Pro-min-vite
Pronac
Pronemia
Pronestyl
Pro-Neurin
Propadrine
Propahist
propantheline bromide
proparacaine hydrochloride
propesin
Prophyllin
propiomazine hydrochloride
Propion Gel

Propion Ophthalmic
propoxyphene hydrochloride
propranolol hydrochloride
Proprone
propylene glycol
propylhexedrine
ProReNata
Proseca
Proserum 5
Proserum 25
ProSobee
Prostaphlin
Prostigmin
Protalba-R
Protamide
Protamine Zinc
Protef Suppositories
Protegel
protein
Protein Mild
proteolytic
Proternol
Pro-Tet Tetanus Immune Globulin
Protinal
Protinex
Protium
Protobol
Protopam
Prototabs
protoveratrine
protoveratrine a
Protozime
protozoacides
protriptyline hydrochloride
Proval #3
Provera
Provest
Providex

Provimalt
Provimin
Prov-U-Sep
Prozine
Prozyme
Prucara
Prulet
Prunicodeine
Prunisatin
Prydonnal Spansule
Prydon Spansule
Pryilgin
pseudoephedrine
pseudoephedrine hydrochloride
pseudomonas polysaccharide
psyllium
Pthalox
Pulsaphen
Purified Cortrophin
Purinethol
Purodigin
P-V-Tussin
Pyelokon-R
Pylora
Pylorpine
Pyma
Pymadex
Pyma Timed Capsules
Pyocidin
Pyracodeine
Pyracort
Pyraldine
Pyral Vials
Pyramine
Pyraneurin
Pyrapap
Pyraphed
Pyrazinamide
Pyrdex
Pyribenzamine

Pyridium
Pyridostigmine bromide
pyridoxine
pyridoxine hydro-
chloride
pyrilamine maleate
pyrilamine tannate
pyrimethamine
Pyrizine
Pyro
Pyrralan
pyrrobutamine
Pyrroxate
pyrvinium pamoate
Pytosin Solution

Q

Q Caps
Quaalude
Quada Creme
Quadamine
Quadetts
Quadrabarb
Quadraflor
Quadramine
Quadramoid
Quadra-Sed
Quadrates
Quadrinal
Quadrops
Quadsul
Qualico Antiseptic Soap
Quanti-Vite
Quatrasal
Quelicin
Quelidrine
Questran
Quiactin
Qui-A-Zone

Quibron
Quide Tablets
Quiess
Quilene
Quimotrase Opthalmic
Quinaglute
Quinamm
Quinetas
quinethazone
Quinette
Quinidex Extentabs
Quinidine
quinidine gluconate
quinidine polygalactu-
ronate
quinidine sulfate
Quinine
quinine sulfate
Quinital
Quin-O-Creme
Quinodon
Quinolor
Quinora
Quinsone Ointment
Quintess
Quintess-N
Quotane Ointment

R

RBC Plus
R. I. P. Estrone
R. S. P. Tablets
R V P
rabies anti-serum
rabies vaccine
racephedrine
racephedrine hydro-
chloride
Racet

Racet LCD Cream
Radiocaps-131
Ragus
Raphetamine 1%
Ratiodrine
Ratio Tablets
Raudixin
Rauja
Raulin
Rauprote
Raurine
Rau-sed
Rauserpine
Rautensin
Rautrax
Rautrax-N
Rautrax-N Modified
Rauval
Rauvera
Rauverid
Rauwiloid
Rauwiloid + Veriloid
rauwolfia
Rauwolfia & Veratrum
rauwolfia serpentina
Rauw-Tina
Rauzide
Recortex
Recotabs
Rectalad Enema
Rectalad-Migraine
Rectalgan
Rectal Medicone
Rectodyne
Rectules
Redexcel
Redifact Forte
Redisol
Reditrin
Redoderlein
Regitine
Regroton

Regulin
Regumen
Reidacol
Reithritol
Rela
Renacidin
Renalgin
Renaltabs
Renasul
Renelate
Renese
Renese-R
Renografin
Renovist
Repoise
Resercen
Reserpatabs
reserpine
Reserpine w/Mebaral
Reser-Plus
Reserpoid
Resinat
Resion
Resistovites
resorcin
resorcinol
resorcinol monoacetate
Resorcitate Lotion
Resource Baking Mix
Respaire
Respet
Respicol
Respihaler DECADRON
Respihaler ProDECA-
    DRON
Respiratory U B A
Respirex
Respi-Sed
Resulin Lotion
Resulin Ointment
Resulin Soap
Resyll

Retet
Reticulex
Reticulogen
Retrografin
Retropaque
Reumalate
Revac Supprettes
Revicaps
Rexamycin
Rezamid Cream
Rezifilm
Rezipas
R-gene 5%
Rheomacrodex
Rhinall
Rhin-a-spray
Rhinazine
Rhinex
Rhinogesic
Rhinspec
Rhubamint
Rhulicream
Rhulihist
Rhulispray
Rhulitol
Rhus Tox Antigen
Rhutox Lotion
Riatrin
Ribocee
Riboderm
riboflavin
Ribozyme
ricinoleic acid
Ridupois
Rinkel Special Mixtures
Rinofeds
Rinohist
Riopan
Risa-125
Risa-131
Ritalin
Rith-A-Tal

Rith-A-20
Ritonic
Robalate
Robam
Robaxin
Robaxisal
Robaxisal-PH
Ro-Bile
Robinul
Robitussets
Robitussin
Roccal 10%
Ro-Cillin
rocky mountain spotted
    fever vaccine
RoCYTE
RoeriBeC
Rogenic
Rolicton
Romach Tablets
Romatinic
Rondec DSC
Rondec T
Rondectorant
Rondomycin
Roniacol
Ronium
Ronuvex
rose petal preparations
Rosenvold Disposable
    Eye Shield
Ro-Sulfa
Ro-Tabs
Roter Tablets
Rotoxamine
Rubeovax
rubella virus vaccine
Rubesol-LA Injectable
Rubicrest Crystal-
    line B_{12}
Rubiguent
Rubraferate

Rubrafolin
Rubragran
Rubramin
Rubraton
Rufolex
Rugar (Radiopaque Medium)
Ruhexatal w/Reserpine
Rulivan
Ruphon
Ruscorbic
rutin
Ruvite
RVPaque
RVPellent
RVPlus
Rydiamin
Rynalert
Rynatan
Rynatuss

S

S.B.P. Tablets
S-44 T.D.
SMA
S-A-C Tablets
Saferon
Safflor
Salatar
Salcedrox
Salcort
Salcort-Delta
Sal-Ethyl Carbonate
Saleto
Salgelate
Sal Hepatica
Salicionyl, G.E.S.
Salicresin
salicylamide

salicylazosulfapyridine
salicylic acid
Salicylic Acid & Sulfur Soap
Salicylic Acid Soap 3 1/2%
salicylsalicylic acid
Salimeph Forte
Salimeph-C/Colchicine
Salinidol Ointment
Salisicol
Salithol
Sali-Zem No. 2
Salpaba
Salpacine
Sal-Phenesin
Salphenyl
Salpix Contrast Medium
Salrin
Sal-Su-Tar
Salsuxin
Saluron
Salutensin
Salyrgan-Theophylline
Sandril
Sandril c̄ Pyronil
Sanguis
Sanicide
Sansert
Santal Oil
Santocal
sarapin
Sarocycline
Sarogesic
Sarogest
Sarolax
Saroxin
Sarpanol
SAStid
Satervite
Savacort-50
Savaplex

Saxin Saccharin
Scadan
Scarlet Red Ointment
Schieffelin Emulsion Base
Schieffelin Neutracolor
Schieffelin Qualatum
Schirmer Tear Test
Sclerex
Scolate
Scopettes
scopolamine
scopolamine hydro-bromide
Scorbisal
Seba-Nil
Sebaveen Shampoo
Sebella
Sebical
Sebical Tar Shampoo
Sebizon Lotion
Sebucare
Sebulex
Sebutone
Secastat
Seco-8
secobarbital
Secomat
Seconal
Secophen
Sedaclar
Sedadrops
Sedalgesic
Sedalixir
Sedalotion
Sedamyl
Sed-A-Nat
Sedapap
Sedaphen
Sed-A-Plex
Sedaserp
Sedatans

Sedatole
Sedatromine
Sedatussin
Sedophylline
Sedoral
Sedragesic
Sed-Tens Ty-Med
Sedtran
Sedutain
selenium sulfide
Selsun
Semaldyne
Sembex
Semcof
Semestrin
Semets
Semoxydrine
Senagest
Senagrada
Senathalin
Senazol
Senilan
Senilex
senna concentrate
Senntab
Senokap DSS
Senokot
Sensi-Kit
Ser-Ap-Es
Serax
Serbio
SERC
Sereenal
Serenium
Serfin
Serfolia
Sergynol
Serobacterin Vaccine
Seromycin
Serpanray
Serpasil
Serpasil-Apresoline

Serpasil-Esidrix
Serpate
Sertabs
Sertina
Setamine
Seven-O-Seven
Sevetol
Sheramin
Shermaplex
Shervac, Oral Respira-
    tory Vaccine
Sibena
Siblin
Sidolax
Sidonna
Sigamine
Sigesic
Sigmagen
Signatal
Signef "Supps"
Signemycin
Sigtab
Silain
Silain-Gel
Silbar
Silicote Cream
silicone preparation
Silikalin
Silvol
simethicone
Similac
Similac Isomil
Similac Isomil 20
Similac PM 60/40
Similac 13
Similac 20
Similac 27
Similac w/Iron
Similac w/Iron 20
Similac w/Iron 24
Simron
Sinacol

Sinahist
Sinaphen
Sinaxar
Sinequan
Singoserp
Singoserp-Esidrix
Sinodec
Sinografin
Sinovan Timed
Sintrom
Sinubid
Sinulin
Sinusule
Sinutab
Sippyplex Powder
Sitabs
sitosterols
Skelaxin
Skim Infant Formula
Skiodan Sodium
Slimzen Forte
S-L Ointment
Slowten
smallpox vaccine
S-M-S Tablets
So-Banic
Sobee
So-Cort
Sodestrin
sodium acetrizoate
sodium acetylsalicylate
sodium acid phosphate
sodium aminosalicylate
sodium amobarbital
sodium ampicillin
sodium bicarbonate
sodium borate
sodium butabarbital
Sodium Chloride
sodium citrate
sodium cloxacillin
    monohydrate

49

sodium dehydrocholate
sodium diatrizoate
sodium dicloxacillin
monohydrate
sodium diethyl bar-
biturate
sodium diphenyl-
hydantoin
sodium fluoride
Sodium Iodide I 131
sodium iodipamide
sodium isobutylally
barbiturate
sodium lauryl sulfate
sodium lauryl sulfo-
acetate
sodium levothyroxine
Sodium Phosphate (p^{32})
sodium oxychlorosene
sodium pentobarbital
sodium perborate
sodium phenylenthyl
barbiturate
sodium phosphate
sodium polystyrene
sulfonate
sodium propionate
Sodium Saccharin
Sodium Salicylate
sodium secobarbital
sodium succinate
Sodium Sulamyd
sodium sulfobromo-
phthalein
sodium tetradecyl sul-
fate
sodium thiopental
sodium thiosulfate
sodium warfarin
Sof-Cil
SOF-2
Softique Bath Beads

Softran
Solacen
Solagest
Solar Cream
Solbar
Solfo-Serpine
Solfoton
Solganal
Solimer Douche
Solonate
Solu-B
Solu-B w/Ascorbic Acid
Solu-Barb 1/4
Solu-Cortef
Solu-Medrol
Solumycin
Solusponge
Solu-Tuss
Solu-Zyme
Solvilith
Soma
Somacort
Somagen
Sombitol
Somide
Somnafac
Somnos
Som Ophyllin
Sonasal w/Pred.
Sonazar
Sonilyn
Soniphen
Soothogel Cream
So-Otic Drops
Sopen-V
Sopor
Sopronol
Soquette
Sorbezol
Sorbi-Cyte Forte
Sorbitinic
Sorbitrate

Sorboquel
Sorbutuss
Soropon
Sosol
So-Tab
So-Topic Cream
Sotradecol
Soyalac
Soyaloid
soybean preparation
Soyboro Powder
Soy-Dome
Soy-Sitz
Spacolin
Spalix
Spandecon
Spanestrin
Spanestrin "p"
Span-FF
Span-RD
Spantran
Spantuss
Spar-Cal
Sparine
Spartase
Spartocin
Spasdex
Spasmacol
Spasmasorb
Spasmid-PB
Spasmo-Forte
SpasmOR
Spasodil
Spasticol P.B.
Spasticol S.A.
Spastosed
Spaszyme
Spaz-uro
Sperotabs
Spiritex
spironolactone
Sporostacin

Spotstik
S-P-T
S-R
stanozolol
Staphage Lysate
Staphcillin
Staphylococcus Ambo-
toxoid
Staphylococcus Tox-
oid-Vaccine
Staphylo-Strepto Sero-
bacterin
Statomin
Statuss
Steclin
Stelazine
Stemutrolin
Stenediol
Stental Extentabs
Stera-Form Cream
Steramine Otic
Sterane
Sterapred
Sterapred UNI-PAK
Sterasal-K
Sterazolidin
Steri-Amps
Sterilized Water
Sterneedle
Stero-Darvon w/A.S.A.
Sterolone
Sterosan Cream
Sterotate
Stilbetin
Stil Forte
Stilphostrol
Stimdex
Stimula Ointment
Stimulon
StomAseptine
Stoxil
Strascogesic

streptokinase-strepto-
dornase
Streptomagma
Strepto-Staphylo Vatox
Stresscaps
Strexate
Strontolac
Stuart Amino Acids
Stuart Formula Tablets
Stuart Hematinic
Stuartinic
Stuart Prenatal
Stuart Prenatal w/Folic
Acid
Stuart V-C-M
Suavitil
Sublimaze
Suby's Solution "G"
Sucaryl
succinylcholine
chloride
Sucostrin
Sudafed
Sudolin
sugar (invert)
Sugracillin
Suladyne
Sul-Caine Drops
Sule (placebo)
Sulfabid
sulfacetamide
Sulfacet-HC
Sulfacet-R Lotion
sulfachlorpyridazine
sulfadiazine
sulfadimethoxine
sulfaethidole
Sulfagram
sulfaguanidine
Sulfallantoin
sulfameter
sulfamethizole

sulfamethoxazole
sulfamethoxypyridazine
Sulfamylon Cream
sulfanilamide
sulfaphenazole
Sulfa-Plex Cream
Sulfased
Sulfa-Statin
sulfas-triple (prepa-
rations)
Sulfasuxidine
sulfated oil surfactants
Sulfathalidine
sulfathiazole
Sulfavitin Ointment
Sul-Fed
Sulfem Vaginal Cream
Sulfid Forte
sulfinpyrazone
sulfisomidine
sulfisoxazole
sulfonamides
Sulfonsol
Sulforcin Base
Sulforcin Lotion
Sulfose Suspension
Sulfstat Forte
Sulfstat 1 Gram
Sulf-10 Ophthalmic
Sulf-30 Ophthalmic
sulfur
sulfur, precipitated
sulfur (colloidal)
Sulfur Diasporal Lotion
Sulfur Soap 10%
Sulfurine
Sulla
Sulpan
Sulphocol
Sul-Spansion
Sul-Spantab
Sultacof

Sultein
Sulthane
Sultril
Sultrin Triple Sulfa
    Cream
Sultrin Triple Sulfa
    Vaginal Tablets
Sultussin
Sumycin
SunDare Lotion
SunStick
SunSwept Cream
Supac
Super A Vitamin
Super D Cod Liver Oil
Super Doss
Super D Perles
Super Hydramin Powder
Super Ironized Yeast
SuperPAS
Super Plenamins
Super Rhi-Lief
Supertah
Supertah-HC Ointment
Supertah S/S
Super Ulex
Supervim Drops
Suprex-C
Surbex-T
Surbex-T Solution
    w/D5-W
Surfacaine
Surfadil
Surfak
Surg-C
Surgel
SURGICEL Absorbable
    Hemostat
Surital
Sus-Phrine
Sustagen
Sustinex

sutilains
Suvren
Sybotan
Sylapar
Syllamalt
Symmetrel
Symptomax
Synalar Creams
Synalar-HP
Synalar Ointments
Synalar Solution
Synalgos
Synasal
Snyate-M
Syncelax
Syncelose
Syncillin
Syncuma
Syncurine Decamethoni-
    um Bromide
Syndecon
Syndrox
Synephricol
Synestrol
Syniodin
Synirin
Synkamin
Synkayvite
Synogen
Synophedal
Synophylate
Snytetrin
Synthaloids
Synthetar
Synthroid
Syntocinon
Syrasulfas
Syrcodate
Syrcohist
syrosingopine
Sytobex
Sytobex-H

T

T-125
T-250
T C S
T. D. Therals
TEM
T. H. & M.
TSG
Tabalin A
Tab-Lase
Taborea
Tacaryl
TACE 12 mg.
TACE 25 mg.
TACE w/Androgen
TACE w/Ergonovine
Tacol
Tadona
Taf-Tab
Tagathen
Tag-39
Tain
Taka-Diastase
Takazyme
Talam
talbutal
Tal-Estamine
Taline
Taloin
Talwin
Tamponets
Tandearil
Tanicaine
tannic acid
Tanorex
Tanurol
Tao
Tao-AC
Tapazole

Ta-Poff
tar, coal
Taractan
Tarbonis
Tarcortin Cream
Tar Distillate "Doak"
Tar-Doak Lotion
Tarpaste
Tauracrine
Taurocolate
Taurophyllin
Ta-Verm
Tavilen-Plus
Taystron
Tear-Efrin
Tearisol
Tedfern
Tedral
Tedral SA
Tedral-25
Teebacin
Teebaconin
Teedees 10
Teedees 15
Teeds Lozenges
Teenac
Teen Shampoo
Tegopen
Tegretol
Tegumin
Teldrin
Telepaque
Telgra
Temaril
Temlo
Tempotriad
Tempra
Tenalgic
Tenda Cream
Tenda-HC
Ten-50-Five Injection
Tenlap

Tenol
Tensilon
Tensodin
Tentabs
Tenuate Dospan
Tenuate 25 mg.
Teon Time Caps
Tepanil
Tepanil Ten-Tab
Teragen
Teranium
Terfonyl
Tergemist
Tergesten
Terphan
Terpicol
terpin hydrate
Terra-Cortril
Terracydin
Terramycin
Terrastatin
Tersaseptic
Tersa-Tar
Teslac
Tesogen
Teson L.A.
Tesone "50"
Tessalon
Testand-B
Tes-Tape
Testarr Fortified Flakes
TestaSpan
Testavol-S
Test-Estrin Buccal
Test-Estrin Injectable
testolactone
testosterone
Testostroval P.A.
Testralate-200
Testrine
Testrogyn
Testro-Med

Tet Capsules
tetanus antitoxin
tetanus immune glob-
  ulin
Tetanus & Diphtheria
  Toxoids Combined
Tetanus Toxoid
tetracaine hydrochloride
Tetrachel
Tetrachel-S
tetracycline
tetracycline hydro-
  chloride
tetracycline phosphate
Tetracydin
Tetracyn
Tetradene
tetrahydrozoline hydro-
  chloride
TetraMax
Tetrasorb-125
Tetraspect
Tetrastatin
Tetrasule
Tetrate "30"
Tetrate "80"
Tetrazets
Tetrex
Tetrex bidCAPS
Tetrex-APC
Tetrex-F
Texacort
Texacort Scalp Lotion
Thalfed
THAM-E
Thantis Lozenges
Thedrinal
Thedrizem
Theelandrol
Theelin
Theelin R-P
Theelol

Thekobarb
Thendelate
thenyldiamine hydro-
  chloride
Theobarb
Theobid
theobromine
Theocalcin
Theocardone No. 1
Theodide
Theofed
Theofort
Theogen
Theo-Guaia
Theokin
Theolaphen
Theolix
Theolixir
Theominal
Theo-Nar
Theonatal-E
Theo-Organidin
theophylline
Theo-Serp
Theptine
Therabex
Therabile
Theracebrin
Thera-Combex
Thera-Combex H-P
  Kapseals
Thera-Deimal
Theragran
Theragran-M
Thera-Mineral
Therapads
Therapas
Therapeutin
Thera Spancap
Theratuss
Thera-Zymacap
Therevac w/Benzocaine

Theridol
Thermodex
Theron
Thex
Thia-Bex
Thiacide
Thia Injectable
thiamine
thiamylal sodium
Thiatron
Thi-Bee
Thi-Cin
thiethylperazine
thihexinol methyl-
  bromide
Thiliron
thimerosal
Thiodex
Thiodyne
Thioguanine
Thiomerin Injection
Thionicavin
Thiopentarsen
thipropazate dihydro-
  chloride
thioridazine
Thiosul
Thiosulfil
Thiosulfil-A-Forte
Thiosulfil Forte
thiotepa
thiothixene
thioxanthene
Thioxin
thiphenamil hydro-
  chloride
Thipyri
Thizodrin
Thora-Dex
Thorazine
Thorexin
Thormal

Thoryza
3X-Statuss
thrombin
Thrombin Sterile
  Powder
Thrombolysin
Thymoboral
thymol
Thymolidine Compound
  Solution
Thyrar
Thyrest
Thyrobex
thyroglobulin
thyroid
Thytropar
thyrotropic hormone
thyroxine
Tigacol
T-I-Gammagee
Tigan
Tinactin
Tindal
Tinver
Titan
titanium dioxide
Titralac
Titroid-200
Tocopherex
Tofrānil
Toin Unicelles
Tokols
Tolachol
Tolagesic
To Lakol Bath Oil
Tolar-8
Tolavad
Tolax
tolazamine
tolazoline hydro-
  chloride
tolbutamide

Toldex
Toleron
Tolferain
Tolfrinic
Tolinase
tolnaftate
Tolseram
Tolserol
Tolu Balsam Syrup
Tonigestine
Tonillone
Tonnostan
Tono-B Wafers
Topic
Topigel
Topisol
Topocide
Torecan
Tossecol
Totacillin
Totalex
Totamin
Tota-Vi-Caps
Totocal
Tracervial-131
Tracne Cream
Trac Tabs
Trac Tabs 2X
Tral Gradumet
Tralmag
tralnitrate phosphate
Tranco-gesic
Trancopal
Trancoprin
Tranite D-Lay
Tranmep
Tranquinal
Transact
Transentine
Transerpin
tranylcypromine sulfate

Traumaide
Trates
Travad Disposable
    Enema
Travase Ointment
Trecator-SC
Trela
Tremin
Tre-o-caps
Treofer
Tre-o-tabs
Trepidone
Trest
Trevidal
Trexinest
Treyhist
triacetin
triacetyloleandomycin
Tri-Alum-Alac
triamcinolone
triamcinolone aceto-
    nide
triamcinolone diace-
    tate
triamcinolone hex-
    acetonide
Triaminic
Triaminic-HC
Triaminicin
Triaminicol
triamterene
Triavil
Triaxin
Tri-Barbs
Triburon
Trib Vaginal Cream
Trichinella Extract
trichlocarban
trichlormethiazide
trichomonacide
Trichotine

triclobisonium chloride
Tricofuron Vaginal
    Suppositories
Tricreamalate
Tridal
tridihexethyl chloride
Tridione
Tri-Droxal
Trienzyme
triethanolamine salicy-
    late
triethylene melamine
Triethylenemelamine
    (TEM)
triethylenethiophos-
    phoramide
trifluoperazine
triflupromazine
Tri-Genik
Trigesic
trihexyphenidyl
Tri-Immunol
Tri-Isohalant
Triketol
Trikon
Trilafon
Trilamine
Trilene
Trilox
Trimagill
trimeprazine tartrate
Trimester
trimethadione
trimethobenzamide
    hydrochloride
Trimeton
Trimo-San
Trinachlor
Trinade
Trinalis Supprettes
Trind
Trind-DM

Trinotic
Trinsicon
Trinsicrest
Triogen
Triomet-131
Triophen
Triosorb-131
trioxsalen
Tripac
Tripac Troches
tripelennamine hydro-
   chloride
Triple Alamine
Triple Antibiotic
   Ointment
Triple Sulfoid
triprolidine hydro-
   chloride
Tripsul
Triptein
Triquin
Tri-Salve
Trisem
Trisert
Trisilobarb
Trisocort Spraypak
Trisogel
Trisohist
Tri-Solgen
Trisomin
Trisoralen
Trisorbin
Trist-A-Lin
Tristerone
Tri-Sulfamine
Trisulfaminic
trisulfapyrimidine
Trisulfazine
Trisulfidon
Tri-Sul L.A. Liquid
Trisul Suspension
Trisureid

Tri-Suspension
Tri-Uro
Triva
Triva Jel
Trivased
Tri Vida F
Tri-Vi-Flor
Tri-Vi-Sol
Trizyme
Trobex
Trocaine
Trocinate
Trolar
troleandomycin
tromethamine
Tromine
Tronothane
Troph-Iron
Trophite
Tropinal
Tropsor
Trovit
Trulase
Trushay Hand Lotion
Trydecyl Cream
trypsin
Tryptar
TSG-GG
TSG-KI
T-Spray
Tuamine
Tuberculin
tuberculin, old
Tuberculin, Tine Test
tuberculin P.P.D.
Tubex
Tucks Cream
Tucks Ointment
Tuinal
Turgasept
Tusergen
Tusquelin

Tussagesic
Tussaminic
Tussapap
Tussar-2
Tussend
Tussimer
Tussionex
Tussi-Organidin
Tussomyl
Tuss-Ornade
Tusstrol
Twel-Viron
Twiston R-A
Twiston Tablets
Twix
Two-Dyne
2/G
2G/DM
tybamate
Tybatran
Tycopan
Tylandril
Tylenol
Tylosterone
tyloxapol
Tympagesic
Tympanide
Tyoben
typhoid vaccine
Tyrobenz
Tyrotrace
Tyvid
Tyzine
Tyzomint

U

ULO
U.R.I. Capsules
U-Cys-Tine

Udi-Globin
Ulacort
Ulcimins
Ulcinal
Ulcort
Ulcortar
Ulex
Ulgestin
Ulmets
Ulsa-Jel w/Mineral Oil
Ultandren
Ultar
Ulti-ject
Ultracaine
Ultran
Ultrogen
Ulvical
"ULVICAL Plus"
Unatal
undecoylium chloride-
    iodine
undecylenate
undecylenate, zinc
undecylenic acid
Undecylic Ointment
Undelex
Unguentum Bossi
Unibase
Unicap
Unidote, Universal
    Antidote
Unigen
Unigesic
Unipen
Unisulf
Unitensen
Unitensen-Phen
Unitensen-R
UORsul Capsules
Upset Antacid-Liquid
Uracel

Uracil Mustard
Uralene
Uratin
Urazium
Urbalax
urea
Ureaphil
Urease-Dunning
Urecholine
Uremide
Urestrin
Urifon
Uripan
Uriplex
Urised
Urisedamine
Uritabs
Urithol
Uritone
Uritral
Urobiotic
Urobiotic-250
Urochron
Urolocaine
Urological Solution G
Urometh
Uropeutic
Uro-Phosphate
Uroqid
Uroqid-Acid
Uroqid-Amide
Urostat
Urostat-2X
Uro-Ves
Ursinus Inlay-Tabs
Ūtrasul
Uval

V

V & M
Vacagen
Vacon
Vacuetts
Vad Sofcream
Vag-Astring
Vaga-Trol
Vagestrol
Vagicream
Vagimine
Vaginostic
Vagi-Plex
Vagisan
Vagisec
Vagiserts
Vagitric
Vagitrol
Valacaps
Valacet
Valachol
Valdrene
Valenol
Valergen 10 mg.
Valerone #2
valethamate bromide
Valisone Cream
Valium
Vallestril
Valmid
Valoctin
Valpin
Valtuss
Vancocin
vancomycin
Vannor
Vanodonnal
Vanoxide

Vanquish
Vanseb Cream Shampoo
Vaponefrin
Vapo-N-Iso
V-Applicators
Varidase
Vasal
Vascutum
Vasitol
Vasocidin
Vasocon-A
Vasocort
Vasodilan
Vaso-80 Unicelles
Vasoglyn
Vasolator
Vasoplex
Vasopred
Vasospan
Vasosulf
Vasotherm
Vasotrate
Vasoxyl
Vastran AMP
Vastran Tablets
V-Cillin
V-Cillin K
vegetable oil (prepa-
    rations)
Velban
Velvachol
Velvetia Cream
Venibar
Venthera
Ventilade
Ventrex
Ventrilex
Veracillin
Veralba
Verased
Veratrite
veratrum viride

Verclysyl 10% in Water
Vercyte
Verdefam
Verequad
Veresconite
Vergo
Veritag
Vermidol
Vermizine
Vernitest
Verophylin
versenate, calcium
    disodium
Vertavis
Vertavis-Phen
Ver-Var
Vesprin
Vi-Alpha
Vi-Aquamin
Viaten
Viatric
Vibedoz
Vi-B-Min Plex
Vibramycin
Vicalmin
Vicaltein
Vi-Citrimin
Vicon-C
Vicon-T
Vi-Daylin ADC
Vi-Daylin Chewable
Vi-Daylin/F ADC
Vi-Daylin w/Fluoride
    Chewable Tablets
Videc
Viderol
Vides C.T. w/Fluoride
Vi-Dexemin
Vi-Dom-"A"
Vi-Dom-A-C
Vidox
Vi-Drape

Vifort
Vi-Hormex
Vi-Magna
Vimah
Vi-Mix Drops
Vimplex LF
vinblastine sulfate
vincristine sulfate
Vinethene
Vingesic
Vio-A
Vio-B
Viobamate
Vio-Bec
VioBin
Vio-Bone
Vio-C w/B
Viocin
Vio-Dex
Vio Fernisone
Vio-Ferronate
Vioform Inserts
Vioform-Hydrocortisone
Vio-Geric H
Vio-Hydrosone
Viokase
Viol
Vio-Lax
Vio-Mineral
Viomycin
Vio-Prenate
Vio-Sal
Vio-Serpine
Viosterol
Viotag
Vio-Thene
Vi-Penta F Zestabs
Vi-Penta Infant Drops
Viplets
Vi-Protinal
Virac
Virac VSA

Viridite
Viril-Lam
Viron #2
Visciodol
Visine Eye Drops
Vi-Sorbin
Vistaril
Vistex
Vi-Syneral
Vitab
Vita Cap M
Vitacoms
Vitacrest
Vitadec
Vitadex-B
Vitagett
Vitahormone
Vita-Kaps
Vitakins
Vita-Lam
Vitalyne
Vita M
Vita-Metrazol
vitamin
vitamin A
vitamin B_1
vitamin B_2
vitamin B_6
vitamin B_{12}
vitamin B complex
vitamin C
vitamin D
vitamin E
vitamin K
vitamin K_1
vitamin P
Vitamoids
Vitapherol
Vitaplex
Vita-Ray
Vitarex
Vitaroid

Vitasol
Vita Zol Elixir
Viteral
Viteron M
Viterra
Vi-Testrin
Vitikon
Vit-Min-I-Fact
VitORmains
VitORmelts-F
VitORsperse
Vitron
Vitron C-Plus
Vitules
Vi-Twel
Vi-Tyke
Vivactil
V-Kor
Vlemasque
Vlem-Dome
Volaxin
Vontrol
VoSol-HC Otic
VoSol Otic
Vymin
Vytone Cream

W

Walco-Nesin
Walco Pepo-Pips
Walcosol
WANS
Warexin
Wescolates
Wescophen-S
Wesmatic
Wesprin
Westhiazole

Wet-Tone Sterile
Ophthalmic
White's Ointment
Whole Infant Formula
Wibi
Wigraine
Wilpo
WinGel
Winstrol
witch hazel
Wolfina
Wright's Liquor
Carbonis Detergens
W-T Lotion
Wyamine
Wyanoid Ointment
Wyanoids HC
Wybiotic
Wychol
Wycillin
Wydase
Wynestron

X

xanthine oxidase
inhibitor
xanthine preparation
Xerac
X-M Cream
X-Nog
X-Prep Liquid
Xylocaine
Xylocaine Hydrochloride
for Spinal Anesthesia
Xylocaine Hydrochloride
4% Solution
Xylocaine Ointment
Xylocaine Viscous

xylometazoline hydro-
chloride
Xynisone

Y

yeast
Yestaga w/Cascara
Ylestrol
Yodoxin
yohimbine
yohimbine hydro-
chloride
Yuvral

Z

Zactane
Zactirin
Zactirin Compound-100
Zamitam

Zamitol
Zanchol
Zarontin
ZeaSORB
Zemarine
Zem-Dab
Zentinic
Zentron
Zephiran
Zermasol
Zerominic
Zeste
Zetar
Zetar Decolorized
Ze-Tar-Quin Cream
Zetar Shampoo
Zetone
Ziboral
Zilagen
zinc
zinc gluconate
zinc oxide
zinc pyrithione
zinc sulfate
Zinc Sulfide

Zincofax
Zinc-Phen
Ziradryl
zirconium oxide
Zirium
ZN-PLUS
Zolacin
zolamine hydro-
chloride
Zolediazine
Zoptic Eye Lotion
Zurpan
Zyanoids
Zyljectin
Zyloprim
Zymabasic
Zymacap
Zymacrest
Zymadrops
Zymafolic
Zymalixir
Zymasyrup
Zymatinic
Zymenol
Zymogest

PART 2

Medical
Terms

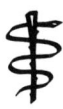

A

ab-a-li-en-a-tion
a-ban-don-ment
ab-ap-i-cal
ab-ap-tis-ton
a-bar-og-no-sis
ab-ar-tic-u-lar
a-ba-si-a
a-bate-ment
a-bat-tage
ab-at-toir
ab-ax-i-al
ab-do-men
ab-dom-i-no-an-te-ri-or
ab-dom-no-cen-te-sis
ab-dom-i-no-hys-ter-ec-
 to-my
ab-dom-i-no-hys-ter-ot-
 o-my
ab-dom-i-no-per-i-ne-al
ab-dom-i-no-pos-te-ri-or
ab-dom-i-nos-co-py
ab-dom-i-nous
ab-dom--i-no-u-ter-ot-o-
 my
ab-dom-i-no-ves-i-cal
ab-du-cens
ab-du-cent
ab-duct
ab-duc-tion
ab-duc-tor
ab-em-bry-on-ic
ab-en-ter-ic
ab-er-rant
ab-er-ra-tion
ab-er-rom-e-ter
a-bey-ance
ab-i-ent
A-bi-es

ab-i-et-ic
ab-i-et-ic ac-id
a-bi-o-gen-e-sis
a-bi-o-log-ic
a-bi-on-er-gy
a-bi-o-sis
a-bi-ot-ro-phy
ab-ir-ri-tant
ab-ir-ri-ta-tion
ab-lac-ta-tion
a-blast-in
ab-la-ti-o
ab-la-tion
ab-le-pha-ri-a
a-bleph-a-ron
a-bleph-a-ry
a-blep-si-a
ab-lu-ent
ab-lu-tion
ab-mor-tal
ab-nerv-al
ab-neu-ral
ab-nor-mal
ab-o-ma-si-tis
ab-o-ma-sum
ab-o-rad
ab-o-ral
a-bort
a-bor-ti-cide
a-bor-tient
a-bor-ti-fa-cient
a-bor-tin
a-bor-tion
a-bor-tive
a-bor-tus
a-bou-li-a
a-bou-lo-ma-ni-a
a-bra-chi-a
a-bra-chi-o-ceph-a-lus
a-bra-chi-us
ab-ra-dant
ab-ra-sion

ab-ra-sive
ab-ra-sor
a-bras-tol
ab-re-ac-tion
a-brin
L—a-brine
a-bro-si-a
ab-rup-ti-o
ab-scess
ab-scis-sa
ab-scis-sion
ab-scon-si-o
ab-sence
ab-sen-tee-ism
ab-sinthe
ab-sin-thic ac-id
ab-sin-thin
ab-sinth-ism
ab-sin-thi-um
ab-sin-thol
ab-so-lute
ab-sorb
ab-sor-bance
ab-sor-be-fa-cient
ab-sorb-ent
ab-sorp-ti-om-e-ter
ab-sorp-tion
ab-sorp-tiv-i-ty
ab-sti-nence
ab-strac-tion
Abt's meth-od
ab-ter-mi-nal
a-bu-li-a
a-bu-lo-ma-ni-a
a-buse
a-but-ment
a-ca-cia
a-cal-ci-co-sis
a-cal-cu-li-a
a-camp-si-a
a-can-thes-the-si-a
a-can-thi-on

63

a-can-tho-a-mel-o-blas-to-ma
A-can-tho-ceph-a-la
a-can-tho-ceph-a-li-a-sis
A-can-tho-chei-lo-ne-ma
a-can-tho-chei-lo-ne-mi-a-sis
a-can-thoid
a-can-tho-ker-a-to-der-mi-a
ac-an-thol-y-sis
ac-an-tho-ma
a-can-tho-pel-vis
A-can-tho-phis
ac-an-tho-sis
a-can-thro-cyte
a-can-thro-cy-to-sis
a-can-thu-lus
a-cap-ni-a
a-cap-su-lar
a-car-di-a
a-car-di-a-cus
a-car-di-o-he-mi-a
a-car-di-o-ner-vi-a
a-car-di-o-tro-phi-a
a-car-di-us
ac-a-ri-a-sis
a-car-i-cide
ac-a-rid
Ac-a-ri-na
a-car-i-no-sis
a-car-i-o-sis
ac-a-ro-der-ma-ti-tis
ac-a-roid
ac-a-ro-pho-bi-a
ac-a-ro-tox-ic
a-car-pi-a
a-car-pous
Ac-a-rus
a-car-y-ote
a-cat-a-lep-si-a
a-cat-a-ma-the-si-a

a-cat-a-pha-si-a
ac-a-tap-o-sis
ac-a-tas-ta-si-a
ac-a-thex-i-a
ac-a-thex-is
ac-a-thi-si-a
a-cau-dal
ac-cel-er-ans
ac-cel-er-ant
ac-cel-er-a-tion
ac-cel-er-a-tor
ac-cel-er-a-tor u-ri-nae
ac-cel-er-in
ac-cel-er-om-e-ter
ac-cen-tu-a-tor
ac-cep-tor
ac-ces-so-ri-us
ac-ces-so-ry
ac-ci-dent
ac-ci-den-tal-ism
ac-ci-dent—prone
ac-cip-i-ter
ac-cli-ma-ti-za-tion
ac-cli-ma-tion
ac-co-lé
ac-com-mo-da-tion
ac-com-plish-ment quo-tient
ac-couche-ment
ac-cou-cheur
ac-cou-cheuse
ac-cre-men-ti-tion
ac-cre-ti-o cor-dis
ac-cre-tion
ac-cu-mu-la-tor
A.C.D. so-lu-tion
a-ce-li-a
a-ce-naes-the-si-a
ac-e-naph-thene
a-ce-nes-the-si-a
a-cen-tric
ac-e-pha-li-a

a-ceph-a-lism
a-ceph-a-lo-bra-chi-a
a-ceph-a-lo-bra-chi-us
a-ceph-a-lo-car-di-a
a-ceph-a-lo-car-di-us
a-ceph-a-lo-chei-rus
a-ceph-a-lo-chi-ri-a
a-ceph-a-lo-chi-rus
a-ceph-a-lo-cyst
a-ceph-a-lo-cys-tis pla-na
a-ceph-a-lo-gas-ter
a-ceph-a-lo-gas-te-ri-a
a-ceph-a-lo-po-di-a
a-ceph-a-lo-po-di-us
a-ceph-a-lo-ra-chus
a-ceph-a-lor-rha-chi-a
a-ceph-a-lor-rha-chus
a-ceph-a-lo-sto-mi-a
a-ceph-a-los-to-mus
a-ceph-a-lo-tho-ra-ci-a
a-ceph-a-lo-tho-rax
a-ceph-a-lus
a-ceph-a-ly
ac-er-ate
a-cer-bi-ty
a-cer-bo-pho-bi-a
ac-er-dol
a-cer-ic
a-cer-o-pho-bi-a
a-cer-vu-line
a-cer-vu-lus
a-ces-cent
a-ces-o-dyne
a-ces-to-ma
ac-e-tab-u-lec-to-my
ac-e-tab-u-lo-plas-ty
ac-e-tab-u-lum
ac-e-tal
ac-et-al-de-hyde
ac-et-am-ide
ac-et-a-mi-no-flu-o-rene
p—a-cet-a-mi-no-phe-nol

ac-et-an-i-lid
ac-e-tan-nin
ac-et-ar-sol
ac-et-ar-sone
ac-e-tate
a-cet-a-zole-am-ide
a-cet—di—a-mer-sul-fon-a-mides
a-ce-tic ac-id
a-ce-tic ac-id am-ide
a-ce-tic al-de-hyde
a-ce-tic an-hy-dride
a-ce-tic e-ther
a-ce-tic fer-men-ta-tion
a-cet-i-fi-ca-tion
ac-e-tim-e-ter
ac-e-tin
ac-e-to-a-ce-tic ac-id
ac-e-to-a-ce-tic es-ter
A-ce-to-bac-ter
a-cet-o-in
ac-e-tol
ac-e-tol-y-sis
a-cet-o-mel
ac-e-to-me-naph-thone
ac-e-to-mer-oc-tol
ac-e-tom-e-ter
ac-e-to-mor-phine
ac-e-to-nae-mi-a
ac-e-ton-asth-ma
ac-e-tone
ac-e-to-ne-mi-a
ac-e-to-ni-trile
ac-e-to-num
ac-e-to-nu-ri-a
a-cet-o-nyl
ac-et-o-phe-net-i-din
ac-e-to-phe-none
a-cet-o-sal
ac-e-tous
ac-et-ox-ime

ac-et-par-a-phe-net-i-dine
a-cet-ri-zo-ic ac-id
a-ce-tum
ac-e-tyl
ac-e-tyl-a-ce-tic ac-id
ac-e-tyl-a-mi-no-hy-drox-y-phen-yl-ar-son-ic ac-id
a-cet-y-la-tion
ac-e-tyl—be-ta—meth-yl-cho-line
ac-e-tyl-car-bro-mal
ac-e-tyl-cho-line
a-cet-y-lene
a-cet-y-lide
a-cet-y-li-za-tion
ac-e-tyl-meth-yl-car-bi-nol
ac-e-tyl-mor-phine
ac-e-tyl-phe-nyl-hy-dra-zine
ac-e-tyl-sal-i-cyl-ic ac-id
ac-e-tyl-sal-ol
ac-e-tyl-sul-fon-a-mide
ac-e-tyl-tan-nic ac-id
ach-a-la-si-a
ache
a-chei-li-a
a-chei-lus
a-chei-ri-a
a-chei-rus
a-chieve-ment age
a-chieve-ment quo-tient
Ach-il-le-a
ach-il-le-in
Achilles
a-chil-lo-bur-si-tis
a-chil-lo-dyn-i-a
ach-il-lor-rha-phy
ach-il-lot-o-my
a-chi-lus

a-chi-ri-a
a-chlor-hy-dri-a
a-chlo-rides
a-chlor-op-si-a
a-chlo-ro-blep-si-a
ach-lu-o-pho-bi-a
a-cho-li-a
ach-o-lu-ri-a
a-chon-dro-pla-si-a
a-chor
A-chor-da-ta
ach-o-re-sis
A-cho-ri-on
a-chre-o-cy-the-mi-a
a-chro-a-cy-te
a-chro-a-cy-to-sis
a-chroi-o-cy-the-mi-a
a-chro-ma-cyte
a-chro-mat-o-cyte
a-chro-ma-si-a
a-chro-mate
a-chro-mat-ic
a-chro-ma-tin
a-chro-ma-tism
a-chro-ma-tol-y-sis
a-chro-ma-to-phil
a-chro-ma-top-si-a
a-chro-ma-to-sis
a-chro-ma-tous
a-chro-mic
a-chro-ma-tu-ri-a
a-chro-mi-a
a-chro-mic
A-chro-mo-bac-te-ri-a-ce-ae
a-chro-mo-der-mi-a
a-chro-mo-trich-i-a
a-chron-y-chous
ach-ro-o-am-y-loid
a-chro-o-cy-to-sis
a-chro-o-dex-trin

65

a-chyl-a-ne-mi-a
a-chy-li-a
ach-y-lo-sis
a-chy-mi-a
a-cic-u-lar
ac-id
ac-id al-bu-min
ac-id al-co-hol
ac-id-am-in-u-ri-a
ac-i-de-mi-a
ac-id—fast
ac-id—form-ing
ac-id fuch-sin
a-cid-i-fi-ca-tion
ac-i-dim-e-ter
ac-id in-tox-i-ca-tion
ac-id-ism
a-cid-i-ty
ac-id num-ber
a-cid-o-cyte
ac-i-do-cy-to-pe-ni-a
ac-i-do-cy-to-sis
ac-i-do-gen-ic
ac-i-dom-e-ter
ac-i-do-pe-ni-a
a-cid-o-phil
a-cid-o-phil-i-a
ac-i-doph-i-lism
ac-i-do-re-sist-ant
ac-i-do-sis
ac-i-dos-te-o-phyte
ac-id-proof
ac-id—re-sist-ant
ac-id tide
a-cid-u-late
ac-i-du-ric
ac-id-yl
a-cid-y-la-ted
ac-i-e-sis
ac-i-ne-si-a
ac-i-ni
ac-i-no-tu-bu-lar

ac-i-nus
ack-ee poi-son-ing
a-cla-di-o-sis
A-cla-di-um
ac-la-sis
a-clas-tic
a-cleis-to-car-di-a
ac-mas-tic
ac-me
ac-ne
ac-ne-form
ac-ne-mi-a
ac-ni-tis
ac-o-as-ma
a-coe-li-a
ac-o-ine
ac-o-kan-ther-in
a-co-la-si-a
a-co-lous
a-co-mi-a
a-con-a-tive
ac-o-nine
a-con-i-tase
ac-o-nite
ac-o-nit-ic ac-id
a-con-i-tine
Ac-o-ni-tum
a-con-u-re-sis
a-co-pro-sis
ac-o-re-a
a-co-ri-a
ac-o-rin
a-cor-mus
Ac-o-rus
Acosta's dis-ease
a-cos-tate
a-cou-aes-the-si-a
a-cou-es-the-si-a
ac-ou-la-li-on
a-cou-me-ter
ac-ou-oph-o-ny
a-cous-ma

a-cous-mat-ag-no-sis
a-cous-mat-am-ne-si-a
a-cous-tic
a-cous-ti-co-pho-bi-a
a-cous-tics
ac-ou-tom-e-ter
ac-quired
ac-ral
a-cra-ni-a
a-cra-si-a
a-cra-ti-a
a-crat-u-re-sis
ac-re-mo-ni-o-sis
ac-ren-ceph-a-lon
ac-ri-bom-e-ter
ac-rid
ac-ri-dine
ac-ri-fla-vine
ac-ri-nyl sul-fo-cy-a-nate
a-crit-i-cal
a-crit-o-chro-ma-cy
ac-ro-aes-the-si-a
ac-ro-ag-no-sis
ac-ro-an-es-the-si-a
ac-ro-ar-thri-tis
ac-ro-as-phyx-i-a
ac-ro-a-tax-i-a
ac-ro-blast
ac-ro-ce-pha-li-a
ac-ro-ceph-a-lop-a-gus
ac-ro-ceph-a-lo-syn-dac-
    tyl-i-a
ac-ro-ceph-a-ly
ac-ro-chor-do-ma
ac-ro-chor-don
ac-ro-ci-ne-sis
ac-ro-con-trac-ture
ac-ro-cy-a-no-sis
ac-ro-der-ma-ti-tis
ac-ro-dig-i-ta-lin
ac-ro-dol-i-cho-me-li-a
ac-ro-dont

ac-ro-dyn-i-a
ac-ro-e-de-ma
ac-ro-es-the-si-a
ac-ro-ger-i-a
ac-rog-no-sis
ac-ro-hy-per-hi-dro-sis
ac-ro-hy-po-ther-my
ac-ro-ker-a-to-sis
   ver-ru-ci-for-mis
a-cro-le-in
ac-ro-mac-ri-a
ac-ro-ma-ni-a
ac-ro-mas-ti-tis
ac-ro-meg-a-loid-ism
ac-ro-meg-a-ly
ac-ro-mel-al-gi-a
ac-ro-met-a-gen-e-sis
ac-ro-mic-ri-a
a-cro-mi-o-cla-vic-u-lar
a-cro-mi-o-cor-a-coid
a-cro-mi-o-hu-mer-al
a-cro-mi-on
a-cro-mi-o-tho-rac-ic
a-crom-pha-lus
ac-ro-my-o-to-ni-a
ac-ro-nar-cot-ic
ac-ro-neu-rop-a-thy
ac-ro-neu-ro-sis
a-cron-y-chous
ac-ro-nyx
ac-ro-os-te-ol-y-sis
ac-ro-pach-y
ac-ro-pach-y-der-ma
ac-ro-pa-ral-y-sis
ac-ro-par-es-the-si-a
ac-ro-pa-thol-o-gy
a-crop-a-thy
a-crop-e-tal
ac-ro-pho-bi-a
ac-ro-pig-men-ta-tion
ac-ro-pig-men-ta-ti-o
   re-tic-u-lar-is

ac-ro-pos-thi-tis
ac-ro-scle-ro-der-ma
ac-ro-scle-ro-sis
ac-rose
ac-ro-some
ac-ro-sphe-no-syn-dac-
   tyl-i-a
ac-ros-te-al-gi-a
ac-ro-ter-ic
Ac-ro-the-ci-um
   floc-co-sum
a-crot-ic
ac-ro-tism
ac-ro-tro-pho-neu-ro-sis
a-cryl-ic ac-id
a-cryl-ic al-de-hyde
a-cryl-ics
ac-ry-lo-ni-trile
ACS
ACTH
ac-ti-di-one
ac-tin
ac-tin-ic
ac-tin-ide
ac-tin-i-form
ac-tin-i-o-he-ma-tin
ac-tin-ism
ac-tin-i-um
ac-ti-no-bac-il-lo-sis
Ac-ti-no-ba-cil-lus
ac-ti-no-chem-is-try
ac-ti-no-der-ma-ti-tis
ac-tin-o-gen
ac-tin-o-graph
ac-tin-o-lite
ac-ti-nol-o-gy
ac-tin-o-lyte
ac-ti-nom-e-ter
ac-ti-no-my-ce-li-al
Ac-ti-no-my-ces
Ac-ti-no-my-ce-ta-ce-ae
Ac-ti-no-my-ce-ta-les

ac-ti-no-my-ce-tin
ac-ti-no-my-co-ma
ac-ti-no-my-co-sis
ac-ti-no-my-co-tin
ac-ti-non
ac-ti-no-neu-ri-tis
ac-ti-no-phy-to-sis
ac-tin-o-rho-dine
ac-tin-o-ru-bin
ac-ti-nos-co-py
ac-ti-no-ther-a-py
ac-tion
ac-ti-thi-az-ic ac-id
ac-ti-va-tion
ac-ti-va-tor
ac-tive
ac-tiv-i-ty
ac-to-my-o-sin
ac-tu-al
a-cu-es-the-si-a
a-cu-i-ty
a-cu-le-ate
a-cu-me-ter
a-cu-mi-nate
ac-u-pres-sure
ac-u-punc-ture
a-cus
ac-u-sec-tor
a-cus-ti-cus
a-cute
a-cute-ness
a-cu-ti-cos-tal
a-cy-a-no-blep-si-a
a-cy-a-nop-si-a
a-cy-a-not-ic
a-cy-cli-a
a-cy-clic
ac-y-e-sis
ac-yl
ac-yl-a-tion
a-cys-ti-a
a-dac-ry-a

a-dac-tyl-i-a
ad-a-man-tine
ad-a-man-ti-no-car-ci-
no-ma
ad-a-man-ti-no-ma
ad-a-man-to-blast
ad-a-man-to-blas-to-ma
ad-ams-ite
ad-ap-ta-tion
a-dapt-er
ad-ap-tom-e-ter
ad-at-om
ad-ax-i-al
ad de-liq
ad-de-pha-gi-a
ad-der
ad-dict
ad-di-ment
Addis' meth-od
ad-dis-in
Ad-di-son-ism
ad-di-tion
ad-du-cent
ad-duct
ad-duc-tion
ad-duc-tor
A-de-cid-u-a-ta
a-de-lo-mor-phous
a-del-pho-site
a-del-pho-tax-is
ad-en-al-gi-a
ad-e-nase
ad-en-as-the-ni-a
ad-en-drit-ic
ad-en-ec-to-my
ad-en-ec-to-pi-a
A-den fe-ver
a-de-ni-a
a-den-i-form
ad-e-nine
ad-e-ni-tis
A-de-ni-um

ad-e-no-ac-an-tho-ma
ad-e-no-a-me-lo-blas-
to-ma
ad-e-no-an-gi-o-sar-co-ma
ad-e-no-can-croid
ad-e-no-car-ci-no-ma
ad-e-no-cele
ad-e-no-cel-lu-li-tis
ad-e-no-chon-dro-ma
ad-e-no-cys-to-ma
ad-e-no-cys-to-sar-co-ma
ad-e-no-fi-bro-ma
ad-e-no-fi-bro-sis
ad-e-no-gen-e-sis
ad-e-nog-e-nous
ad-e-no-hy-per-sthe-ni-a
ad-e-no-hy-poph-y-sis
ad-e-noid
ad-e-noi-dec-to-my
ad-e-noid-es per-i-to-
ni-tis
ad-e-noid-ism
ad-e-noi-di-tis
ad-e-no-lei-o-my-o-fi-
bro-ma
ad-e-no-li-po-ma
ad-e-no-li-po-ma-to-sis
ad-e-no-log-a-di-tis
ad-e-no-lym-phi-tis
ad-e-no-lym-pho-cele
ad-e-no-lym-pho-ma
ad-e-no-ma
ad-e-no-ma-la-ci-a
ad-e-no-ma-tome
ad-e-no-ma-to-sis
ad-e-nom-a-tous
ad-e-no-mere
ad-e-no-my-o-hy-per-
pla-si-a
ad-e-no-my-o-ma
ad-e-no-my-o-me-tri-tis
ad-e-no-my-o-sar-co-ma

ad-e-no-my-o-sis
ad-e-no-myx-o-chon-dro-
sar-co-ma
ad-e-no-myx-o-ma
ad-e-no-myx-o-sar-co-ma
ad-e-non-cus
ad-e-nop-a-thy
ad-e-no-phar-yn-gi-tis
ad-e-no-phleg-mon
ad-e-no-sal-pin-gi-tis
ad-e-no-sar-co-ma
ad-e-no-sar-co-rhab-do-
my-o-ma
ad-e-no-scle-ro-sis
ad-e-nose
a-den-o-sine
a-den-o-sine-di-phos-
phate
a-den-o-sine-mon-o-
phos-phate
a-den-o-sine-mon-o-
phos-phor-ic ac-id
a-den-o-sine-tri-phos-
pha-tase
a-den-o-sine-tri-phos-
phate
a-den-o-sine-tri-phos-
phor-ic ac-id
ad-e-no-sis
ad-e-no-tome
ad-e-not-o-my
A-den ul-cer
ad-e-nyl
ad-e-nyl-ic ac-id
ad-e-nyl-py-ro-phos-pha-
tase
ad-e-nyl-py-ro-phos-
phate
ad-e-nyl-py-ro-phos-
phor-ic ac-id
ad-e-pha-gi-a

ad-eps
a-der-mi-a
a-der-min
a-der-mo-gen-e-sis
a-der-mo-tro-phi-a
Ad-hat-o-da
ad-he-sion
ad-he-si-ot-o-my
ad-he-sive
a-di-ac-tin-ic
a-di-ad-o-cho-ki-ne-sis
Ad-i-an-tum
a-di-a-pho-ret-ic
a-di-as-to-le
a-di-a-ther-mic
a-di-a-thet-ic
a-dic-i-ty
ad-i-ent
Adie's syn-drome
a-dip-ic
a-dip-ic ac-id
ad-i-po-cele
ad-i-po-cel-lu-lar
ad-i-po-cere
ad-i-po-fi-bro-ma
ad-i-pol-y-sis
ad-i-po-ma
ad-i-po-ne-cro-sis
    ne-o-na-to-rum
ad-i-po-pex-is
ad-i-po-sa dys-tro-phi-a
    gen-i-ta-lis
ad-i-pose
ad-i-po-sis
ad-i-pos-i-tas cer-e-bral-is
ad-i-po-si-tis
ad-i-pos-i-ty
ad-i-po-so-gen-i-tal
ad-i-po-su-ri-a
a-dip-sa
a-dip-si-a
ad-i-tus

ad-just-ment
ad-jus-tor
ad-ju-vant
ad lib
ad-me-di-al
ad-mi-nic-u-lum
ad-mis-sion rate
ad-na-sal
ad-nate
ad nau-se-am
ad-ner-val
ad-nex-a
ad-nex-i-tis
ad-nex-o-gen-e-sis
ad-o-don-ti-a
ad-o-les-cence
ad-o-les-cent mam-mo-
    pla-si-a
a-don-i-din
a-do-nin
A-do-nis
ad-o-ral
ad-or-bit-al
ADP
ad-re-nal
ad-re-nal cor-tex
ad-re-nal cor-ti-cal ex-
    tract
ad-re-nal-ec-to-my
ad-ren-al-in-e-mi-a
ad-ren-al-in-u-ri-a
ad-re-nal-ism
ad-re-na-li-tis
ad-ren-al-og-ra-phy
ad-ren-arch-e
ad-ren-er-gic
ad-re-ner-gic block-ing
    a-gent
ad-ren-o-chrom
ad-ren-o-cor-ti-co-
    mi-met-ic

ad-ren-o-cor-ti-co-
    tro-phic
ad-ren-o-cor-ti-co-
    tro-pic
ad-ren-o-cor-ti-co-
    tro-pin
ad-re-no-gen-i-tal
ad-re-no-gram
ad-re-no-lyt-ic
ad-ren-o-pause
ad-re-nos-te-rone
ad-re-no-tox-in
ad-ren-o-trope
ad-ren-o-tro-pic
ad-ren-o-tro-pin
ad-re-not-ro-pism
a-dro-mi-a
ad-ru-e
ad-sor-bate
ad-sorb-ent
ad-sorp-tion
ad-ster-nal
ad-ter-mi-nal
ad-tor-sion
a-dult
a-dul-ter-ant
a-dul-ter-a-tion
ad-vance
ad-ven-ti-ti-a
ad-ven-ti-tious
ad-y-na-mi-a
Aeby's plane
A-ë-des
ae-doe-o-ceph-a-lus
ae-lu-rop-sis
ae-quum
a-er-ate
a-er-a-tion
a-er-e-mi-a
a-er-en-do-car-di-a
a-er-en-ter-ec-ta-si-a
a-e-ri-al

a-er-if-er-ous
a-er-i-form
a-er-o-an-a-er-o-bic
A-er-o-bac-ter
a-er-obe
a-er-o-bic
a-er-o-bi-ol-o-gy
a-er-o-bi-o-scope
a-er-o-bi-o-sis
a-er-o-cele
a-er-o-col-pos
a-er-o-cys-tos-co-py
a-er-o-don-tal-gi-a
a-er-o-don-ti-a
a-er-o-duc-tor
a-er-o-dy-nam-ics
a-er-o-em-bo-lism
a-er-o-em-phy-se-ma
a-er-o-gen
a-er-o-gen-e-sis
a-er-o-gram
a-er-og-ra-phy
a-er-o-hy-drop-a-thy
a-er-o-i-on-i-za-tion
a-er-o-i-on-o-ther-a-py
a-er-o-mam-mog-ra-phy
a-er-o-med-i-cine
a-er-om-e-ter
a-er-o-neu-ro-sis
a-er-op-a-thy
a-er-o-pause
a-er-o-per-i-to-ne-um
a-er-o-pha-gi-a
a-er-o-phil
a-er-o-pho-bi-a
a-er-o-phore
a-er-o-phyte
a-er-o-pi-e-so-ther-a-py
a-er-o-ple-thys-mo-graph
a-er-o-pleu-ra
a-er-o-scope
a-er-os-co-py

a-er-o-si-al-oph-a-gy
a-er-o-si-nus-i-tis
a-er-o-sis
a-er-o-sol
a-er-o-stat-ics
a-er-o-tax-is
a-er-o-ther-a-peu-tics
a-er-o-ther-mo-ther-a-py
a-er-o-ti-tis me-di-a
a-er-o-to-nom-e-ter
a-er-ot-ro-pism
a-er-o-tym-pa-nal
a-er-o-u-re-thro-scope
ae-ru-go
Aesculapius
aes-ti-val
aes-tus
ae-ther
Ae-thu-sa
ae-ti-o-por-phy-rin
a-fe-brile
a-fe-tal
af-fect
af-fect-a-bil-i-ty
af-fec-ta-tion
af-fec-tion
af-fec-tiv-i-ty
af-fec-to-mo-tor
af-fekt-ep-i-lep-sie
af-fer-ent
af-fil-i-a-tion
af-fi-nal
af-fi-nin
af-fin-i-ty
af-fir-ma-tion
af-flux
af-fu-sion
a-fi-brin-o-gen-e-mi-a
a-foe-tal
af-ri-dol
af-tan-nin
aft-er-birth

aft-er-brain
aft-er-care
aft-er-cat-a-ract
aft-er-cur-rent
aft-er-damp
aft-er-dis-charge
aft-er-ef-fect
aft-er-gild-ing
aft-er-hear-ing
aft-er-im-age
aft-er-im-pres-sion
aft-er-pains
aft-er-per-cep-tion
aft-er-po-ten-tial
aft-er-sen-sa-tion
aft-er-sound
aft-er-stain
aft-er-taste
aft-er-treat-ment
aft-er-vi-sion
a-func-tion
a-ga-lac-ti-a
ag-a-lor-rhe-a
a-gam-ete
a-gam-ic
a-gam-ma—glob-u-lin-e-
    mi-a
a-gam-o-cy-tog-o-ny
Ag-a-mo-fi-la-ri-a
a-gam-o-gen-e-sis
ag-a-mog-o-ny
a-gam-o-spore
ag-a-mous
a-gar
a-gar—a-gar
a-gar-ic
a-gar-ic ac-id
a-gar-i-cin
A-gar-i-cus
a-gar-y-thrine
a-gas-tric
a-gas-tro-neu-ri-a

A-ga-ve
Ag-chy-los-to-ma
a-gen-e-sis
a-gen-i-o-ce-pha-li-a
a-gen-i-tal-ism
a-gen-o-so-mi-a
a-gen-o-so-mus
a-gent
a-ge-ra-si-a
a-geu-si-a
ag-ger
ag-glom-er-ate
ag-glu-ti-na-tion
ag-glu-ti-nin
ag-glu-tin-o-gen
ag-glu-ti-noid
ag-glu-ti-no-phore
ag-glu-tin-o-scope
ag-gre-gate
ag-gre-ga-tion
ag-gres-sin
ag-gres-sion
ag-i-ta-tion
a-gi-ta-tor caud-ae
ag-i-to-graph-i-a
ag-i-to-la-li-a
ag-i-to-pha-si-a
Ag-kis-tro-don
a-glan-du-lar
a-glau-cop-si-a
ag-li-a
a-glo-mer-u-lar
a-glos-si-a
a-glos-so-sto-mi-a
a-glos-sus
a-glu-cone
ag-lu-ti-tion
a-gly-cae-mic
a-gly-ce-mic
a-gly-cone
a-gly-co-su-ric
Ag-ly-pha

ag-ma-tine
ag-mi-nate
ag-na-thi-a
ag-na-tho-ceph-a-lus
ag-na-thus
ag-ne-a
ag-noe-a
ag-no-gen-ic
ag-no-si-a
ag-nos-ter-ol
ag-om-phi-a-sis
a-gon-ad-ism
ag-o-nal
a-go-ni-a
ag-o-ni-a-din
ag-o-nist
ag-o-ny
ag-o-ra-pho-bi-a
a-gram-ma-pha-si-a
a-gram-ma-tism
a-gran-u-lo-cyte
a-gran-u-lo-cy-the-mi-a
a-gran-u-lo-cy-to-sis
a-gran-u-lo-plas-tic
a-gran-u-lo-sis
a-graph-i-a
ag-ri-mo-ny
ag-ri-us
Ag-ro-bac-te-ri-um
ag-ro-ma-ni-a
a-gryp-ni-a
ag-ryp-not-ic
a-gua-miel
a-gue
a-gyi-o-pho-bi-a
a-gy-ri-a
a-hyp-ni-a
aich-mo-pho-bi-a
Ai-lan-thus
ail-ing
ail-ment
ai-lu-ro-pho-bi-a

ain-hum
air my-e-log-ra-phy
air sick-ness
air-way
a-ja-cine
a-jac-o-nine
aj-mal-i-cine
aj-ma-line
aj-mal-i-nine
a-ka-mu-shi
a-kan-thes-the-si-a
a-kar-y-o-cyte
a-kar-y-ote
ak-a-thi-si-a
a-ker-a-to-sis
a-kin-aes-the-si-a
ak-i-ne-si-a
a-kin-es-the-si-a
ak-i-net-ic
A-kis spi-no-sa
ak-o-asm
a-la
al-a-bam-ine
al-a-bas-ter
al-a-bas-trine
a-lae
a-la-li-a
a-lan-gine
al-a-nine
a-lan-tic
a-lan-tol
a-lan-to-lac-tone
al-a-nyl
al-a-nyl-gly-cine
a-las-trim
a-la-tus
al-ba
al-bas-pi-din
Albert's stain
al-bes-cent
al-bi-cans
al-bi-du-ri-a

al-bi-fac-tion
al-bi-nism
al-bi-no
al-bi-no-ism
al-bi-nu-ri-a
al-bo-ci-ne-re-ous
al-bu-gin-e-a
al-bu-gin-e-ous
al-bu-gi-ni-tis
al-bu-go
al-bu-men
al-bu-min
al-bu-mi-nate
al-bu-mi-nif-er-ous
al-bu-mi-nim-e-ter
al-bu-mi-nog-e-nous
al-bu-mi-noid
al-bu-mi-nol-y-sin
al-bu-mi-nom-e-ter
al-bu-mi-nose
al-bu-min-u-ret-ic
al-bu-mi-nu-ri-a
al-bu-mi-nu-ric
al-bu-moid
al-bu-mo-scope
al-bu-mose
al-bu-mo-su-ri-a
al-bu-tan-nin
Al-ca-lig-e-nes fe-cal-is
al-cap-to-nu-ri-a
al-che-my
al-co-gel
al-co-hol
al-co-hol-ase
al-co-hol-ate
al-co-hol-a-ture
al-co-hol-ic
al-co-hol-ism
al-co-hol-om-e-ter
al-co-hol-o-phil-i-a
al-co-hol-u-ri-a
al-co-hol-y-sis

al-co-sol
al-de-hyde
al-do-bi-on-ic ac-id
al-do-hex-ose
al-dol
al-dol-ase
al-don-ic ac-id
al-do-pen-tose
al-dose
al-do-side
al-dos-ter-one
al-do-tet-rose
al-dox-ime
al-drin
a-lec-i-thal
a-lem-bic
A-lep-po but-ton
al-e-trin
al-e-tris
al-eu-drin
al-eu-ke-mi-a
al-eu-ki-a he-mor-
    rhag-i-ca
a-leu-ro-nat
a-leu-rone
a-lex-i-a
a-lex-in
a-lex-i-phar-mac
a-ley-dig-ism
Al-gae
al-ga-ro-ba
al-ge-don-ic
al-ge-si-a
al-ge-sim-e-ter
al-ges-the-si-a
al-get-ic
al-gid
al-gin-ate
al-gin-ic ac-id
al-gi-o-mo-tor
al-gi-o-mus-cu-lar
al-go-gen-e-sis

al-go-gen-ic
al-go-lag-ni-a
al-gom-e-ter
al-go-pho-bi-a
al-gor
al-go-spasm
al-i-ble
al-i-bour wa-ter
al-i-cy-clic
a-lien-a-tion
a-lien-ist
al-i-ment
al-i-men-ta-ry
al-i-men-ta-tion
al-i-men-to-ther-a-py
al-i-na-sal
al-i-phat-ic
al-i-quot
al-i-sphe-noid
a-liz-a-rin
al-ka-le-mi-a
al-ka-les-cent
al-ka-li
al-ka-lim-e-ter
al-ka-line
al-ka-line tide
al-ka-lin-i-ty
al-ka-lin-ize
al-ka-li-nu-ri-a
al-ka-li-pe-ni-a
al-ka-lize
al-ka-loid
al-ka-lo-sis
al-ka-lo-ther-a-py
alk-a-mine
al-kane
al-ka-net
al-kan-nin
al-ka-nol
al-ka-nol-a-mine
al-kap-ton
al-kap-to-nu-ri-a

al-ka-ver-vir
al-ke-ken-gi
al-kene
al-ke-nol
al-ker-mes
alk-ox-ide
alk-ox-yl
al-kyl
al-kyl-a-mine
al-kyl-ate
al-kyl-a-tion
al-kyl-ol-a-mine
al-kyl-o-gen
al-kyne
al-ky-nol
al-la-ches-the-si-a
al-laes-the-si-a
al-lan-to-cho-ri-on
al-lan-to-en-ter-ic
al-lan-to-gen-e-sis
Al-lan-toi-de-a
al-lan-toi-do-an-gi-op-a-
    gous
al-lan-to-in
al-lan-tois
al-las-so-ther-a-py
al-lax-is
al-le-gor-i-za-tion
al-lelé
al-lel-o-cat-a-lyt-ic
al-le-lo-morph
al-lel-o-tax-is
al-lene
al-len-the-sis
al-ler-gen
al-ler-gid
al-ler-gin
al-ler-gist
al-ler-gi-za-tion
al-ler-go-der-mi-a
al-ler-go-sis
al-ler-gy

Al-les-che-ri-a
al-les-the-si-a
al-le-thrin
al-li-cin
al-li-ga-tion
al-li-ga-tor for-ceps
al-lit-er-a-tion
Al-li-um
al-lo-chei-ri-a
al-lo-ches-the-si-a
al-lo-che-zi-a
al-lo-cho-les-ter-ol
al-lo-cor-tex
al-loe-o-sis
al-lo-er-o-tism
al-lom-e-try
al-lo-mor-phism
al-lo-mor-pho-sis
al-lo-path
al-lop-a-thy
al-loph-a-sis
al-lo-plasm
al-lo-plast
al-lo-plas-ty
al-lo-pol-y-ploid
al-lo-preg-nane
al-lo-psy-che
al-lo-psy-chic
al-lo-rhyth-mi-a
al-lose
al-lo-some
al-lo-ste-a-to-des
al-lo-syn-ap-sis
al-lo-therm
al-lot-ri-o-don-ti-a
al-lot-ri-o-geu-si-a
al-lo-tri-o-lith
al-lot-ri-o-pha-gi-a
al-lot-ri-u-ri-a
al-lo-trope
al-lo-troph-ic
al-lot-ro-py

al-lo-tryl-ic
al-lox-an
al-lox-an-ic ac-id
al-lox-an-tin
al-lox-a-zine
al-lox-u-ri-a
al-lox-y-pro-te-ic ac-id
al-loy
all-spice
al-lyl
al-lyl-a-mine
al-lyl-bar-bi-tur-ic ac-id
al-lyl-ene
al-lyl-i-so-pro-pyl-bar-bi-
    tur-ic ac-id
N—al-lyl-nor-mor-phine
al-ma-gu-cin
al-mond
al-mond—eyed
a-lo-chi-a
Al-o-e
al-oe—em-o-din
al-oes
al-o-et-ic
al-o-e-tin
a-lo-gi-a
al-o-in
al-o-pe-ci-a
al-pha
al-pha—hy-poph-a-mine
al-pha—i-o-dine
al-pha—lo-be-line
al-pha-naph-thol
al-pha—naph-thyl-thi-o-u-
    re-a
al-pha-pro-dine hy-dro-
    chlo-ride
al-pha-to-coph-er-ol
al-pho-der-mi-a
al-phos
al-pho-sis
al-pho-zone

al-phus
Al-sto-ni-a
al-sto-nine
al-ter-ant
al-ter-a-tion cav-i-taire
al-ter-a-tive
al-ter-e-go-ism
Al-ter-na-ri-a
al-ter-nar-ic ac-id
al-ter-nat-ing
al-ter-na-tion
al-ter-na-tor
al-the-a
al-ti-tude sick-ness
al-tri-gen-der-ism
al-trose
al-um
a-lu-min-a
a-lu-mi-num
a-lu-si-a
al-ve-at-ed
al-ve-in
al-ve-o-la-bi-al
al-ve-o-lar
al-ve-o-late
al-ve-o-lec-to-my
al-ve-o-li
al-ve-o-lin-gual
al-ve-o-li-tis
al-ve-o-lo-cla-si-a
al-ve-o-lo-con-dyl-e-an
al-ve-o-lo-den-tal
al-ve-o-lo-la-bi-al
al-ve-o-lo-lin-gual
al-ve-o-lon
al-ve-ol-o-plas-ty
al-ve-o-lo-sub-na-sal
al-ve-o-lot-o-my
al-ve-o-lus
al-ve-ol-y-sis
al-ve-us
al-vi

al-vi-no-lith
al-vus
a-lym-phi-a
a-lym-pho-cy-to-sis
a-lys-mus
al-ys-o-sis
a-lys-sous
am-a-dou
a-mai-o-sis
a-mal-gam
a-mal-gam-ate
a-mal-gam-a-tion
a-man-din
Am-a-ni-ta
Am-a-ni-ta phal-loi-des
a-man-i-tin
a-ma-ra
am-a-ranth
am-a-rine
am-a-roid
am-a-se-sis
a-mas-ti-a
am-a-tho-pho-bia
am-a-tive-ness
am-a-tol
am-au-ro-sis
am-au-rot-ic
am-a-xo-pho-bi-a
am-ber
am-ber-gris
am-bi-dex-trous
am-bi-lat-er-al
am-bi-le-vous
am-bi-oc-u-lar-i-ty
am-bi-o-pi-a
am-bi-sex-u-al
am-bi-sin-is-ter
am-bi-tend-en-cy
am-biv-a-lence
am-bi-vert
am-bly-a-cou-si-a
am-bly-chro-ma-si-a

Am-bly-om-ma
am-bly-ope
am-bly-o-pi-a
am-bly-o-pi-at-rics
am-bly-o-scope
am-bo-cep-toid
am-bo-cep-tor
am-bo-sex-u-al
am-bo-tox-oid
Am-boy-na but-ton
am-bre-in
Am-bro-si-a
am-bu-lance
am-bu-la-to-ry
am-bus-tion
a-me-ba
am-e-bi-a-sis
a-me-bi-cide
a-me-bid
a-me-bo-cyte
a-me-boid
a-me-boid-ism
am-e-bo-ma
a-me-bu-la
am-e-bu-ri-a
a-mei-o-sis
am-el-e-ia
a-mel-i-fi-ca-tion
a-mel-o-blast
a-mel-o-blas-to-ma
a-mel-o-blas-to-sar-co-ma
a-me-lo-gen-e-sis
a-me-lus
a-me-ni-a
a-men-o-ma-ni-a
a-men-or-rhe-a
a-ment
a-men-ti-a
am-er-i-ci-um
am-er-is-tic
a-me-si-al-i-ty
a-me-tab-o-lous

74

a-me-tri-a
a-me-tro-he-mi-a
am-e-tro-pi-a
am-i-an-thi-nop-sy
am-i-an-thoid
am-i-an-tho-sis
a-mi-cet-in
a-mi-cro-bic
a-mi-cron
a-mi-cro-scop-ic
a-mic-u-lum
am-i-dase
am-ide
am-i-din
am-i-dine
a-mi-do-az-o-tol-u-ene
a-mi-do-ben-zene
am-i-dol
am-i-done hy-dro-chlo-ride
a-mi-do-py-rine
am-i-dox-ime
a-mim-i-a
a-mi-na-crine
am-i-na-tion
a-mine
a-mi-no-a-ce-tic ac-id
a-mi-no-ac-e-to-phe-none
a-mi-no ac-id
a-mi-no-a-cid-u-ri-a
a-mi-no-ac-ri-dine
a-mi-no al-co-hol
a-mi-no-az-o-tol-u-ene
a-mi-no-az-o-tol-u-ol
a-mi-no-ben-zene
a-mi-no-flu-o-rene
a-mi-no-glu-cose
a-mi-no-lip-id
a-mi-no-meth-an-am-i-dine
a-mi-no-pent-a-mide
a-mi-no-pep-ti-dase

a-mi-no-pep-to-drate
a-mi-no-phyl-line
a-mi-no-pol-y-pep-ti-dase
a-mi-no-pro-te-ase
a-mi-no-pu-rine
a-mi-no-py-rine
a-mi-no-quin naph-tho-ate
a-mi-no-sal-i-cyl-ic ac-id
a-mi-no-suc-cin-am-ic ac-id
a-mi-no su-gar
a-mi-no-su-ri-a
a-mi-no-tol-u-ene
am-i-nu-ri-a
a-mi-o-sis
am-i-thi-o-zone
a-mi-to-sis
am-me-ter
am-mi-din
am-mine
am-mism
am-moi-din
am-mo-nate
am-mo-na-tion
am-mo-ni-a
am-mo-ni-ac
am-mo-ni-e-mi-a
am-mon-i-fi-ca-tion
am-mo-ni-um
am-mo-ni-u-ri-a
am-mo-no base
am-mo-nol-y-sis
am-mon-o-tel-ic
am-mo-ther-a-py
am-ne-mon-ic
am-ne-si-a
am-ni-a
am-ni-o-cho-ri-al
am-ni-o-em-bry-on-ic
am-ni-o-gen-e-sis

am-ni-og-ra-phy
am-ni-on
am-ni-or-rhe-a
Am-ni-o-ta
am-ni-o-ti-tis
am-ni-o-tome
am-ni-ot-o-my
a-moe-ba
a-mok
a-mor
a-mo-ral-i-a
a-mor-phic
a-mor-phin-ism
a-mor-phous
a-mor-phus
a-mo-ti-o ret-i-nae
am-per-age
am-pere
am-pere-me-ter
am-pher-ot-o-ky
am-phet-a-mine
am-phi-ar-thro-sis
am-phi-as-ter
Am-phib-i-a
am-phib-i-ous
am-phi-blas-tic
am-phi-blas-tu-la
am-phi-bles-tro-des
am-phi-chro-ic
am-phi-coe-lous
am-phi-cra-ni-a
am-phi-cre-a-tine
am-phi-cre-at-i-nine
am-phi-cyte
am-phi-des-mic
am-phi-di-ar-thro-sis
am-phi-er-o-tism
am-phi-gas-tru-la
am-phi-gen-e-sis
am-phig-o-ny
am-phi-kar-y-on
am-phi-mix-is

am-phi-mor-u-la
am-phi-ox-us
Am-phi-sto-ma-ta
am-phi-tene
am-phi-the-a-ter
am-phit-o-ky
am-phit-ri-chous
am-pho-di-plo-pi-a
am-pho-lyte
am-phor-ic
am-pho-ril-o-quy
am-pho-roph-o-ny
am-pho-ter-ic
am-phot-er-o-di-plo-pi-a
am-pli-fi-ca-tion
am-pli-fi-er
am-pli-tude
am-pul
am-pul-la
am-pul-lu-la
am-pu-ta-tion
am-pu-tee
a-muck
a-mu-si-a
am-y-cho-pho-bi-a
am-y-dri-a-sis
a-my-e-len-ceph-a-lus
am-y-e-li-a
am-y-el-in-at-ed
a-my-e-lus
a-myg-da-la
a-myg-da-lase
a-myg-dal-ic ac-id
a-myg-da-lin
a-myg-da-loid
a-myg-da-loid-ec-to-my
a-myg-da-lo-lith
am-yl
am-y-la-ceous
am-yl al-co-hol
am-yl-ase
am-yl-ene

am-yl ni-trate
am-y-lo-bar-bi-tone
am-y-lo-dex-trin
am-y-lo-dys-pep-si-a
a-myl-o-gen
am-y-loid
am-y-loi-do-sis
am-y-lol-y-sis
am-y-lon
am-y-lo-pec-tin
am-y-lop-sin
am-yl-ose
am y lum
am-y-lu-ri-a
a-my-o-es-the-si-a
a-my-o-pla-si-a
a-my-o-sta-si-a
a-my-o-tax-i-a
a-my-o-to-ni-a
a-my-o-to-ni-a con-
   gen-i-ta
a-my-o-tro-phi-a
am-y-rin
Am-y-ris
a-myx-i-a
a-myx-or-rhe-a
a-nab-a-sine
an-a-bi-ot-ic
an-a-bol-er-gy
a-nab-o-lin
an-ab-o-lism
an-a-camp-tics
An-a-car-di-a-ce-ae
an-a-car-dic ac-id
an-a-cat-a-did-y-mus
an-a-ce-li-a-del-phous
an-a-cid-i-ty
a-nac-la-sis
a-nac-li-sis
an-ac-me-sis
an-a-cou-si-a
a-nac-ro-a-si-a

an-a-crot-ic in-ci-su-ra
a-nac-ro-tism
an-a-cu-si-a
an-a-de-ni-a
an-a-did-y-mus
an-a-dip-si-a
an-aer-obe
an-aer-o-bi-ase
an-aer-o-bi-o-sis
an-aer-o-gen-ic
an-aer-o-phyte
an-a-gen-e-sis
an-a-go-ge
an-a-gog ic
an-a-gy-rine
an-a-kat-a-did-y-mus
an-a-lep-sis
an-a-lep-tic
an-al-ge-si-a
an-al-ge-sic
an-al-ler-gic
an-a-log
a-nal-o-gy
a-nal-y-sand
a-nal-y-sis
an-a-lyst
an-a-lyt-ic
an-a-ly-zer
an-am-ne-sis
an-am-ni-ot-ic
an-a-mor-pho-sis
an-an-a-ba-si-a
an-an-a-phy-lax-is
an-an-as-ta-si-a
a-nan-cas-ti-a
an-an-dri-a
an-an-gi-o-pla-si-a
an-an-gi-o-plas-tic
an-a-pau-sis
an-a-pei-rat-ic
an-a-phal-an-ti-a-sis
an-a-phase

76

an-a-phi-a
an-a-pho-re-sis
an-a-pho-ri-a
an-aph-ro-dis-i-a
an-aph-ro-dis-i-ac
an-a-phy-lac-tic
an-a-phy-lac-tin
an-a-phy-lac-to-gen
an-a-phy-lac-toid
an-a-phyl-a-tox-in
an-a-phy-lax-is
an-a-pla-si-a
an-a-plas-mo-sis
an-a-plas-tic
an-a-plas-ty
an-a-ple-ro-sis
an-a-poph-y-sis
an-a-rith-mi-a
an-ar-thri-a
an-a-sar-ca
an-a-schist-ic
an-a-stal-sis
a-nas-ta-sis
an-as-tig-mat-ic
a-nas-to-mo-sis
a-nas-to-mot-i-ca
an-as-tral
a-nat-a-bine
a-nat-o-mist
a-nat-o-my
an-a-tox-in
an-a-tro-pi-a
an-au-di-a
an-a-vac-cine
an-a-ven-in
an-az-o-tu-ri-a
an-chor-age
an-chy-lops
an-co-ne-us
an-co-noid
An-cy-los-to-ma

An-cy-los-to-ma
  braz-i-li-en-se
An-cy-los-to-ma
  can-i-num
An-cy-los-to-ma
  du-o-de-nale
an-cy-los-to-mi-a-sis
an-dra-nat-o-my
an-dri-at-rics
an-dro-blas-to-ma
an-dro-ga-lac-to-ze-mi-a
an-dro-gam-one
an-dro-gen
an-dro-gen-e-sis
an-drog-e-nous
an-dro-gyne
an-drog-y-nism
an-drog-y-ny
an-droid
an-dro-ma-ni-a
an-drom-e-do-tox-in
an-dro-mor-phous
an-droph-i-lous
an-dro-pho-bi-a
an-dros-tane
an-dro-stene-di-ol
an-dro-stene-di-one
an-dros-ter-one
a-ne-de-ous
a-ne-lec-trot-o-nus
a-ne-mi-a
an-e-mom-e-ter
A-nem-o-ne
a-nem-o-nin
a-ne-mo-pho-bi-a
an-en-ce-pha-li-a
an-en-ceph-a-lus
an-en-ter-ous
an-ep-i-a
an-ep-i-plo-ic
an-er-ga-si-a
an-er-gy

an-er-oid
an-e-ryth-ro-blep-si-a
an-e-ryth-ro-cyte
an-e-ryth-ro-pla-si-a
an-e-ryth-rop-si-a
an-es-the-ki-ne-sis
an-es-the-si-a
an-es-the-sim-e-ter
an-es-the-si-ol-o-gy
an-es-the-si-om-e-ter
an-es-thet-ic
an-es-the-tize
an-es-trum
an-e-thole
a-ne-thum
an-e-to-der-ma
an-eu-ploid
a-neu-ri-a
an-eu-rin
an-eu-rysm
an-eu-rys-mec-to-my
an-eu-rys-mo-graph
an-eu-rys-mo-plas-ty
an-eu-rys-mor-rha-phy
an-eu-rys-mot-o-my
an-eu-tha-na-si-a
an-frac-tu-os-i-ty
an-frac-tu-ous
an-gei-al
an-gel-i-ca
an-gel-ic ac-id
an-gi-ec-ta-sis
an-gi-ec-tid
an-gi-ec-to-my
an-gi-ec-to-pi-a
an-gi-i-tis
an-gi-na
an-gi-no-pho-bi-a
an-gi-o-blast
an-gi-o-blas-to-ma
an-gi-o-car-di-o-gram
an-gi-o-car-di-og-ra-phy

an-gi-o-car-di-op-a-thy
an-gi-o-cav-er-no-ma
an-gi-o-cav-ern-ous
an-gi-o-chei-lo-scope
an-gi-o-cho-li-tis
an-gi-o-chon-dro-ma
an-gi-o-der-ma pig-men-
   to-sum
an-gi-o-der-ma-ti-tis
an-gi-o-di-a-ther-my
an-gi-o-dys-tro-phi-a
an-gi-o-e-de-ma
an-gi-o-el-e-phan-ti-a-sis
an-gi-o-en-do-the-li-o-ma
an-gi-o-fi-bro-blas-to-ma
an-gi-o-fi-bro-ma
an-gi-o-gen-e-sis
an-gi-o-gli-o-ma
an-gi-o-gli-o-ma-to-sis
an-gi-og-ra-phy
an-gi-o-hy-per-to-ni-a
an-gi-o-hy-po-to-ni-a
an-gi-oid
an-gi-o-ker-a-toi-di-tis
an-gi-o-ker-a-to-ma
an-gi-o-li-po-ma
an-gi-o-lith
an-gi-ol-o-gy
an-gi-o-lu-poid
an-gi-ol-y-sis
an-gi-o-ma
an-gi-o-ma-la-ci-a
an-gi-o-ma-to-sis
an-gi-o-meg-a-ly
an-gi-om-e-ter
an-gi-o-my-o-lip-o-ma
an-gi-o-my-o-ma
an-gi-o-my-op-a-thy
an-gi-o-my-o-sar-co-ma
an-gi-o-neu-rec-to-my
an-gi-o-neu-ro-ma
an-gi-o-neu-ro-my-o-ma

an-gi-o-neu-ro-sis
an-gi-o-no-ma
an-gi-o-pa-ral-y-sis
an-gi-o-pa-re-sis
an-gi-op-a-thy
an-gi-o-pla-ni-a
an-gi-o-plas-ty
an-gi-o-pneu-mog-ra-phy
an-gi-o-poi-e-sis
an-gi-o-poi-et-ic
an-gi-o-pres-sure
an-gi-or-rha-phy
an-gi-or-rhex-is
an-gi-o-sar-co-ma
an-gi-o-scle-ro-sis
an-gi-o-scope
an-gi-o-sco-to-ma
an-gi-o-sis
an-gi-o-spasm
an-gi-o-sperm
an-gi-o-stax-is
an-gi-o-ste-no-sis
an-gi-os-te-o-sis
an-gi-o-tel-ec-ta-si-a
an-gi-o-ten-ic
an-gi-o-ti-tis
an-gi-ot-o-my
an-gi-ot-o-nase
an-gi-o-ton-ic
an-gi-ot-o-nin
an-gi-o-tribe
an-gi-o-troph-ic
an-gi-ox-yl
an-gi-tis
an-gle
an-go-phra-si-a
an-gor
an-gos-tu-ra
ang-strom
An-guil-lu-la
an-guil-lu-li-a-sis
an-gu-la-tion

an-gu-lus
an-ha-la-mine
an-ha-line
an-ha-lon-i-dine
an-ha-lo-nine
an-he-do-ni-a
an-hem-a-to-poi-e-sis
an-he-ma-to-sis
an-he-mo-lyt-ic
an-hi-dro-sis
an-hy-drase
an-hy-dra-tion
an-hy-dre-mi-a
an-hy-dride
an-hy-drite
an-hy-dro-git-a-lin
an-hy-dro-hy-drox-y-
   pro-ges-ter-one
an-hy-drous
an-hyp-no-sis
a-ni-a-ci-no-sis
an-i-an-thi-nop-sy
an-ic-ter-ic
an-id-e-us
an-i-lide
an-i-line
a-ni-lin-gus
an-il-ism
a-nil-i-ty
an-i-ma
an-i-mal
an-i-mal-cule
an-i-mas-tic
an-i-ma-tion
an-i-ma-tism
an-i-mism
an-i-mus
an-i-on
an-i-rid-i-a
an-is-al-de-hyde
an-ise
an-is-ei-kom-e-ter

an-i-sei-ko-ni-a
a-nis-ic ac-id
an-i-so-chro-ma-si-a
an-i-so-chro-mi-a
an-i-so-co-ri-a
an-i-so-cy-to-sis
an-i-so-dac-ty-lous
an-i-so-dont
an-i-so-ga-mete
an-i-sog-a-my
an-i-sog-na-thous
an-i-so-gyn-e-co-mas-ti-a
an-i-sole
an-i-so-me-li-a
an-i-so-me-ri-a
an-i-so-me-tro-pi-a
a-nis-o-my-cin
an-i-so-pi-a
an-i-so-sphyg-mi-a
an-i-sos-then-ic
an-i-so-ton-ic
an-i-sot-ro-py
a-ni-sum
an-i-su-ri-a
a-ni-trog-e-nous
an-kle
an-ky-lo-bleph-a-ron
an-ky-lo-chei-li-a
an-ky-lo-col-pos
an-ky-lo-dac-tyl-i-a
an-ky-lo-don-ti-a
an-ky-lo-glos-si-a
an-ky-lo-kol-pos
an-ky-losed
an-ky-lo-sis
an-ky-lo-tome
an-ky-lot-o-my
an-la-ge
an-neal
an-nec-tent
An-nel-i-da
an-ne-lism

an-nu-late
an-nu-lose
an-nu-lo-spi-ral
an-nu-lus
an-o-chro-ma-si-a
a-no-ci-as-so-ci-a-tion
a-no-ci-cep-tor
a-no-ci-the-si-a
a-no-coc-cyg-e-al
an-o-dal
an-ode
an-o-der-mous
an-od-mi-a
an-o-don-ti-a
an-o-don-tous
an-o-dyne
an-o-dyn-i-a
an-o-e-si-a
an-o-et-ic
a-noi-a
a-nom-a-lo-scope
a-nom-a-ly
a-no-mi-a
an-o-mous
an-o-nych-i-a
a-non-y-ma
an-o-op-si-a
a-no-per-i-ne-al
A-noph-e-les
an-o-phel-i-cide
an-o-phel-i-fuge
A-noph-e-li-ni
an-o-pho-ri-a
an-oph-thal-mi-a
an-oph-thal-mos
an-o-pi-a
a-no-plas-ty
An-o-plu-ra
an-op-si-a
an-or-chism
an-or-chus
a-no-rec-tal

a-no-rec-to-plas-ty
an-o-rex-i-a
an-or-gas-my
an-or-thog-ra-phy
an-or-tho-pi-a
an-or-tho-sis
a-no-scope
an-os-mi-a
an-o-sog-no-si-a
a-no-spi-nal
an-os-to-sis
an-o-ti-a
an-o-tro-pi-a
an-o-tus
a-no-ves-i-cal
an-ov-u-lar
an-o-vu-la-to-ry
an-ox-e-mi-a
an-ox-i-a
an-sa
an-sae
an-sate
an-ser-ine
an-si-form
ant-ac-id
an-tag-o-nism
an-tag-o-nist
ant-al-ka-line
ant-aph-ro-dis-i-ac
an-te-au-ral
an-te-bra-chi-um
an-te ci-bum
an-te-cu-bi-tal
an-te-cur-va-ture
an-te-flex-ion
an-te-hy-poph-y-sis
an-te mor-tem
an-te-na-ri-al
an-te-na-tal
an-te par-tum
an-te-ri-or
an-ter-o-dor-sal

an-ter-o-ex-ter-nal
an-ter-o-grade
an-ter-o-in-fe-ri-or
an-ter-o-in-te-ri-or
an-ter-o-in-ter-nal
an-ter-o-lat-er-al
an-ter-o-me-di-an
an-ter-o-pa-ri-e-tal
an-ter-o-pi-tu-i-tar-y
an-ter-o-pos-te-ri-or
an-ter-o-su-pe-ri-or
an-te ver-sion
ant-he-lix
ant-hel-min-tic
an-the-ma
an-the-mis
ant-hem-or-rhag-ic
an-ther
an-tho-cy-a-nin
An-tho-my-ia
an-tho-pho-bi-a
an-thra-ce-mi-a
an-thra-cene
an-thra-coid
an-thra-co-ne-cro-sis
an-thra-co-sil-i-co-sis
an-thra-co-sis
an-thra-gal-lol
an-thra-glu-co-rhe-in
an-thra-lin
an-thra-nil-ic ac-id
an-thra-nol
an-thra-pur-pu-rin
an-thra-qui-none
an-thra-ro-bin
an-thrax
an-throne
an-thro-pho-bi-a
an-thro-po-bi-ol-o-gy
an-thro-po-gen-e-sis
an-thro-poid
An-thro-poi-de-a

an-thro-pol-o-gy
an-thro-pom-e-ter
an-thro-pom-e-try
an-thro-po-mor-phic
an-thro-poph-a-gy
an-thro-po-phil-ic
an-thro-po-pho-bi-a
an-thro-po-so-ma-
    tol-o-gy
ant-hyp-not-ic
an-ti-ac-id
an-ti-ag-glu-ti-nin
an-ti-ag-gres-sin
an-ti-al-bu-mate
an-ti-al-bu-min
an-ti-a-lex-in
an-ti-am-bo-cep-tor
an-ti-am-yl-ase
an-ti-an-a-phy-lax-is
an-ti-a-ne-mi-a
an-ti-a-ne-mic
an-ti-an-ti-bod-y
an-ti-ar-ach-nol-y-sin
an-ti-a-rin
an-ti-a-ris
an-ti-ar-thrit-ic
an-ti-bac-te-ri-al
an-ti-bi-o-sis
an-ti-bi-ot-ic
an-ti-blas-tic
an-ti-bod-y
an-ti-bra-chi-um
an-ti-car-cin-o-gen
an-ti-car-i-ous
an-ti-cat-a-lyst
an-ti-ca-thex-is
an-ti-cath-ode
an-ti-ceph-a-lin
an-ti-chei-rot-o-nus
an-ti-chlor
an-ti-chol-in-er-gic
an-ti-cho-lin-es-ter-ase

an-ti-chro-mat-ic
an-ti-co-ag-u-lant
an-ti-col-la-gen-ase
an-ti-com-ple-ment
an-ti-con-cep-tive
an-ti-con-cus-sion
an-ti-con-vul-sive
an-ti-cus
an-ti-cu-tin
an-ti-di-a-bet-ic
an-ti-di-ar-rhe-al
an-ti-di-u-ret-ic
an-ti-dote
an-ti-drom-ic
an-ti-dys-en-ter-ic
an-ti-e-met-ic
an-ti-en-zyme
an-ti-fe-brile
an-ti-fer-ment
an-ti-fi-bri-nol-y-sin
an-ti-fi-bro-ma-to-gen-ic
an-ti-ga-lac-tic
an-ti-gen
an-ti-ge-nic-i-ty
an-ti-he-lix
an-ti-he-mo-lyt-ic
an-ti-he-mo-phil-ic
    fac-tor
an-ti-hem-or-rhag-ic
an-ti-hem-or-rhoi-dal
an-ti-hi-drot-ic
an-ti-his-ta-mine
an-ti-hor-mone
an-ti-hy-a-lu-ron-i-dase
an-ti-hy-drop-ic
an-ti-in-fec-tive
an-ti-ke-to-gen-e-sis
an-ti-li-pase
an-ti-lip-fa-no-gen
an-ti-lu-et-ic
an-ti-lyt-ic
an-ti-ma-lar-i-al

an-ti-mel-lin
an-ti-men-or-rhag-ic
an-ti-mere
an-ti-me-tab-o-lite
an-ti-me-tro-pi-a
an-ti-mo-nic
an-ti-mo-nous
an-ti-mo-ny
an-ti-mo-nyl
an-ti-my-cin A
an-ti-my-cot-ic
an-ti-nar-cot-ic
an-ti-neu-ral-gic
an-ti-neu-rit-ic
an-tin-i-on
an-tin-va-sin 1
an-ti-o-be-sic
an-ti-o-don-tal-gic
an-ti-op-so-nin
an-ti-ox-i-dant
an-ti-par-a-lyt-ic
an-ti-par-a-sit-ic
an-ti-pep-sin
an-ti-pep-tone
an-ti-per-i-od-ic
an-ti-per-i-stal-sis
an-ti-phag-o-cyt-ic
an-ti-phlo-gis-tic
an-ti-phone
an-ti-phthi-ri-ac
an-ti-plas-min
an-ti-plas-tic
an-ti-pneu-mo-coc-cic
an-tip-o-dal
an-ti-pro-throm-bin
an-ti-pro-ton
an-ti-pru-rit-ic
an-ti-py-o-gen-ic
an-ti-py-ret-ic
an-ti-py-rine
an-ti-py-rin-o-ma-ni-a
an-ti-ra-bic

an-ti-ra-chit-ic
an-ti-ren-nin
an-ti-re-tic-u-lar
an-ti-rhe-o-scope
an-ti-rheu-mat-ic
an-ti—Rh se-rum
an-ti-ri-bo-fla-vin
an-ti-ri-cin
an-ti-sca-bet-ic
an-ti-scor-bu-tic
an-ti-sep-sis
an-ti-sep-tic
an-ti-sep-tol
an-ti-se-rum
an-ti-si-al-a-gogue
an-ti-si-al-ic
an-ti-so-cial
an-ti-spas-mod-ic
an-ti-spas-tic
an-ti-spi-ro-che-tic
an-ti-ster-num
an-ti-strep-to-coc-cic
an-ti-strep-to-dor-nase
an-ti-strep-to-he-mo-
   ly-sin
an-ti-strep-to-ki-nase
an-ti-strep-to-ly-sin
an-ti-su-dor-if-ic
an-ti-syph-i-lit-ic
an-ti-the-nar
an-ti-ther-mic
an-ti-ther-min
an-ti-throm-bin
an-ti-throm-bo-plas-tin
an-ti-tox-i-gen
an-ti-tox-in
an-ti-trag-i-cus
an-ti-tra-gus
an-ti-tris-mus
an-ti-trope
an-ti-tryp-sin
an-ti-tus-sive

an-ti-ty-phoid
an-ti-u-re-ase
an-ti-ve-ne-re-al
an-ti-ven-in
an-ti-vi-ral
an-ti-vi-rot-ic
an-ti-vir-u-lin
an-ti-vi-rus
an-ti-vi-ta-min
an-ti-viv-i-sec-tion
an-ti-xen-ic
an-ti-xe-roph-thal-mic
an-ti-xe-rot-ic
an-ti-zy-mot-ic
ant-lo-pho-bi-a
an-trec-to-my
an-tri-tis
an-tro-at-ti-cot-o-my
an-tro-cele
an-tro-na-sal
ant-ro-phose
an-tro-scope
an-tros-to-my
an-tro-tym-pan-ic
an-trum
a-nu-cle-ar
an-u-ri-a
an-u-rous
a-nus
an-vil
anx-i-e-ty
a-or-ta
a-or-tal-gi-a
a-or-ti-co-re-nal
a-or-ti-tis
a-or-tog-ra-phy
a-or-tot-o-my
a-pal-les-the-si-a
a-pan-cre-a
a-pan-dri-a
ap-an-thro-pi-a
a-par-a-lyt-ic

ap-ar-thro-sis
a-pas-ti-a
ap-a-thism
ap-a-thy
ap-a-tite
a-pei-ro-pho-bi-a
a-pel-lous
ap-en-ter-ic
a-pe-ri-ent
a-pe-ri-od-ic
a-per-i-stal-sis
a-per-i-tive
ap-er-tom-e-ter
ap-er-tu-ra
ap-er-ture
a-pex
a-pha-gi-a
a-pha-ki-a
aph-a-lan-gi-a
aph-al-ge-si-a
a-phan-i-sis
a-pha-si-a
a-phelx-i-a
a-phe-mi-a
aph-e-pho-bi-a
aph-e-ter
a-phil-an-thro-py
Aph-i-o-chae-ta
a-pho-ni-a
a-phose
a-phra-si-a
aph-ro-dis-i-a
aph-ro-dis-i-ac
aph-ro-dis-i-o-ma-ni-a
aph-ro-ne-si-a
aph-tha
aph-thenx-i-a
aph-thon-gi-a
aph-tho-sis
aph-thous
a-pi-cec-to-my
ap-i-ci-tis

ap-i-co-ec-to-my
ap-i-co-lo-ca-tor
ap-i-col-y-sis
a-pi-cot-o-my
ap-i-lo-ca-tor
ap-i-nol
a-pi-ol
a-pi-o-ther-a-py
a-pi-pho-bi-a
A-pis
A-pi-um
a-pla-cen-tal
ap-la-nat-ic
a-pla-si-a
a-plas-tic
a-pleu-ri-a
ap-ne-a
ap-neu-mi-a
ap-neu-sis
ap-o-at-ro-pine
ap-o-cam-no-sis
ap-o-car-te-re-sis
ap-o-chro-mat-ic
ap-o-clei-sis
ap-o-co-de-ine
ap-o-crine
ap-o-cy-nam-a-rin
ap-o-cyn-e-in
a-poc-y-nin
a-poc-y-num
ap-o-de-mi-al-gi-a
a-po-di-a
ap-o-en-zyme
a-po-er-y-thein
ap-o-fer-ment
ap-o-fer-ri-tin
a-pog-a-my
ap-o-mix-is
ap-o-mor-phine
ap-o-myt-to-sis
ap-o-nal
a-pon-eu-ror-rha-phy

a-pon-eu-ro-ses
a-pon-eu-ro-sis
a-pon-eu-ro-si-tis
a-pon-eu-rot-o-my
a-pon-i-a
a-poph-y-sate
a-poph-y-sis
a-poph-y-si-tis
ap-o-plas-mi-a
ap-o-plec-ti-form
ap-o-plex-y
a-pop-nix-is
ap-o-qui-nine
ap-or-rhip-sis
a-po-si-a
ap-o-sid-er-in
ap-o-si-ti-a
ap-o-some
a-pos-po-ry
a-pos-ta-sis
a-pos-thi-a
a-poth-e-car-y
ap-ox-e-me-na
ap-ox-e-sis
ap-o-zy-mase
ap-pa-ra-tus
ap-pend-age
ap-pen-dec-to-my
ap-pen-di-ci-tis
ap-pen-di-clau-sis
ap-pen-di-co-lith
ap-pen-di-cos-to-my
ap-pen-dix
ap-per-cep-tion
ap-per-son-i-fi-ca-tion
ap-pe-tite
ap-pe-ti-zer
ap-pla-nate
ap-pli-ca-tor
ap-po-si-tion
ap-proach
ap-prox-i-mal

ap-prox-i-mate
ap-prox-i-ma-tion
a-prac-tog-no-si-a
a-prax-i-a
a-proc-ti-a
a-pro-sex-i-a
a-pro-so-pi-a
ap-sel-a-phe-si-a
ap-si-thy-ri-a
ap-sych-i-a
ap-ty-a-lism
a-pus
a-py-e-tous
a-py-rene
a-py-rex-i-a
aq-ua
aq-uae-duc-tus
aq-ue-duct
a-que-ous
aq-uo—i-on
ar-a-bic ac-id
ar-a-bin
a-rab-i-nose
a-rab-i-tol
a-rach-ic
ar-a-chid-ic
a-rach-i-don-ic ac-id
ar-a-chin
a-rach-ne-pho-bi-a
A-rach-ni-da
a-rach-nid-ism
ar-ach-ni-tis
a-rach-no-dac-ty-ly
a-rach-noid
a-rach-noi-de-a
a-rach-noi-di-tis
a-rach-noid—u-re-ter-
    os-to-my
ar-ach-nol-y-sin
a-ra-phi-a
a-ra-ro-ba
ar-bor-i-za-tion

ar-bor vi-tae
ar-bu-tin
ar-cade
ar-cha-ic
ar-che-go-ni-um
ar-chen-ter-on
ar-che-o-ki-net-ic
ar-che-py-on
ar-che-type
ar-chi-a-ter
ar-chi-coele
ar-chi-gas-ter
ar-chi-gas-tru-la
ar-chi-neph-ron
ar-chi-pal-li-um
ar-chi-tec-ton-ic
ar-cho-plasm
ar-chos
ar-chu-si-a
ar-ci-form
arc-ta-tion
ar-cu-ate
ar-cu-a-tion
ar-cus
a-re-a
ar-e-a-tus
ar-e-cin
a-rec-o-line
a-re-flex-i-a
a-re-gen-er-a-tion
ar-e-na-ceous
ar-e-na-tion
ar-ene
a-re-o-la
ar-gam-bly-o-pi-a
Ar-gas per-si-cus
Ar-gas-i-dae
ar-ge-ma
ar-gen-taf-fin
ar-gen-taf-fi-no-ma
ar-gen-tic
ar-gen-to-phile

ar-gen-tous
ar-gen-tum
ar-gil-la-ceous
ar-gi-nase
ar-gi-nine
ar-gi-nyl
ar-gol
ar-gon
Argyll Robertson
    pupil
ar-gyr-i-a
ar-gy-ro-len-tis
ar-gy-ro-phile
ar-gy-ro-sis
a-rhin-en-ce-pha-li-a
a-rhin-i-a
a-ri-bo-fla-vi-no-sis
ar-i-cine
a-ris-to-gen-ic
A-ris-to-lo-chi-a
a-ris-to-lo-chine
ar-ith-met-ic mean
a-rith-mo-ma-ni-a
ar-ky-o-chrome
ar-ma-men-tar-i-um
Ar-mil-li-fer ar-mil-
    la-tus
Ar-mil-li-fer mon-il-i-
    for-mis
arm-pit
ar-ni-ca
ar-ni-cin
ar-o-mat-ic
ar-rec-tor
ar-rest
ar-rhe-no-blas-to-ma
ar-rhe-not-o-ky
ar-rhin-en-ce-pha-li-a
ar-rhin-i-a
ar-rhyth-mi-a
ar-row-root
ars a-man-di

ar-sa-nil-ic ac-id
ar-se-nate
ar-se-nic
ar-sen-ic ac-id
ar-sen-i-cal
ar-sen-i-co-der-ma
ar-sen-i-cum
ar-se-nide
ar-se-ni-ous
ar-se-nite
ar-se-niu-ret-ted
ar-se-no-ther-a-py
ar-se-nous
ar-se-num
ar-sine
ar-sin-ic ac-id
ar-son-val-i-za-tion
ars-phen-a-mine
ars-thin-ol
ar-te-fact
ar-ter-ec-to-my
ar-ter-en-ol
ar-te-ri-a
ar-te-ri-al-i-za-tion
ar-te-ri-arc-ti-a
ar-te-ri-a-sis
ar-te-ri-ec-ta-sis
ar-te-ri-ec-to-my
ar-te-ri-ec-to-pi-a
ar-te-ri-o-cap-il-lar-y
ar-te-ri-o-fi-bro-sis
ar-te-ri-o-gram
ar-te-ri-o-graph
ar-te-ri-og-ra-phy
ar-te-ri-o-la
ar-te-ri-ole
ar-te-ri-o-lith
ar-ter-i-o-li-tis
ar-te-ri-o-lo-ne-cro-sis
ar-te-ri-o-lo-scle-ro-sis
ar-te-ri-o-ma-la-ci-a
ar-te-ri-o-ne-cro-sis

ar-te-ri-op-a-thy
ar-te-ri-o-pla-ni-a
ar-te-ri-o-plas-ty
ar-te-ri-o-pres-sor
ar-te-ri-o-punc-ture
ar-te-ri-o-re-nal
ar-te-ri-or-rha-phy
ar-te-ri-or-rhex-is
ar-te-ri-o-scle-ro-sis
ar-te-ri-o-spasm
ar-te-ri-o-ste-no-sis
ar-te-ri-os-to-sis
ar-te-ri-o-strep-sis
ar-te-ri-o-tome
ar-te-ri-ot-o-my
ar-te-ri-o-ve-nous
ar-te-ri-o-ver-sion
ar-te-ri-tis
ar-ter-y
ar-thral-gi-a
ar-threc-to-my
ar-thre-de-ma
ar-thres-the-si-a
ar-thrit-ic
ar-thrit-i-des
ar-thri-tis
ar-throc-a-ce
ar-thro-cele
ar-thro-cen-te-sis
ar-thro-chon-dri-tis
ar-thro-cla-si-a
ar-thro-de-sis
ar-thro-di-a
ar-thro-dyn-i-a
ar-thro-dys-pla-si-a
ar-throe-de-ma
ar-thro-em-py-e-sis
ar-thro-en-dos-co-py
ar-thro-er-ei-sis
ar-throg-ra-phy
ar-thro-gry-po-sis
ar-thro-ka-tad-y-sis

ar-thro-lith
ar-throl-o-gy
ar-throl-y-sis
ar-throm-e-ter
ar-thron-cus
ar-throp-a-thy
ar-thro-phyte
ar-thro-plas-ty
Ar-throp-o-da
ar-thror-rha-gi-a
ar-thro-scope
ar-thros-co-py
ar-thro-sis
ar-thro-spore
ar-thros-to-my
ar-thro-tome
ar-throt-o-my
ar-thro-tro-pi-a
ar-throus
ar-tic-u-lar
ar-tic-u-lar-is ge-nus
ar-tic-u-late
ar-tic-u-la-ti-o
ar-tic-u-la-tion
ar-tic-u-la-tor
ar-tic-u-lus
ar-ti-fact
ar-ti-fi-cial
ar-y-ep-i-glot-tic
ar-yl
ar-yl-ene
ar-y-te-no-ep-i-glot-tic
a-ryt-e-noid
ar-y-te-noi-dec-to-my
ar-y-te-noi-di-tis
ar-y-te-noi-do-pex-y
ar-y-vo-cal-is
as-a-fet-i-da
as-a-phi-a
a-sar-ci-a
as-a-ron
as-a-rum

as-bes-tos
as-bes-to-sis
as-ca-ri-a-sis
as-car-i-cide
As-car-i-dae
as-car-i-dol
As-ca-ris
As-ca-ris lum-bri-coides
as-cend-ing
Aschheim—Zondek test
as-ci-tes
as-cle-pain
as-cle-pi-ad-in
as-cle-pi-as
As-co-my-ce-tes
a-scor-bate
a-scor-bic ac-id
as-co-spore
as-cus
a-se-mi-a
a-sep-sis
a-sex-u-al
a-si-a-li-a
a-si-at-i-co-side
Asklepios
a-so-cial
a-so-ma
a-so-ni-a
as-pal-a-so-ma
as-par-a-gin
as-par-a-gin-ase
as-par-a-gin-ic ac-id
as-par-a-gi-nyl
as-par-tase
as-par-tic ac-id
a-spas-tic
a-spe-cif-ic
as-per-gil-lic ac-id
as-per-gil-lin
as-per-gil-lo-sis
As-per-gil-lus
a-sper-ma-tism

a-sper-mi-a
a-sper-ma-to-gen-e-sis
as-per-ous
as-phyx-i-a
as-phyx-i-ant
as-pi-din
as-pid-i-um
as-pi-do-sper-ma
as-pi-do-sper-mine
as-pi-ra-tion
as-pi-ra-tor
as-pi-rin
As-pis
a-spo-ro-gen-ic
a-spo-rous
a-spor-u-late
as-sault
as-say
as-sim-i-la-tion
as-so-ci-a-tion
as-so-nance
as-sue-tude
As-ta-cus
a-sta-si-a
as-ta-tine
as-ta-xan-thin
a-ste-a-to-sis
as-ter
a-ster-e-og-no-sis
as-te-ri-on
a-ster-nal
a-ster-ni-a
as-ter-oid
as-the-ni-a
as-the-no-bi-o-sis
as-the-no-co-ri-a
as-the-nom-e-ter
as-the-no-pho-bi-a
as-the-no-pi-a
as-the-no-sper-mi-a
as-the-nox-i-a
asth-ma

a-stig-ma-graph
a-stig-ma-tism
a-stig-ma-tom-e-ter
as-tig-mat-o-scope
a-stig-mom-e-ter
a-stig-mo-scope
a-stom-a-tous
a-sto-mi-a
as-trag-a-lec-to-my
as-trag-a-lus
as-tra-pho-bi-a
as-trin-gent
as-tro-blast
as-tro-blas-to-ma
as-tro-cytes
as-tro-cy-to-ma
as-trog-li-a
as-trog-li-o-ma
as-troid
as-tro-ma
as-tro-pho-bi-a
as-tro-sphere
a-styph-i-a
a-stys-i-a
a-syl-la-bi-a
a-syl-lum
a-sym-met-ric
a-sym-me-try
a-sym-phy-tous
a-symp-to-mat-ic
as-ymp-tot-ic
a-syn-chro-nism
a-syn-cli-tism
a-syn-de-sis
a-syn-ech-i-a
a-syn-er-gy
a-syn-e-si-a
as-y-no-di-a
a-sys-tem-at-ic
a-sys-to-li-a
a-tac-tic
a-tac-ti-form

a-tac-til-i-a
a-tav-i-cus
at-a-vism
a-tax-a-pha-si-a
a-tax-i-a
a-tax-i-a-graph
a-tax-i-o-pho-bi-a
a-tax-o-phe-mi-a
at-e-lec-ta-sis
a-tel-en-ce-pha-li-a
a-te-li-o-sis
at-e-lo-car-di-a
at-e-lo-ceph-a-lous
at-e-lo-chei-li-a
at-e-lo-chei-ri-a
at-e-lo-glos-si-a
at-e-log-nath-i-a
at-e-lo-mit-ic
at-e-lo-my-e-li-a
at-e-lo-po-di-a
at-e-lo-pro-so-pi-a
at-e-lo-ra-chid-i-a
at-e-lo-sto-mi-a
at-e-pho-bi-a
a-the-li-a
ath-er-o-gen-e-sis
ath-er-o-ma
ath-er-o-ma-to-sis
ath-er-o-scle-ro-sis
ath-e-to-sis
ath-lete's foot
a-threp-si-a
a-thy-mic
a-thy-re-o-sis
at-lan-to-ax-i-al
at-lan-to-ep-i-stroph-ic
at-lan-to—oc-cip-i-tal
at-las
at-lo-ax-oid
at-lod-y-mus
at-mol-y-sis
at-mom-e-ter

at-mos-phere
a-to-ci-a
at-om
at-om-i-za-tion
a-to-ni-a
at-o-ny
at-o-pen
a-top-ic
a-top-og-no-si-a
at-o-py
a-tox-ic
a-tox-yl
a-tra-che-li-a
a-trach-e-lo-ceph-a-lus
a-tre-mi-a
a-tre-si-a
a-tre-to-ceph-a-lus
a-tre-to-cor-mus
a-tre-to-cys-ti-a
a-tre-to-gas-tri-a
a-tre-to-le-mi-a
a-tre-to-me-tri-a
at-re-top-si-a
a-tret-or-rhin-i-a
a-tre-to-sto-mi-a
a-tret-u-re-thri-a
a-tri-a
at-ri-cho-sis
at-ri-chous
a-tri-o-sep-to-pex-y
a-tri-o-ven-tric-u-lar
a-tri-o-ven-tric-u-lar-is
    com-mu-nis
a-tri-um
at-ro-pho-der-ma
at-ro-pho-der-ma-to-sis
at-ro-phy
at-ro-pine
at-ro-pin-ize
at-ro-scine
at-tar
at-ten-tion

at-ten-u-a-tion
at-tic
at-ti-co-an-trot-o-my
at-ti-co-mas-toid
at-ti-cot-o-my
at-ti-tude
at-ton-i-ty
at-trac-tion
at-tri-tion
a-typ-i-cal
au-di-mu-tism
au-di-o-gen-ic
au-di-o-gram
au-di-ol-o-gy
au-di-om-e-ter
au-di-om-e-try
au-di-o-vis-u-al
au-di-tion
au-di-tog-no-sis
au-di-to-psy-chic
au-di-to-ry
au-di-to-sen-so-ry
aug-ment
aug-men-tor
aug-na-thus
au-lo-pho-bi-a
au-lo-phyte
au-ra
aurae
au-ral
au-ran-ti-a
au-ran-ti-am-a-rin
aur-an-ti-a-sis cu-tis
au-ran-ti-um
au-rate
au-ric
au-ri-cle
au-ric-u-la
au-ric-u-la-re
au-ric-u-lar-is
au-ric-u-lo-fron-tal-is
au-ric-u-lo-tem-po-ral

86

au-ric-u-lo-ven-tric-u-lar
au-ris
au-rist
au-ro-ra-pho-bi-a
au-ro-ther-a-py
au-ro-thi-o-glu-cose
au-ro-thi-o-glyc-an-ide
au-rous
au-rum
aus-cul-ta-tion
au-ta-coid
au-te-cious
au-te-me-si-a
au-tism
au-tis-tic
au-to-ac-ti-va-tion
au-to-ag-glu-ti-na-tion
au-to-ag-glu-ti-nin
au-to-al-go-lag-ni-a
au-to-a-nal-y-sis
au-to-an-am-ne-sis
au-to-an-ti-bi-o-sis
au-to-an-ti-bod-y
au-to-au-di-ble
au-to-blast
au-to-ca-tal-y-sis
au-to-ca-ta-lyt-ic
au-to-ca-thar-sis
au-to-cho-le-cys-to-du-o-de-nos-to-my
au-to-cho-le-cys-to-trans-verse-co-los-to-my
au-toch-tho-nous
au-toc-la-sis
au-to-clave
au-to-con-den-sa-tion
au-to-con-duc-tion
au-to-cy-to-tox-in
au-to-di-ges-tion
au-to-ech-o-la-li-a
au-to-ech-o-prax-i-a
au-toe-cic

au-to-ec-ze-ma-ti-za-tion
au-to-e-mas-cu-la-tion
au-to-er-o-tism
au-to-e-rot-i-cism
au-to-fel-la-ti-o
au-tog-a-my
au-tog-e-nous
au-to-graft
au-to-graph
au-to-he-mol-y-sis
au-to-he-mo-ther-a-py
au-to-hy-drol-y-sis
au-to-hyp-no-tism
au-to-hyp-no-sis
au-to-im-mun-i-za-tion
au-to-in-fec-tion
au-to-in-fu-sion
au-to-in-oc-u-la-tion
au-to-in-tox-i-cant
au-to-in-tox-i-ca-tion
au-to-i-so-ly-sin
au-to-kin-e-sis
au-tol-o-gous
au-tol-y-sate
au-to-ly-sin
au-tol-y-sis
au-to-mat-ic
au-tom-a-tin
au-tom-a-tin-o-gen
au-tom-a-tism
au-tom-a-ti-za-tion
au-tom-a-ton
au-to-my-so-pho-bi-a
au-to-ne-phrec-to-my
au-to-no-ma-si-a
au-to-nom-ic
au-ton-o-mous
au-to—ox-i-da-tion
au-top-a-thy
au-to-pha-gi-a
au-to-phil-i-a
au-to-pho-bi-a

au-to-pho-no-ma-ni-a
au-toph-o-ny
au-to-plas-ty
au-to-pneu-mo-nec-to-my
au-to-pro-tol-y-sis
au-top-sy
au-to-psy-che
au-to-psy-chic
au-to-psy-cho-sis
au-to-ra-di-og-ra-phy
au-to-re-in-fu-sion
au-to-sen-si-ti-za-tion
au-to-site
au-to-some
au-to-sug-ges-tion
au-to-syn-de-sis
au-to-syn-noi-a
Autotechnicon
au-tot-o-my
au-to-top-ag-no-si-a
au-to-trans-form-er
au-to-trans-fu-sion
au-to-trans-plan-ta-tion
au-to-troph
au-to-vac-ci-na-tion
au-to-vac-cine
aux-an-o-dif-fer-en-ti-a-tion
aux-an-o-gram
aux-a-nog-ra-phy
aux-e-sis
aux-et-ic
aux-in
aux-o-bar-ic
aux-o-car-di-a
aux-o-chrome
aux-o-cyte
aux-o-drome
aux-om-e-ter
av-a-lanche
a-val-vu-lar
a-vas-cu-lar-i-za-tion

A-ve-na
a-ve-nin
av-er-age
a-vi-an pneu-mo-en-
    ceph-a-li-tis
a-vi-an pseu-do-plague
a-vi-a-tor's ear
av-i-din
a-vid-i-ty
a-vir-u-lent
a-vi-tam-ic ac-id
a-vi-ta-min-o-sis
a-vo-ca-li-a
Avogadro's law
av-oir-du-pois
a-vul-sion
ax-an-thop-si-a
ax-i-a-tion
ax-il-la
ax-is
ax-o-den-drit-ic
ax-o-fu-gal
ax-oid
ax-o-lem-ma
ax-o-mat-ic
ax-om-e-ter
ax-on
ax-o-neme
ax-o-nom-e-ter
ax-on-ot-me-sis
ax-op-e-tal
ax-o-plasm
az-a-gua-nine
a-za-ser-ine
a-ze-o-trope
az-ide
az-ine
az-o-ben-zene
az-o-car-mine G
az-o com-pound
az-o-der-min
az-o dyes

az-o-lit-min
a-zo-o-sper-mi-a
az-o-pro-te-in
az-o-ru-bin S
az-o-te-mi-a
az-o-tized
Az-o-to-bac-ter
az-o-tom-e-ter
az-o-tor-rhe-a
az-o-tu-ri-a
az-u-lene
az-ure
az-u-rin
a-zu-ro-phile
az-y-go-ag-na-thus
az-y-gos
a-zy-mi-a
a-zym-ic

B

Ba-be-si-a
bab-e-si-a-sis
Babinski's sign
Bac-cha-ris
bac-ci-form
bac-il-lar-y
bac-il-le-mi-a
ba-cil-li-form
ba-cil-lo-pho-bi-a
bac-il-lu-ri-a
Ba-cil-lus
back-ache
back-bone
back-ward-ness
bac-te-re-mi-a
bac-te-ri-a
Bac-te-ri-a-ce-ae
bac-te-ri-cid-al
bac-te-ri-cide

bac-te-ri-ci-din
bac-te-rid
bac-te-ri-form
bac-ter-i-o-chlor-o-phyll
bac-te-ri-oc-la-sis
bac-te-ri-o-er-y-thrin
bac-te-ri-o-flu-o-res-cin
bac-te-ri-o-gen-ic
bac-te-ri-o-he-mo-ly-sin
bac-te-ri-oid
bac-te-ri-ol-o-gist
bac-te-ri-ol-o-gy
bac-te-ri-o-ly-sin
bac-te-ri-ol-y-sis
bac-te-ri-o-phage
bac-te-ri-o-pha-gol-o-gy
bac-te-ri-o-pho-bi-a
bac-te-ri-o-pro-te-in
bac-te-ri-op-so-nin
bac-te-ri-os-co-py
bac-te-ri-os-ta-sis
bac-te-ri-o-stat
bac-te-ri-o-ther-a-py
bac-te-ri-o-tox-in
bac-te-ri-o-trop-ic
bac-te-ri-ot-ro-pin
Bac-te-ri-um
bac-te-ri-u-ri-a
bac-ter-oid
Bac-ter-o-i-des
baf-fle
ba-tas-so-sis
Bag-dad boil
Ba-hi-a ul-cer
bak-er
bal-ance
bal-a-nism
bal-a-ni-tis
bal-a-no-plas-ty
bal-a-no-pos-thi-tis
bal-a-no-pre-pu-tial
bal-a-nor-rha-gi-a

bal-an-or-rhe-a
Bal-an-tid-i-um coli
bal-a-nus
bald-ness
Bal-kan frame
bal-lism
bal-lis-mus
bal-lis-to-car-di-o-graph
bal-lis-to-pho-bi-a
ball mill
bal-loon-ing
bal-lotte-ment
bal-ne-ol-o-gy
bal-ne-o-ther-a-py
bal-sam
bal-sam-weed
band-age
bar-ag-no-sis
bar-ba
bar-bi-tal
bar-bi-tone
bar-bit-u-rate,
    bar-bi-tu-rate
bar-bi-tu-ric ac-id
bar-bi-tu-rism
bar-bo-tage
bar-es-the-si-a
bar-es-the-si-om-e-ter
bar-i-to-sis
ba-ri-um
bar-ley
bar-o-cep-tor
bar-o-don-tal-gi-a
bar-og-no-sis
bar-o-graph
bar-o-ma-crom-e-ter
ba-rom-e-ter
bar-o-pho-bi-a
bar-o-scope
bar-o-si-nus-i-tis
bar-o-tal-gi-a
bar-o-ti-tis

bar-o-trau-ma
bar-ren-ness
bar-ri-er
bar-tho-lin-i-tis
Bar-to-nel-la
bar-to-nel-lo-sis
bar-y-la-li-a
bar-y-pho-ni-a
ba-sal met-a-bol-ic rate
bas-cu-la-tion
bas-cule move-ment
bas-e-doid
base-ment
bas—fond
ba-si-al-ve-o-lar
ba-si-bran-chi-al
ba-si-chro-ma-tin
ba-sic-i-ty
ba-si-cra-ni-al
ba-sid-i-o-ge-net-ic
Ba-sid-i-o-my-ce-tes
ba-sid-i-o-phere
ba-sid-i-o-spore
ba-sid-i-um
ba-si-fa-cial
ba-si-hy-al
bas-ilar
ba-si-lat-er-al
ba-sil-ic
ba-sil-ic vein
ba-sil-o-breg-mat-ic
ba-sil-o-men-tal
ba-sil-o-pha-ryn-ge-al
ba-si-na-sal
ba-si-o-al-ve-o-lar
ba-si-oc-cip-i-tal
ba-si-oc-cip-i-tal bone
ba-si-on
ba-si-o-tribe
ba-si-o-trip-sy
ba-si-pho-bi-a
ba-si-pre-sphen-oid

ba-si-rhi-nal
ba-sis
ba-si-sphe-noid
ba-si-syl-vi-an
ba-si-tem-po-ral
ba-si-ver-te-bral
bas-ket
ba-so-phil
ba-so-phil-i-a
ba-so-phil-ic
ba-soph-i-lism
ba-soph-i-lous
ba-so-pho-bi-a
ba-so-plasm
bas-si-net
bath-es-the-si-a
bath-o-pho-bi-a
bath-y-car-di-a
bath-y-chro-mic ef-fect
bat-o-pho-bi-a
bat-ter-y
bat-yl al-co-hol
Bauru ulcer
bay-ber-ry
bdel-yg-mi-a
bead-ed
beat-ing
bed-bug
bed-fast
bed-pan
bed-rid-den
bed-sore
be-hen-ic ac-id
bej-el
bel
bel-la-don-na
bel-la-don-nine
bell—crowned
Bellevue bridge
Belling's stain
bel-lones
Bell's pal-sy

bel-ly
bel-ly-ache
bel-o-ne-pho-bi-a
Bence Jones pro-tein
Bence Jones's cyl-in-ders
bends
Benedict's test
Benedikt syn-dro-me
be-nign
be-nig-nant
Bennhold's test
ben-ton-ite
ben-zac-o-nine
benz-al-de-hyde
ben-zal-dox-ime
ben-zal-ko-ni-um
    chlo-ride
ben-zan-thra-cenes
ben-zene
ben-ze-tho-ni-um
    chlo-ride
ben-zi-dine
benz-im-id-a-zole
ben-zo-ate
ben-zo-caine
ben-zo-ic ac-id
ben-zo-di-ox-ane
ben-zo-in
ben-zol
ben-zo-naph-tha-lene
ben-zo-ni-trile
ben-zo-phe-none
ben-zo-py-rene
ben-zo-qui-none a-ce-tic
    ac-id
ben-zo-sul-fi-mide
Benzyl ben-zo-ate
    lo-tion
ber-ber-ine
ber-ga-mot oil
ber-i-ber-i
Berkefeld fil-ter

berke-li-um
Berlin blue
Ber-ti-el-la mu-cro-nat-a
be-ryl-li-o-sis
be-ryl-li-um
bes-i-clom-e-ter
Besnier—Boeck dis-ease
Best's car-mine
Best's dis-ease
bes-ti-al-i-ty
be-ta
be-ta-cism
be-ta-ine
be-ta-par-ti-cle
be-ta-to-pic
be-ta-tron
be-tel
Betz cells
be-va-tron
bev-el
be-zoar
bhang
bi-ased er-rors
bi-ased sam-ple
bi-a-stig-ma-tism
bi-ax-i-al
bib-li-o-clast
bib-li-o-klep-to-ma-ni-a
bib-li-o-ma-ni-a
bib-li-o-pho-bi-a
bi-cap-i-tate
bi-car-bon-ate
bi-car-di-o-gram
bi-ceph-a-lous
bi-ceps
bi-chlo-ride
bi-chro-mate
bi-cor-nate
bi-cus-pid
bi-dac-ty-ly
Biebrich scar-let
bi-e-lec-trol-y-sis

Biermer's dis-ease
Biernacki's sign
Biesiadecki's fos-sa
Biett's dis-ease
bi-fid
bi-fo-cal
bi-for-min
bi-fur-ca-tion
Bigelow's meth-od
bi-gem-i-nal
bi-gem-i-ny
bi-labe
bi-lat-er-al
bile salts
Bil-har-zi-a
bil-i-ar-y
bil-i-cy-a-nin
bil-i-fla-vin
bil-i-ful-vin
bil-i-fus-cin
bi-lig-u-late
bil-i-hu-min
bil-i-leu-kan
bil-i-neu-rine
bil-ious
bil-ious-ness
bil-i-pha-in
bil-i-pra-sin
bil-i-pur-pu-rin
bil-i-ru-bic ac-id
bil-i-ru-bin
bil-i-ru-bi-ne-mi-a
bil-i-ru-bin—glo-bin
bil-i-ru-bi-nu-ri-a
bil-i-u-ri-a
bil-i-ver-din
bil-i-xan-thine
bi-lo-bate
bi-loc-u-lar
bi-man-u-al
bi-na-ry
bi-na-sal

90

bin-au-ral
bind-er
bi-o—as-say
bi-o-aut-og-ra-phy
bi-o-blast
bi-o-cat-a-lyst
bi-o-chem-i-cal
bi-o-chem-is-try
bi-o-chem-or-phic
bi-o-chem-or-phol-o-gy
bi-o-chrome
bi-o-cli-ma-tol-o-gy
bi-o-cy-tin
bi-o-di-al-y-sate
bi-o-di-al-y-sis
bi-o—e-lec-tric-i-ty
bi-o-en-er-get-ics
bi-o-flav-o-noids
bi-o-gen-e-sis
bi-o-ge-net-ic
bi-og-e-ny
bi-o-ki-net-ics
bi-o-log-i-cal as-say
bi-o-log-i-cals
bi-ol-o-gist
bi-ol-o-gy
bi-o-lu-mi-nes-cence
bi-o-math-e-mat-ics
bi-o-me-chan-ics
bi-om-e-ter
bi-om-e-try
bi-o-mi-cros-co-py
bi-o-pho-tom-e-ter
bi-o-phys-ics
bi-op-sy
bi-o-psy-chol-o-gy
bi-ose
bi-o-sta-tis-tics
bi-o-syn-the-sis
bi-o-ta
bi-ot-ic
bi-ot-ics

bi-o-tin
bi-o-type
bi-o-ty-pol-o-gy
bip-a-ra
bi-par-a-sit-ic
bi-pa-ri-e-tal
bip-a-rous
bi-ped
bi-ped-al
bi-pen-ni-form
bi-po-lar-i-ty
bi-po-ten-ti-al-i-ty
bi-re-frac-tive
bi-re-frin-gence
bi-rhin-i-a
bi-ri-mose
birth-mark
birth rate
bi-sex-u-al
bis-fe-ri-ous
Biskra but-ton
Bismarck brown Y
bis-muth
bis-mu-thi-a
bis-muth-o-sis
bis-sa
bis-sa-bol
bis-sy-no-sis
bis-tort
bis-tou-ry
bi-sul-fide
bi-sul-fite
bi-tar-trate
bite-wing
bi-thi-o-nol
Bitot's spots
bit-ters
bi-tu-men
bi-u-rate
bi-u-ret
bi-u-ret re-ac-tion
bi-va-lent

bi-valve
bi-ven-ter
black-damp
Black Death
black-head
black-leg
black-out
black-tongue
black-water fe-ver
blad-der
Blakemore's op-er-a-tion
Blalock—Taussig
    op-er-a-tion
blas-te-ma
blas-tin
blas-to-chyle
blas-to-coele
blas-to-cyst
Blas-to-cys-tis
    ho-mi-nis
blas-to-derm
blas-to-gen-e-sis
blas-tog-e-ny
blas-to-ki-ne-sis
blas-tok-o-lin
blas-tol-y-sis
blas-to-ma
blas-tom-a-to-gen-ic
blas-to-mere
Blas-to-my-ces bras-i-
    lien-sis
Blas-to-my-ces der-ma-
    ti-ti-dis
Blas-to-my-ce-tes
blas-to-my-ce-tic
Blas-to-my-coi-des
blas-to-my-co-sis
blas-to-neu-ro-pore
blas-to-pore
blas-to-sphere
blas-to-spore
blas-tot-o-my

blas-tu-la
Bla-tel-la ger-man-ica
Blat-ta or-i-en-tal-is
bleb
bleed-er
bleed-ing
bleed-ing time
blem-ma-trope
blend-ing
blen-noph-thal-mi-a
blen-nor-rha-gi-a
blen-nor-rhe-a
bleph-a-ra
bleph-a-ral
bleph-a-rec-to-my
bleph-ar-e-de-ma
bleph-ar-e-lo-sis
bleph-a-rism
bleph-a-ri-tis
bleph-a-ro-ad-e-no-ma
bleph-a-ro-ath-er-o-ma
bleph-a-ro-blen-nor-rhe-a
bleph-a-ro-chal-a-sis
bleph-a-ro-chrom-hi-dro-sis
bleph-a-ro-clei-sis
bleph-a-roc-lo-nus
bleph-a-ro-con-junc-ti-vi-tis
bleph-a-ro-di-as-ta-sis
bleph-a-ro-dys-chroi-a
bleph-a-ro-me-las-ma
bleph-a-ron
bleph-a-ron-cus
bleph-a-ro-pa-chyn-sis
bleph-a-ro-phi-mo-sis
bleph-a-roph-ry-plas-ty
bleph-a-ro-phy-ma
bleph-a-ro-plast
bleph-a-ro-plas-ty
bleph-a-ro-ple-gi-a
bleph-a-rop-to-sis

bleph-a-ro-py-or-rhe-a
bleph-a-ror-rha-phy
bleph-a-ro-spasm
bleph-a-ro-sphinc-ter-ec-to-my
bleph-a-ro-stat
bleph-a-ro-ste-no-sis
bleph-a-ro-sym-phy-sis
bleph-a-ro-syn-ech-i-a
bleph-a-rot-o-my
blep-so-path-i-a
blind-ness
blind spot
blink-ing
blis-ter
blis-ter-ing
bloat
block
block-ing
blood
blood—brain bar-ri-er
blood count
blood groups
blood-less
blood-let-ting
blood poi-son-ing
blood pres-sure
blood ur-e-a ni-tro-gen
blow-fly
blue ba-by
blue drum
Blumberg's sign
Blu-mer's shelf
blunt—hook
Blyth's test
Bobroff's op-er-a-tion
Bochdalek's tri-an-gle
Bock-hart's im-pe-ti-go
Bodansky's meth-od
bod-y
Boeck's sar-coid
Bohler's splint

Bohmer's he-ma-tox-y-lin
Bohr ef-fect
boil
bole
Bo-ley gauge
Bollinger's gran-ules
Bolt-worth skate
bo-lus
bone on-lay
bone wax
Bonnet's op-er-a-tion
Bonnet's sign
Bonnier's syn-drome
boom-slang
boos-ter dose
bo-rate
bo-rat-ed
bo-rax
bor-bo-ryg-mus
Bor-deaux mix-ture
Bor-deaux red
bor-der
Bordet—Gengou me-di-um
bo-ric ac-id
bo-ro-cal-cite
bo-ro-cit-ric ac-id
bo-ro-glyc-er-in
bo-ron
bo-ro-sal-i-cyl-ic ac-id
Bor-re-li-a dut-ton-ii
Bor-re-li-a nov-yi
Bor-re-li-a re-cur-ren-tis
Bor-re-li-a re-frin-gens
Bor-re-li-a vin-cen-ti-i
boss
Boston's sign
bot
bot-a-ny
bot-fly
Both res-pi-ra-tor
both-ri-old

both-ri-um
bot-o-gen-in
bot-ry-oid
bots
Bottcher's cells
bot-tle
bot-u-lism
bou-gie
bouil-lon
bour-donne-ment
Bourgery's lig-a-ment
Bourneville's dis-ease
Bouveret's syn-drome
Boveri's test
bo-vine
bow-el
bow-leg
Bowman's cap-sule
Bowman's mem-brane
box-er's ear
Boyer's op-er-a-tion
Boyle's law
Bozeman's cath-e-ter
Bozeman's po-si-tion
Bozzolo's dis-ease
brace
bra-chi-a
bra-chi-al ar-ter-y
bra-chi-al-gi-a
bra-chi-a-lis
bra-chi-form
bra-chi-o-cyl-lo-sis
brach-i-o-ra-di-al-is
bra-chi-ot-o-my
bra-chi-um
brach-y-ceph-a-ly
bra-chych-il-y
brach-y-chi-rous
brach-y-dac-ty-ly
brach-y-glos-sal
brach-yg-nath-ous
brach-y-ker-kic

brach-y-me-tap-o-dy
brach-y-mei-o-sis
brach-y-mor-phic
brach-y-pel-lic
brach-y-pel-vic
brach-y-pha-lan-gi-a
brach-y-po-dous
brach-y-pro-sop-ic
brach-y-rhin-i-a
brach-y-rhyn-chus
brach-y-skel-ic
brach-y-staph-y-line
brach-y-sta-tic con-trac-tion
brach-y-u-ran-ic
Brackett's op-er-a-tion
Bradford frame
brad-y-ar-thri-a
brad-y-aux-e-sis
brad-y-car-di-a
brad-y-crot-ic
brad-y-di-as-to-le
brad-y-glos-si-a
brad-y-ki-ne-si-a
brad-y-la-li-a
brad-y-lex-i-a
brad-y-pha-si-a
brad-y-phre-ni-a
brad-y-pne-a
brad-y-pra-gi-a
brad-y-prax-i-a
brad-y-rhyth-mi-a
brad-y-tel-e-o-ki-ne-sis
Braille sys-tem
brain sand
brain stem
bran-chi-al
branch-ing
bran-chi-og-e-nous
bran-chi-o-ma
bran-chi-o-mere
bran-chi-om-er-ism

bran-dy
brass poi-son-ing
Braun's graft
Braun's hook
Braun's test
brawn-y
Braxton Hicks's con-trac-tions
Braxton Hicks's sign
Braxton Hicks's ver-sion
break-bone fe-ver
breast
breast-bone
breath
breath-ing
Breda's dis-ease
breech pres-en-ta-tion
breg-ma
breg-mat-o-dym-i-a
Breisky's meth-od
brems-strahl-en
bren-ner-o-ma
Brenner tu-mor
Breschet's ca-nals
brev-i-col-lis
brev-i-lin-e-al
brev-i-ra-di-ate
bribe
bridge
bridge-work
bri-dle
Briggs's bag
Bright's dis-ease
bright-ness
bril-liance
bril-liant cres-yl blue
bril-liant green
bril-liant vi-tal red
Brill's dis-ease
brim-stone
Brinton's dis-ease
Briquet's syn-drome

Brissaud—Marie
  syn-drome
Brit-ish an-ti—lew-is-ite
broach
Broadbent's ap-o-plex-y
Broadbent's sign
broad—spec-trum
  an-ti-bi-ot-ic
Broca's ar-e-a
Brocq's dis-ease
Broder's clas-si-fi-ca-tion
Brodie's ab-scess
Brodie's tu-mor
Brodmann's map
bro-mate
bro-mat-ed
bro-ma-tom-e-try
bro-ma-to-ther-a-py
bro-ma-to-tox-in
bro-ma-to-tox-ism
bro-me-lin
brom-hi-dro-si-pho-bi-a
brom-hi-dro-sis
bro-mide
bro-mi-dro-sis
bro-mine
bro-min-ism
bro-mism
bro-mite
bro-mo-ben-zyl-cy-a-nide
bro-mo-cre-sol green
bro-mo-cre-sol pur-ple
bro-mo-der-ma
bro-mo-hy-per-hi-dro-sis
bro-mo-ma-ni-a
bro-mo-men-or-rhe-a
bro-mo-phe-nol blue
bro-mop-ne-a
bro-mo-pro-pane
bro-mo-pro-pene
bro-mo-thy-mol blue
brom-te-trag-nost

bronch-ad-e-ni-tis
bron-chi
bron-chi-ec-ta-sis
bron-chi-o-gen-ic
bron-chi-ole
bron-chi-o-lec-ta-sis
bron-chi-o-li-tis
bron-chi-tis
bron-cho-cele
bron-cho-con-stric-tor
bron-cho-dil-a-ta-tion
bron-cho-di-la-tor
bron-cho-e-de-ma
bron-cho-e-soph-a-ge-al
bron-cho-e-soph-a-
  gol-o-gy
bron-cho-e-soph-a-
  gos-co-py
bron-cho-gen-ic
bron-cho-gram
bron-chog-ra-phy
bron-cho-lith
bron-chol-o-gy
bron-cho-mo-ni-li-a-sis
bron-cho-mo-tor
bron-cho-my-co-sis
bron-chop-a-thy
bron-choph-o-ny
bron-cho-plas-ty
bron-cho-pleu-ral
bron-cho-pneu-mo-ni-a
bron-cho-pneu-mo-ni-tis
bron-cho-pul-mo-na-ry
bron-chor-rha-phy
bron-chor-rhe-a
bron-cho-scope
bron-cho-spasm
bron-cho-spi-ro-che-
  to-sis
bron-cho-spi-rog-ra-phy
bron-cho-spi-rom-e-ter
bron-cho-spi-rom-e-try

bron-cho-ste-no-sis
bron-chos-to-my
bron-chot-o-my
bron-cho-ve-sic-u-lar
bron-chus
bron-to-pho-bi-a
bronze di-a-be-tes
brood cyst
Brooke's tu-mor
broth
brow
Brown—Sequard syn-
  drome
brown mix-ture
Bru-cel-la
bru-cel-lo-sis
Bruch's mem-brane
Bruck's dis-ease
Brudzinski's signs
bruise
bruisse-ment
bruit
Brunner's glands
Bruns's syn-drome
Brux-ism
brux-o-ma-ni-a
bryg-mus
bu-bas
bu-bo
bu-bon-ad-e-ni-tis
bu-bon-al-gi-a
bu-bon-ic plague
bu-bon-o-cele
bu-bon-u-lus
bu-car-di-a
buc-ca
buc-ci-na-tor
buc-co-ax-i-al
buc-co-clu-sal
buc-co-cer-vi-cal
buc-co-dis-tal

buc-co-fa-cial ob-tu-ra-tor
buc-co-gin-gi-val
buc-co-la-bi-al
buc-co-lin-gual
buc-co-me-si-al
buc-co-na-sal
buc-co-na-so-pha-ryn-ge-al
buc-co-pha-ryn-ge-al
buc-co-phar-yn-ge-us
buc-co-pulp-al
buc-co-ver-sion
buc-cu-la
Buck's ex-ten-sion
Bucky's di-a-phragm
buc-ne-mi-a
bud
bud-ding
Budinger—Ludloff—Lawen dis-ease
Buerger's dis-ease
bu-fa-gins
bu-fa-lin
buff-er
buff-y coat
bu-fo-tal-in
bu-fo-ten-i-dine
bu-fot-e-nin
bu-fo-tox-in
Bulau drain-age
bulb-ar
bul-bo-cav-er-no-sus
bul-bo-nu-cle-ar
bul-bo-u-re-thral
bulb-ous
bul-bo-ven-tric-u-lar
bul-bus
bul-bus ar-te-ri-o-sus
bul-bus cor-dis
bu-le-sis
bu-lim-i-a

Bu-li-nus
bul-la
bul-late
Bumke's pu-pil
bun-dle
Bun-ga-rus can-di-dus
Bun-ga-rus fas-ci-a-tus
bun-ion
bun-ion-ec-to-my
Bunnell's test
bu-no-dont
Bunsen burn-er
buph-thal-mos
bur-bot
bur-bot—liv-er oil
Burchard's test
bu-ret
burn
bur-nish-er
burr
bur-row
bur-sa
bur-sec-to-my
bur-si-tis
bur-so-lith
Bury's dis-ease
bush-mas-ter
Busse—Buschke's dis-ease
bu-ta-di-ene
bu-tane
Butcher's saw
bu-tene
bu-ten-yl
Butschli's nu-cle-ar spin-dle
but-ter
but-ter yel-low
but-tock
but-ton-hole
but-tress
bu-tyl

bu-tyr-a-ceous
bu-tyr-ic ac-id
bu-tyr-in
bu-tyr-in-ase
bu-tyr-oid
bux-ine
Buzaglo's stain
bys-si-no-sis
bys-soid

C

ca-ble
ca-ca-o but-ter
cac-es-the-si-a
ca-chex-i-a
cach-in-na-tion
ca-chou
cac-o-de-mo-ni-a
cac-o-dyl-ate
cac-o-geu-si-a
ca-coph-o-ny
ca-cos-mi-a
ca-dav-er
ca-dav-er-ine
ca-dav-er-ous
cad-mi-um
ca-du-ca
ca-du-ce-us
ca-du-cous
cae-cum
cae-ru-lo-plas-min
Cae-sar-i-an sec-tion
ca-fard
caf-fe-ine
caf-fe-in-ism
caf-fe-ol
cai-no-pho-bi-a
caked
Cal-a-bar swel-lings

cal-a-mine
cal-a-mus
ca-la-mus scrip-to-ri-us
cal-ca-ne-o-as-trag-a-lar
cal-ca-ne-o-ca-vus
cal-ca-ne-o-cu-boid
cal-ca-ne-o-dyn-i-a
cal-ca-ne-o-na-vic-u-lar
cal-ca-ne-o-val-gus
cal-ca-ne-us
cal-car
cal-car-e-ous
cal-car-i-u-ri-a
cal-ce-mi-a
cal-ci-co-sis
cal-cif-er-ol
cal-cif-ic
cal-ci-fi-ca-tion
cal-cig-er-ous
cal-ci-grade
cal-cim-e-ter
cal-ci-na-tion
cal-ci-no-sis
cal-ci-pe-ni-a
cal-cis
cal-ci-um
cal-ci-u-ri-a
cal-co-glob-u-lin
cal-co-sphe-rite
cal-cu-lo-gen-e-sis
cal-cu-lo-sis
cal-cu-lus
cal-e-fa-cient
calf
cal-i-bra-tion
ca-li-ec-ta-sis
cal-i-for-ni-um
cal-i-pers
cal-is-then-ics
Call—Ex-ner bod-ies
cal-li-pe-di-a
cal-liph-o-ra

Cal-li-phor-i-dae
cal-lo-ma-ni-a
cal-lo-sal
cal-los-i-tas
cal-los-i-ty
cal-lo-so-mar-gin-al
cal-lo-sum
cal-lus
cal-o-mel
cal-or
cal-o-ra-di-ance
cal-o-res-cence
ca-lor-ic
cal-o-rie
cal-o-rif-ic
ca-lor-i-gen-ic
cal-o-rim-e-ter
cal-o-ri-met-ric
    e-quiv-a-lent
cal-o-rim-e-try
cal-va-ri-a
cal-vi-ti-es
cal-vous
ca-lyx
cam-bi-um
cam-er-a
cam-i-sole
cam-pes-ter-ol
cam-phene
cam-phor
cam-pho-ra-ceous
cam-phor-ate
cam-phor-ic ac-id
cam-phor-ism
cam-phor-o-ma-ni-a
cam-pim-e-ter
camp-to-cor-mi-a
camp-to-dac-ty-ly
Can-a-da bal-sam
can-a-dine
ca-nal
can-a-lic-u-li

can-al-ic-u-lo-plas-ty
can-a-lic-u-lus
ca-na-lis
ca-nal-i-za-tion
can-al-og-ra-phy
can-av-a-nine
can-cel-lous
can-cer
can-cer-o-gen
can-cer-ol-o-gist
can-cer-ol-o-gy
can-cer-o-pho-bi-a
can-croid
can-crum-o-ris
Can-di-da al-bi-cans
can-di-did
can-did-u-lin
can-di-ru
can-dle
ca-nel-la
ca-nine
ca-ni-nus
ca-ni-ti-es
can-ker
can-na-bid-i-ol
can-na-bin
can-nab-in-ol
can-nab-i-non
can-na-bis
can-na-bism
can-na-bol
can-ni-bal-is-tic
can-non-bone
can-nu-la
can-tha-ri-a-sis
can-thar-i-des
can-thar-i-dic ac-id
can-thar-i-din
can-thar-i-dism
can-tha-ris
can-thec-to-my
can-thi-tis

can-thol-y-sis
can-tho-plas-ty
can-thor-rha-phy
can-thot-o-my
can-thus
ca-pac-i-tance
ca-pac-i-tor
ca-pac-i-ty
cap-il-lar-ec-ta-si-a
cap-il-la-rim-e-ter
cap-il-lar-i-ty
cap-il-la-ros-co-py
cap-il-lar-y
cap-il-li-ti-um
cap-il-lo-ve-nous
ca-pil-lus
cap-i-tate
cap-i-ta-tum
cap-i-tel-lum
ca-pit-u-lum
cap-rate
cap-re-o-late
cap-ric ac-id
ca-pro-ic ac-id
cap-ro-ate
cap-ryl-ate
ca-pryl-ic ac-id
cap-sa-i-cin
cap-si-cum
cap-su-la
cap-sule
cap-su-lec-to-my
cap-su-li-tis
cap-su-lor-rha-phy
cap-su-lo-tome
cap-su-lot-o-my
cap-ta-tion
cap-ture
ca-put
car-a-pace
car-a-way
car-ba-mate

car-bam-ic ac-id
car-bam-ide
car-ba-mi-no-he-mo-
glo-bin
car-bar-sone
car-ba-sus
car-ba-zot-ic ac-id
carb-he-mo-glo-bin
car-bi-nol
car-bo-cy-clic
car-bo-hy-drase
car-bo-hy-drate
car-bo-hy-dra-tu-ri-a
car-bo-late
car-bol-ic ac-id
car-bo-li-gase
car-bo-lism
car-bo-lized oil
car-bo-lu-ri-a
car-bol-xy-lene
car-bon
car-bon-ate
car-bon-a-ted
car-bon-ic ac-id
car-bon-ic an-hy-drase
car-bo-ni-um
car-bon-i-za-tion
car-bon-om-e-ter
car-bon-u-ri-a
car-bon-yl
Car-bor-un-dum
Car-bo-wax
Car-box-ide
car-box-y-he-mo-glo-bin
car-box-yl
car-box-yl-ase
car-box-y-meth-yl-cel-
lu-lose
car-box-y-my-o-glo-bin
car-box-y-pep-ti-dase
car-box-y-pol-y-pep-
ti-dase

car-bro-mal
car-bun-cle
car-bun-cu-lo-sis
car-byl-a-mine
car-ci-no-gen
car-ci-no-gen-e-sis
car-ci-no-ge-net-ic
car-ci-noid
car-ci-no-ma
car-ci-nom-a-toid
car-ci-nom-a-to-i-des
al-ve-o-gen-i-ca
mul-ti-cen-tri-ca
car-ci-no-ma-to-sis
car-ci-no-sar-co-ma
car-ci-no-sis
car-da-mom
car-di-a
car-di-ac
car-di-ac in-suf-fi-
cien-cy
car-di-a-co ne-gro
car-di-al-gi-a
car-di-am-e-ter
car-di-a-neu-ri-a
car-di-asth-ma
car-di-ec-ta-sis
car-di-ec-to-my
car-di-o-ac-cel-er-a-tor
car-di-o-ac-tive
car-di-o-an-gi-ol-o-gy
car-di-o—a-or-tic
car-di-o-ar-te-ri-al
car-di-o-cele
car-di-o-cen-te-sis
car-di-o-cir-rho-sis
car-di-oc-la-sis
car-di-o-di-la-tor
car-di-o-di-o-sis
car-di-o-dy-nam-ics
car-di-o-dy-na-mom-et-ry
car-di-o-dyn-i-a

97

car-di-o-e-soph-a-ge-al
car-di-o-gen-e-sis
car-di-o-gen-ic
car-di-o-gram
car-di-o-graph
car-di-o-graph-ic
car-di-og-ra-phy
car-di-o-he-pat-ic
car-di-oid
car-di-o-in-hib-i-to-ry
car-di-o-ki-net-ic
car-di-o-ky-mog-ra-phy
car-di-o-lip-in
car-di-o-lith
car-di-ol-o-gist
car-di-ol-o-gy
car-di-ol-y-sis
car-di-o-ma-la-ci-a
car-di-o-meg-a-ly
car-di-o-mel-a-no-sis
car-di-o-men-su-ra-tor
car-di-o-men-to-pex-y
car-di-om-e-ter
car-di-om-e-try
car-di-o-my-o-pex-y
car-di-o-my-ot-o-my
car-di-o-nec-tor
car-di-o-neph-ric
car-di-o-neu-ral
car-di-o-pal-u-dism
car-di-o-path
car-di-o-pa-thol-o-gy
car-di-op-a-thy
car-di-o-per-i-car-di-o-
    pex-y
car-di-o-per-i-car-di-tis
car-di-o-pho-bi-a
car-di-o-phone
car-di-o-plas-ty
car-di-o-ple-gi-a
car-di-o-pneu-mat-ic
car-di-o-pneu-mo-graph

car-di-op-to-sis
car-di-o-pul-mo-nar-y
car-di-o-punc-ture
car-di-o-py-lor-ic
car-di-o-re-nal
car-di-o-re-spir-a-to-ry
car-di-o-roent-gen-
    o-gram
car-di-o-roent-gen-og-
    ra-phy
car-di-or-rha-phy
car-di-or-rhex-is
car-di-os-chi-sis
car-di-o-scope
car-di-o-spasm
car-di-o-spec-tro-gram
car-di-o-spec-tro-graph
car-di-o-ste-no-sis
car-di-o-ta-chom-e-ter
car-di-o-ther-a-py
car-di-ot-o-my
car-di-o-ton-ic
car-di-o-tox-ic
car-di-o-vas-cu-lar
car-di-o-vec-tog-ra-phy
car-di-tis
car-di-val-vu-li-tis
ca-ri-es
ca-ri-na
car-i-o-gen-ic
Carls-bad salt
car-min-a-tive
car-mine
car-na-u-ba wax
car-ni-fi-ca-tion
car-ni-tine
Carnoy's fix-ing flu-id
car-ob gum
car-o-tene
car-o-te-ne-mi-a
ca-rot-e-noid
car-o-te-no-sis

ca-rot-ic
ca-rot-i-co-cli-noid
ca-rot-i-co-tym-pan-ic
ca-rot-id
car-ot-o-dyn-i-a
car-pal
car-pec-to-my
car-phol-o-gy
car-po-met-a-car-pal
car-po-pe-dal
car-po-pha-lan-ge-al
car-pus
Carrel meth-od
car-ri-er
car-ri-er—free
Carrion's dis-ease
car-ti-lage
car-ti-lag-i-nous
car-ti-la-gin-i-fi-ca-tion
car-un-cle
car-y-o-chrome
car-y-o-clas-tic
Casares Gil's stain
cas-ca bark
cas-car-a
cas-car-a sa-gra-da
    flu-id-ex-tract
case his-to-ry
ca-se-ase
ca-se-ate
ca-se-a-tion
ca-se-in
ca-se-in-o-gen
ca-se-ose
ca-se-ous
case-worm
cas-sa-va
Casselberry's po-si-tion
cas-sette
cas-sia
cas-sic ac-id
cast

Castellani's dis-ease
cast-ing
cas-tor oil
cas-to-re-um
cas-trate
cas-tra-tion
cas-tro-phre-ni-a
cas-u-al-ty
cas-u-is-tics
cat-a-ba-si-al
ca-tab-a-sis
ca-tab-o-lism
ca-tab-o-lite
cat-a-clei-sis
cat-a-clo-nus
cat-a-cous-tics
cat-a-crot-ic
cat-ac-ro-tism
cat-a-di-op-tric
cat-a-lase
cat-a-lep-sy
cat-a-lep-ti-form
ca-tal-y-sis
cat-a-lyst
cat-a-ly-za-tion
cat-a-ly-zer
cat-a-me-ni-a
cat-a-mor-pho-sis
cat-a-pha-si-a
ca-taph-o-ra
cat-a-pho-re-sis
cat-a-pho-ri-a
cat-a-phor-ic
cat-a-phy-lax-is
cat-a-pla-si-a
cat-a-plasm
cat-a-plex-y
cat-a-ract
ca-tarrh
cat-a-stal-sis
cat-a-thy-mi-a
cat-a-to-ni-a

cat-a-ton-ic
cat-a-tro-pi-a
cat-e-chol
cat-e-lec-trot-o-nus
cat-er-pil-lar
cat-gut
ca-thar-sis
ca-thar-tic
ca-thect
ca-thep-sin
cath-e-ret-ic
cath-e-ter
cath-e-ter-ize
ca-thex-is
cath-ode
ca-thod-ic
cat-i-on
cat-i-on-ic
cat-o-dont
ca-top-trics
ca-top-tro-scope
cat's—ear
cat's purr
cau-dal
cau-date
cau-da e-qui-na
cau-da pan-cre-a-tis
cau-dad
cau-da-tum
cau-do-ceph-al-ad
caul
cau-li-flow-er ear
cau-line
cau-lo-ple-gi-a
cau-mes-the-si-a
cau-sal-gi-a
caus-tic
cau-ter-ant
cau-ter-i-za-tion
cau-ter-ize
cau-ter-y
cav-al-ry bone

cav-ern
cav-ern-i-tis
cav-er-no-ma
cav-er-nos-to-my
cav-er-no-sum
cav-ern-ous
Ca-vi-a
cav-i-tas
cav-i-ta-tion
Ca-vi-te fe-ver
cav-i-ty
ca-vo-sur-face
ca-vo-val-gus
ca-vum
ca-vus
ca-vy
Cazenave's dis-ease
ce-bo-ce-phal-ic
ce-bo-ceph-a-lus
ce-bo-ceph-a-ly
ce-cec-to-my
ce-ci-tis
ce-co-cele
ce-co-co-los-to-my
ce-co-il-e-os-to-my
ce-co-pex-y
ce-co-pli-ca-tion
ce-cop-to-sis
ce-cor-rha-phy
ce-co-sig-moid-os-to-my
ce-cos-to-my
ce-cot-o-my
ce-cum
ce-dar oil
ce-li-ac
ce-li-a-del-phus
ce-li-ec-ta-si-a
ce-li-o-col-pot-o-my
ce-li-o-en-ter-ot-o-my
ce-li-o-gas-trot-o-my
ce-li-o-hys-ter-ec-to-my
ce-li-o-hys-ter-ot-o-my

ce-li-o-par-a-cen-te-sis
ce-li-os-co-py
ce-li-ot-o-my
ce-li-tis
cell
cel-la
cell mass
cel-lo-bi-ose
cel-lo-dex-trin
cel-loi-din
cel-lu-lase
cel-lu-li-tis
cel-lu-lo-sa chor-i-oi-de-ae
cel-lu-lose
ce-lo-scope
ce-lo-so-ma
ce-lo-so-mus
Cel-si-us
ce-ment
ce-men-ti-cle
ce-men-ti-fi-ca-tion
ce-men-to-blast
ce-men-to-blas-to-ma
ce-men-to-den-ti-nal
ce-men-to-gen-e-sis
ce-men-to-ma
ce-men-to-per-i-os-ti-tis
ce-men-to-sis
ce-men-tum
ce-nes-the-si-a
ce-nes-thop-a-thy
ce-no-gen-e-sis
cen-sor-ship
cen-tau-ry
cen-ter
cen-ter-ing
cen-te-sis
cen-ti-bar
cen-ti-grade
cen-ti-gram
cen-ti-li-ter

cen-ti-me-ter
cen-ti-nor-mal
cen-ti-pede
cen-ti poise
cen-trad
cen-trage
cen-tra-phose
cen-trax-o-ni-al
cen-tren-ce-phal-ic
cen-trif-u-gal
cen-tri-fuge
cen-tri-ole
cen-trip-e-tal
cen-tro-cyte
cen-tro-des-mose
cen-tro-don-tous
cen-tro-lec-i-thal
cen-tro-mere
cen-tro-phose
cen-tro-some
cen-tro-sphere
cen-trum
Cen-tru-roi-des
ceph-al-ad
ceph-a-lal-gi-a
ceph-a-le-a
ceph-al-gi-a
ceph-al-he-ma-to-ma
ceph-al-hy-dro-cele
ce-phal-ic
ceph-a-lin
ceph-a-li-za-tion
ceph-a-lo-cau-dal
ceph-a-lo-cele
ceph-a-lo-cen-te-sis
ceph-a-lo-chord
ceph-a-lo-di-pro-so-pus
ceph-a-lo-gen-e-sis
ceph-a-lo-graph
ceph-a-log-ra-phy
ceph-a-lo-gy-ric
ceph-a-lo-hem-a-to-cele

ceph-a-lo-he-mom-e-ter
ceph-a-loid
ceph-a-lo-me-ni-a
ceph-a-lo-men-in-gi-tis
ceph-a-lom-e-ter
ceph-a-lom-e-try
ceph-a-lo-ni-a
ceph-a-lo—or-bi-tal
ceph-a-lop-a-thy
ceph-a-lo-pel-vic
ceph-a-lo-pha-ryn-ge-us
ceph-a-lo-ple-gi-a
ceph-a-los-co-py
ceph-a-lo-spo-ri-o-sis
Ceph-a-lo-spo-ri-um
ceph-a-lo-tho-rac-ic
ceph-a-lo-tho-ra-cop-a-gus
ceph-a-lo-tome
ceph-a-lot-o-my
ceph-a-lo-trac-tor
ceph-a-lo-tribe
ceph-a-lo-trip-sy
ceph-a-lo-try-pe-sis
ce-ra
cer-a-sin
ce-rate
cer-a-to-cri-coid
cer-a-to-phar-yn-geus
Cer-a-toph-yl-lus fas-ci-a-tus
ce-ra-tum
cer-ca-ri-a
cer-clage
cer-co-mo-nad
Cer-co-mo-nas In-tes-ti-nal-is
ce-re-a flex-i-bil-i-tas
cer-e-bel-lif-u-gal
cer-e-bel-lip-e-tal
cer-e-bel-li-tis
cer-e-bel-lo-ru-bral

cer-e-bel-lo-ru-bro-
  spi-nal
cer-e-bel-lo-spi-nal
cer-e-bel-lum
cer-e-bral
cer-e-bra-tion
cer-e-bric ac-id
cer-e-brif-u-gal
cer-e-brin
cer-e-brip-e-tal
cer-e-bro-med-ul-lar-y
cer-e-bro-phys-i-ol-o-gy
cer-e-bro-pon-tine
cer-e-bro-scle-ro-sis
cer-e-brose
cer-e-bro-side
cer-e-bro-spi-nal
cer-e-bro-to-ni-a
cer-e-bro-to-nin
cer-e-brum
ce-re-ous
cer-e-sin
ce-ri-um
ce-roid
ce-ro-sis
cer-ti-fi-a-ble
ce-ru-men
ce-ru-mi-no-sis
cer-vi-cec-to-my
cer-vi-ci-tis
cer-vi-co-ax-i-al
cer-vi-co-brach-i-al-gi-a
cer-vi-co-buc-cal
cer-vi-co-buc-co-ax-i-al
cer-vi-co-dyn-i-a
cer-vi-co-fa-cial
cer-vi-co-la-bi-al
cer-vi-co-lin-gual
cer-vi-co-pu-bic
cer-vi-co-rec-tal
cer-vi-co-u-ter-ine
cer-vi-co-vag-i-nal

cer-vi-co-vag-i-ni-tis
cer-vi-co-ves-i-cal
cer-vix
ce-ryl
Ce-sar-e-an sec-tion
ce-si-um
Cestan syn-drome
ces-tode
ces-to-di-a-sis
ces-toid
ce-ta-ce-um
ce-tin
cet-ri-mide
cet-yl-al-co-hol
cet-yl-pyr-i-din-i-um
  chlo-ride
ce-vine
Chaddock's re-flex
Chadwick's sign
chae-to-min
cha-fing
Chagas' dis-ease
Cha-gres fe-ver
chain saw
cha-la-za
cha-la-zi-on
chal-co-sis
chal-i-co-sis
chalk
chalk-stone
chal-one
cha-lyb-e-ate
cham-ber
cham-e-ceph-a-lus
cham-e-ceph-a-ly
cham-e-cra-ni-al
cham-e-pro-sop-ic
Champy's fix-ing flu-id
chan-cre
chan-croid
chan-nel
cha-ot-ic

chapped
char-ac-ter
char-as
char-coal
Charcot's joint
Charcot—Marie—Tooth
  dis-ease
Charcot's syn-drome
charge
char-la-tan
char-la-tan-ism
char-ley horse
char-ta
char-treus-in
char-tu-la
chaul-moo-gra-oil
chaul-moo-grate
chaul-moo-gric ac-id
cheek-bone
chees-y
chei-lal-gi-a
chei-lec-to-my
chei-lec-tro-pi-on
chei-li-tis
chei-log-na-tho-pal-a-tos-
  chi-sis
chei-log-na-tho-pros-o-
  pos-chi-sis
chei-log-na-tho-u-ra-nos-
  chi-sis
chei-lo-plas-ty
chei-los-chi-sis
chei-lo-sis
chei-los-to-mat-o-plas-ty
chei-lot-o-my
chei-ma-pho-bi-a
che-late
che-lat-ing a-gent
che-la-tion
chel-i-do-ni-um
chem-i-cal
chem-i-cal war-fare

chem-i-co-cau-ter-y
chem-i-lu-mi-nes-cence
chem-ist
chem-is-try
chem-o-cep-tor
chem-o-co-ag-u-la-tion
chem-o-pro-phy-lax-is
chem-o-re-flex
che-mo-sis
chem-o-stat
chem-o-sur-ger-y
chem-o-tax-is
chem-o-ther-a-py
che-mo-troph
che-mot-ro-pism
Che-no-po-di-um
che-o-plas-ty
cher-o-pho-bi-a
cher-ry
cher-u-bism
chest
Cheyne—Stokes res-
    pi-ra-tion
chi-as-ma
chick-en-pox
chig-ger
chil-blain
child-bed
child-birth
chill
Chi-lo-mas-tix mes-nil-i
Chi-lop-o-da
chi-me-ra
chin
chi-o-na-blep-si-a
chi-o-no-pho-bi-a
chi-rag-ra
chi-ral-gi-a par-es-
    the-ti-ca
chi-rap-si-a
chi-rar-thri-tis
chi-ris-mus

chi-ro-kin-es-thet-ic
chi-rol-o-gy
chi-ro-meg-a-ly
chi-ro-plas-ty
chi-rop-o-dist
chi-rop-o-dy
chi-ro-pom-pho-lyx
chi-ro-prac-tic
chi-ro-scope
chi-ro-spasm
chi-rur-geon
chi-rur-ger-y
chi-tin
chi-to-bi-ose
chlam-y-do-blas-to-my-
    co-sis
chlam-y-do-spore
Chlam-y-do-zo-a-ce-ae
Chlam-y-do-zo-on
chlo-as-ma
chlor-ac-ne
chlo-ral
chlo-ra-ne-mi-a
chlo-rate
chlo-ra-zol
chlo-ra-zol black E
chlor-dane
Chlor-el-la vul-gar-is
chlo-rel-lin
chlor-eph-i-dro-sis
chlor-hem-a-tin
chlor-hy-dri-a
chlo-ride shift
chlo-ri-du-ri-a
chlo-rin-a-tion
chlo-rine
chlo-rite
chlo-ro-ac-e-to-phe-none
chlo-ro-bu-ta-nol
chlo-ro-cre-sol
chlo-ro-cru-or-in
chlo-ro-form

chlor-o-gua-nide hy-dro-
    chlo-ride
chlo-ro-ma
chlo-ro-naph-tha-lene
chlo-ro-per-cha
chlo-ro-phe-nol
chlo-ro-phen-o-thane
chlo-ro-phy-lase
chlo-ro-phyll
chlo-ro-pic-rin
chlo-ro-plast
chlo-ro-plas-tin
chlo-ro-pro-pane
chlo-ro-pro-pene
chlo-rop-si-a
chlo-ro-pu-rine
chlo-ro-quine
    phos-phate
chlo-ror-a-phin
chlo-ro-sis
chlo-ro-stig-ma
chlo-ro-thy-mol
chlo-ro-tri-an-i-sene
chlo-ro-vi-nyl-di-chlo-ro-
    ar-sine
chlo-ro-xy-le-nol
cho-a-na
choke-damp
choked disk
chokes
chok-ing
chol-a-gogue
chol-a-mine
cho-lane
chol-an-e-re-sis
chol-an-gi-ec-ta-sis
chol-an-gi-o-gas-tros-to-
    my
chol-an-gi-og-ra-phy
chol-an-gi-o-li-tis
cho-lan-gi-o-ma
chol-an-gi-os-to-my

chol-an-gi-ot-o-my
chol-an-gi-tis
cho-lan-ic ac-id
chol-an-o-poi-et-ic
cho-late
chol-e-bil-i-ru-bin
chol-e-cal-cif-er-ol
chol-e-chrom-e-re-sis
chol-e-chro-mo-poi-e-sis
chol-e-chry-o-cy-to-sis
chol-e-cy-a-nin
chol-e-cyst
chol-e-cyst-a-gogue
chol-e-cyst-al-gi-a
chol-e-cyst-ec-ta-si-a
chol-e-cyst-ec-to-my
chol-e-cyst-en-ter-or-
rha-phy
chol-e-cyst-en-ter-os-
to-my
chol-e-cys-ti-tis
chol-e-cys-to-co-los-
to-my
chol-e-cys-to-du-o-de-nal
chol-e-cys-to-du-o-de-
nos-to-my
chol-e-cys-to-gas-tros-to-
my
chol-e-cys-to-gram
chol-e-cys-tog-ra-phy
chol-e-cys-to-il-e-os-
to-my
chol-e-cys-to-jej-u-nos-
to-my
chol-e-cys-to-ki-net-ic
chol-e-cys-to-ki-nin
chol-e-cys-to-li-thi-a-sis
chol-e-cys-to-lith-ot-
o-my
chol-e-cys-to-pex-y
chol-e-cys-tor-rha-phy
chol-e-cys-tos-to-my

chol-e-cys-tot-o-my
cho-le-doch-al
cho-led-o-chec-to-my
cho-led-o-chi-tis
cho-led-o-cho-do-chor-
rha-phy
cho-led-o-cho-du-o-de-
nos-to-my
cho-led-o-cho-en-ter-os-
to-my
cho-led-o-cho-gas-tros-to-
my
cho-led-o-cho-lith-i-a-sis
cho-led-o-cho-li-thot-
o-my
cho-led-o-cho-plas-ty
cho-led-o-chor-rha-phy
cho-led-o-chos-to-my
cho-led-o-chot-o-my
cho-led-o-chus
chol-e-glo-bin
chol-e-he-ma-tin
cho-le-ic ac-id
chol-e-lith
chol-e-li-thi-a-sis
chol-e-li-thot-o-my
chol-e-lith-o-trip-sy
cho-lem-e-sis
cho-le-mi-a
chol-e-poi-e-sis
chol-e-poi-et-ic
chol-e-pra-sin
chol-e-pyr-rhin
chol-er-a
chol-er-e-sis
chol-er-ic
chol-er-i-form
chol-er-i-za-tion
chol-er-oid
chol-er-rha-gi-a
cho-les-cin-ti-gram
chol-es-tane

cho-les-ta-nol
cho-les-te-a-to-ma
cho-les-te-a-to-sis
chol-es-tene
cho-les-te-nol
chol-es-ter-ase
cho-les-ter-i-nu-ri-a
cho-les-ter-ol
cho-les-ter-ol-ase
cho-les-ter-ol-e-mi-a
cho-les-ter-ol-o-poi-e-sis
cho-les-ter-o-sis
cho-les-ter-yl
cho-let-e-lin
chol-e-ver-din
cho-lic ac-id
cho-line
cho-line-a-cet-y-lase
cho-lin-er-gic
cho-lin-es-ter-ase
chol-o-chrome
chol-o-gogue
chol-o-lith
chol-or-rhe-a
cho-lu-ri-a
chon-dral
chon-drec-to-my
chon-dri-fi-ca-tion
chon-dri-gen
chon-drin
chon-dri-o-cont
chon-dri-o-gene
chon-dri-o-kin-e-sis
chon-dri-ome
chon-dri-tis
chon-dro-al-bu-mi-noid
chon-dro-an-gi-o-path-i-a
cal-car-e-a sen punc-
ta-ta
chon-dro-blast
chon-dro-blas-to-ma

103

chon-dro-car-ci-no-ma
  (sal-i-var-y—gland-
  type)
chon-dro-cla-sis
chon-dro-clast
chon-dro-cos-tal
chon-dro-cra-ni-um
chon-dro-cyte
chon-dro-der-ma-ti-tis
  nod-u-lar-is hel-i-cis
chon-dro-dys-tro-phi-a
chon-dro-dys-tro-phy
chon-dro-ec-to-der-mal
chon-dro-ep-i-tro-
  chle-a-ris
chon-dro-fi-bro-ma
chon-dro-fi-bro-sar-
  co-ma
chon-dro-gen-e-sis
chon-drog-e-nous
chon-dro-glos-sus
chon-droid
chon-dro-i-tin
chon-dro-i-tin-sul-fu-ric
  ac-id
chon-dro-ma
chon-dro-ma-la-ci-a
chon-dro-ma-to-sis
chon-dro-mat-ous
chon-dro-mere
chon-dro-mu-coid
chon-dro-myx-o-hem-an-
  gi-o-end-o-the-li-o—
  sar-co-ma
chon-dro-myx-o-ma
chon-dro-myx-o-sar-
  co-ma
chon-dro-os-te-o-dys-
  tro-phy
chon-dro—os-te-o-ma
chon-dro—os-te-o-sar-
  co-ma

chon-drop-a-thy
chon-dro-pha-ryn-ge-us
  mus-cle
chon-dro-plas-ty
chon-dro-po-ro-sis
chon-dro-pro-te-in
chon-dro-sar-co-ma
chon-dro-sin
chon-dro-sis
chon-dro-ster-nal
chon-dro-tome
chon-drot-o-my
chor-da ten-di-nea
chor-da tym-pa-ni
chor-da-mes-o-blast
chor-da-mes-o-derm
Chor-da-ta
chor-date
chord-en-ceph-a-lon
chor-di-tis
chor-do-ma
chor-dot-o-my
cho-re-a
cho-re-i-form
cho-re-o-ath-e-toid
cho-re-o-ath-e-to-sis
cho-ri-o-ad-e-no-ma
cho-ri-o-al-lan-to-ic
cho-ri-o-al-lan-to-is
cho-ri-o-cap-il-la-ris
cho-ri-o-car-ci-no—ma
cho-ri-o-cele
cho-ri-o-ep-i-the-li-o-ma
cho-ri-o-ma
cho-ri-o-men-in-gi-tis
cho-ri-on
cho-ri-on-ep-i-the-li-o-ma
cho-ri-o-ni-tis
cho-ri-o-ret-i-nal
cho-ri-o-ret-i-ni-tis
cho-ri-o-ret-in-op-a-thy
chor-i-sis

cho-ris-to-blas-to-ma
cho-ri-sto-ma
cho-roid
cho-roid, choroi-dal
cho-roid-i-tis
cho-roi-do-cy-cli-tis
cho-roi-do-i-ri-tis
cho-roi-do-ret-i-ni-tis
chre-ma-to-pho-bi-a
Christ-mas dis-ease
chro-maf-fin
chro-maf-fi-no-ma
chro-ma-phil
chro-ma-phobe
chro-ma-si-a
chro-mate
chro-ma-te-lop-si-a
chro-mat-ic
chro-ma-tid
chro-ma-tin
chro-ma-to-der-ma-to-sis
chro-ma-to-dys-o-pi-a
chro-ma-tog-e-nous
chro-mat-o-gram
chro-ma-tog-ra-phy
chro-ma-tol-y-sis
chro-mat-o-mere
chro-ma-tom-e-ter
chro-ma-tom-e-try
chro-ma-top-a-thy
chro-ma-to-phil
chro-ma-to-phore
chro-ma-toph-o-rous
chro-ma-to-plasm
chro-ma-top-si-a
chro-ma-top-tom-e-try
chro-ma-to-sis
chrome yel-low
chrom-hi-dro-sis
chro-mic ac-id
chro-mid-i-um
chro-mi-um

Chro-mo-bac-te-ri-um
chro-mo-blast
chro-mo-blas-to-my-
  co-sis
chro-mo-cen-ter
chro-mo-cys-tos-co-py
chro-mo-cyte
chro-mo-gen
chro-mo-gen-e-sis
chro-mo-mere
chro-mo-ne-ma
chro-mo-par-ic
chro-mo-phane
chro-mo-phobe
chro-mo-pho-bic
chro-mo-phore
chro-mo-phor-ic
chro-mo-phose
chro-mo-plasm
chro-mo-plast
chro-mo-pro-te-in
chro-mop-si-a
chro-mop-tom-e-ter
chro-mos-co-py
chro-mo-some
chro-mo-tro-pic ac-id
chro-nax-ie
chron-ax-im-e-ter
chron-ic
chron-o-graph
chron-om-e-try
chron-o-pho-bi-a
chron-o-scope
chron-o-trop-ic
chrys-a-lis
chrys-a-ro-bin
chry-sene
chrys-o-cy-a-no-sis
chrys-o-der-ma
Chrys-o-my-ia
Chry-sops
chry-so-ther-a-py

Chvostek's sign
chyl-an-gi-o-ma
chyle
chy-le-mi-a
chy-li-dro-sis
chy-lo-cele
chy-lo-der-ma
chy-loid
chy-lo-mi-crons
chy-lor-rhe-a
chy-lo-tho-rax
chy-lu-ri-a
chyme
chy-mo-sin
chy-mo-sin-o-gen
chy-mo-tryp-sin
chy-mo-tryp-sin-o-gen
ci-bis-o-tome
ci-bo-pho-bi-a
cic-a-trix
cic-u-tism
cil-i-a
cil-i-ar-i-scope
cil-i-ar-ot-o-my
cil-i-ar-y
Cil-i-a-ta
cil-i-at-ed
cil-i-o-scle-ral
cil-i-um
cil-lo-sis
Ci-mex he-mip-ter-us
Ci-mex lec-tul-ar-i-us
cin-cho-na
cin-cho-nine
cin-cho-nism
cin-cho-phen
cin-e-flu-o-rog-ra-phy
ci-ne-re-a
cin-e-roent-gen-og-ra-phy
cin-gu-lec-to-my
cin-gu-lo-trac-to-my
cin-gu-lum

cin-na-mon
cir-ci-nate
cir-cle
cir-cuit
cir-cu-lar
cir-cu-la-tion
cir-cu-la-to-ry fail-ure
cir-cu-lus
cir-cum-a-nal
cir-cum-ar-tic-u-lar
cir-cum-ci-sion
cir-cum-cor-ne-al
cir-cum-duc-tion
cir-cum-flex
cir-cum-in-su-lar
cir-cum-len-tal
cir-cum-nu-cle-ar
cir-cum-o-ral
cir-cum-po-lar-i-za-tion
cir-cum-scribed
cir-cum-stan-ti-al-i-ty
cir-cum-val-late
cir-cum-vas-cu-lar
cir-cus move-ment
cir-rho-sis
cir-rus
cir-sec-to-my
cir-soid
cir-som-pha-los
cir-soph-thal-mi-a
cir-sot-o-my
cis-sa
cis-tern
cis-ter-na
cis-ves-ti-tism
cit-ral
cit-rate
cit-ric ac-id
cit-rin
cit-ro-gen-ase
cit-ron
cit-ron-el-la oil

ci-trul-line
Cit-rus
cit-to-sis
Clado's band
Clad-o-spor-i-um wer-neck-i
clair-voy-ance
clamp
clang-as-so-ci-a-tion
clap
clap-ping
cla-rif-i-cant
clar-i-fi-ca-tion
Clarke's col-umn
clas-tic
clau-di-ca-tion
claus-tro-pho-bi-a
claus-trum
cla-va
cla-vate
Clav-i-ceps pur-pur-e-a
clav-i-cle
clav-i-cot-o-my
cla-vic-u-late
cla-vic-u-lec-to-my
cla-vus
claw-foot
claw-hand
clear-ance
cleav-age
cleft
clei-do-cos-tal
clei-do-cra-ni-al
clei-do-hu-mer-al
clei-do-hy-oid
clei-do-ic
clei-do-mas-toid
clei-do—oc-cip-i-tal
clei-do-scap-u-lar
clei-do-ster-nal
clei-dot-o-my
clei-thro-pho-bi-a

cle-oid
cli-mac-ter-ic
cli-mate
cli-ma-tol-o-gy
cli-ma-to-ther-a-py
cli-max
clin-ic
clin-i-cal
cli-ni-cian
clin-i-co-hem-a-to-log-ic
clin-i-co-pa-thol-o-gy
clin-i-co-ra-di-o-log-ic
cli-no-ceph-a-lus
cli-no-ceph-a-ly
cli-no-dac-ty-ly
cli-noid
cli-nom-e-ter
cli-no-scope
clis-e-om-e-ter
clit-i-on
clit-o-ral-gi-a
clit-o-ri-dec-to-my
clit-o-ri-di-tis
clit-o-ri-dot-o-my
clit-o-ris
clit-o-rism
clit-o-ri-tis
cli-vus
clo
clo-a-ca
clone
clon-ic
clon-i-co-ton-ic
clon-ism
clon-o-graph
clo-nor-chi-a-sis
Clo-nor-chis sin-en-sis
clo-nus
Clos-trid-i-um bo-tu-li-num
Clos-trid-i-um nov-yi

Clos-trid-i-um per-frin-gens
Clos-trid-i-um tet-a-ni
Clos-trid-i-um wel-chii
clo-sure
clot re-trac-tion
clot-ting time
club-foot
club-hand
clump-ing
clu-ne-al
Clute's in-ci-sion
clut-ter-ing
cly-sis
co-a-cer-vate
co-ad-ap-ta-tion
co-ag-u-la
co-ag-u-lant
co-ag-u-lase
co-ag-u-late
co-ag-u-la-tion
co-ag-u-lum
co-a-les-cence
coal tar
co-ap-ta-tion
co-arc-ta-tion
co-arc-tot-o-my
co-ar-tic-u-la-tion
coat-ing
Coats's dis-ease
co-bal-a-min
co-balt
Co-bra
co-bra lec-i-thid
co-bra-ly-sin
co-ca
co-caine
co-cain-ism
co-cain-o-ma-ni-a
co-car-box-yl-ase
co-car-cin-o-gen
coc-ci

coc-cid-i-a
coc-cid-i-al
Coc-cid-i-oi-des
coc-cid-i-oi-din
coc-cid-i-o-sis
coc-cid-i-um
coc-co-ba-cil-lus
coc-cog-e-nous
coc-cus
coc-cy-al-gi-a
coc-cy-ceph-a-lus
coc-cy-dyn-i-a
coc-cy-gec-to-my
coc-cy-ge-o-fem-o-ral-is
coc-cyg-e-us
coc-cy-go-dyn-i-a
coc-cyx
coch-i-neal
coch-le-a
coch-le-ar nerve
coch-le-o-ves-tib-u-lar
Coch-li-o-my-ia
co-coa
co-con-scious
coc-to-pre-cip-i-tin
coc-to-sta-bile
co-de-car-box-yl-ase
co-de-hy-drase
co-de-hy-dro-gen-ase
co-de-ine
co-ef-fi-cient
coe-len-ter-on
coe-lom
coe-no-cyte
co-en-zyme
coeur en sab-ot
co-fac-tor
co-fer-ment
cof-fee
cof-fer dam
cof-fin
cog-ni-tion

cog-wheel
co-hab-i-ta-tion
co-her-ence
co-he-sion
coil
coi-no-site
co-i-tion
co-i-to-pho-bi-a
co-i-tus in-ter-rup-tus
co-la nut
co-la-tion
col-a-to-ri-um
col-a-ture
col-chi-cine
col-chi-cum
cold—blood-ed
cold-sore
co-lec-to-my
co-le-o-cys-ti-tis
Co-le-op-ter-a
co-le-op-to-sis
co-le-ot-o-my
co-li-bac-il-le-mi-a
co-li-bac-il-lo-sis
co-li-bac-il-lu-ri-a
co-li-ba-cil-lus
col-ic
co-li-ca
col-i-form
col-i-phage
co-li-tis
co-li-u-ri-a
col-la-cin
col-la-gen
col-la-ge-nase
col-la-gen-o-sis
col-lapse
col-lar-bone
col-lar-ette
col-lat-er-al
col-lec-tor
Colles' frac-ture

col-lic-u-lus
col-li-dine
col-li-ga-tive
col-li-ma-tor
col-lin-e-ar
col-li-qua-tion
col-liq-ua-tive
col-li-sion
col-li-tis
col-lo-di-on
col-lo-di-um
col-loid
col-loid-oph-a-gy
coi-lo-ne-ma
col-lum
col-lu-na-ri-um
col-lu-to-ri-um
col-lyr-i-um
col-ma-scope
col-o-bo-ma
co-lo-ce-cos-to-my
co-lo-co-los-to-my
co-lon
col-o-ny
col-o-ny coun-ter
col-o-proc-tos-to-my
col-op-to-sis
col-or-blind-ness
col-o-rec-tos-to-my
col-or-im-e-ter
col-or-im-e-try
col-or in-dex
co-lor-rha-phy
co-lo-sig-moid-os-to-my
col-los-to-my
col-os-tra-tion
co-los-tror-rhe-a
co-los-trum
co-lot-o-my
col-pal-gi-a
col-pa-tre-si-a
col-pec-ta-si-a

col-pec-to-my
col-pi-tis
col-po-cele
col-po-per-i-ne-o-plas-ty
col-po-per-i-ne-or-rha-
phy
col-po-pex-y
col-po-plas-ty
col-por-rha-phy
col-po-scope
col-pos cop-y
col-pot-o-my
co-lum-bi-um
col-u-mel-la
col-umn
co-lum-na
co-ma
com-a-tose
comb-ing
Comby's sign
com-e-do
com-e-do—car-ci-no-ma
com-e-do-nes
com-men-sal-ism
com-mi-nute
com-mi-nut-ed
com-mis-su-ra
com-mis-sure
com-mis-sur-ot-o-my
com-mit-ment
com-mo-ti-o cer-e-bri
com-mo-ti-o ret-i-nae
com-mu-ni-ca-ble
com-mu-ni-cans
com-par-a-scope
com-pat-i-bil-i-ty
com-pen-sa-tion
com-pen-sa-to-ry pause
com-pe-tence
com-plaint
com-ple-ment
com-ple-men-tal

com-ple-men-ta-ry
com-ple-men-toid
com-ple-men-to-phil
com-plex
com-plex-ion
com-pli-ca-tion
com-po-nent
com-po-si-tion
com-po-si-tus
com-pos men-tis
com-pound
com-press
com-pres-sion
com-pres-sor
com-pul-sion
com-pul-sive per-son-
al-i-ty
co-mus
co-na-tion
con-cave
con-cav-i-ty
con-ceive
con-cen-tra-tion
con-cen-tric
con-cep-tion
con-cep-tus
con-cha
con-chi-tis
con-cho-tome
con-com-i-tant
con-cre-ment
con-cres-cence
con-cre-tio cor-dis
con-cre-tion
con-cus-sion
con-den-sa-tion
con-dens-er
con-di-tion-ing
con-dom
con-duct-i-bil-i-ty
con-duc-tion
con-duc-tor

con-du-pli-ca-to
    cor-po-re
con-dyle
con-dy-lec-to-my
con-dy-loid
con-dy-lo-ma
con-dy-lot-o-my
cone
cone-nose
con-fab-u-la-tion
con-fec-tion
con-fer-tus
con-fine-ment
con-flict
con-flu-ence
con-flu-ens si-nu-um
con-flu-ent
con-fo-cal
con-fron-ta-tion
con-fu-sion
con-ge-la-tion
con-ge-ner
con-gen-i-tal
con-ges-tion
con-gi-us
con-glo-bate
con-glom-er-ate
con-glu-tin
con-glu-ti-na-tion
con-glu-ti-nin
Con-go red
con-gress
co-nid-i-o-phore
co-nid-i-o-spore
co-nid-i-um
co-ni-ine
co-ni-ism
co-ni-o-sis
co-ni-o-spor-i-o-sis
co-ni-um
con-i-za-tion
con-ju-ga-ta ve-ra

con-ju-gate
con-ju-ga-tion
con-junc-ti-va
con-junc-ti-vi-tis
con-junc-tiv-o-ma
con-junc-tiv-o-plas-ty
co-no-my-oi-din
con-san-guin-i-ty
con-scious-ness
con-sen-su-al
con-sent
con-serv-a-tive
con-sist-ence
con-sol-i-dant
con-sol-i-da-tion
con-stant
con-stel-la-tion
con-sti-pa-tion
con-sti-tu-tion
con-stric-tor
con-sul-tant
con-sul-ta-tion
con-sump-tion
con-tact
con-tac-tant
con-ta-gious
con-ta-gious-ness
con-tam-i-na-tion
con-tem-pla-tive
con-tent
con-tig-u-ous
con-ti-nence
con-tin-gen-cy
con-tor-tion
con-tour
con-toured
con-tra—an-gles
con-tra-cep-tion
con-tra-cep-tive
con-trac-tile
con-trac-til-i-ty
con-trac-tion

con-trac-ture
con-tra-fis-su-ra
con-tra-in-di-ca-tion
con-tra-lat-er-al
con-tra-stim-u-lant
con-tre-coup
con-trec-ta-tion
con-trol
con-tuse
con-tu-sion
co-nus
con-va-les-cence
con-vec-tion
con-ver-gence
con-ver-sion
con-ver-tin
con-vex
con-vex-o—con-cave
con-vex-o—con-vex
con-vo-lu-ted
con-vo-lu-tion
con-vul-sant
con-vul-sion
Cooley's a-ne-mi-a
co-or-di-na-tion
coot-ie
co-pe-pod
cop-i-o-pi-a
Cop-lin jar
cop-o-dys-ki-ne-si-a
co-po-lym-er-i-za-tion
cop-per
cop-per-as
cop-per-head
co-pre-cip-i-ta-tion
cop-rem-e-sis
cop-ro-lag-ni-a
cop-ro-la-li-a
cop-ro-lith
cop-roph-a-gy
cop-ro-phe-mi-a
cop-ro-phil-i-a

cop-roph-i-lous
cop-ro-pho-bi-a
cop-ro-phra-si-a
cop-ro-por-phy-rin
cop-ro-por-phy-ri-nu-ri-a
cop-ro-stane
cop-ros-ter-ol
cop-ro-zo-ic
cop-u-la
cop-u-la-tion
cor bi-loc-u-lare
cor bi-ven-tric-u-lar-e
cor pul-mon-al-e
cor-a-cid-i-um
cor-a-co-a-cro-mi-al
cor-a-co-bra-chi-a-lis
cor-a-co-cla-vic-u-lar
cor-a-co-hu-mer-al
cor-a-coid
cor-chor-tox-in
cord
cor-dec-to-my
cor-dial
cor-di-form
cor-di-tis
cor-do-pex-y
cor-dot-o-my
cor-e-cli-sis
cor-ec-ta-sis
cor-ec-tome
cor-ec-to-pi-a
cor-e-di-al-y-sis
cor-e-di-as-ta-sis
co-re-duc-tase
co-rel-y-sis
cor-e-mor-pho-sis
cor-en-cli-sis
cor-e-om-e-ter
cor-e-on-ci-on
cor-e-plas-ty
cor-e-ste-no-ma
cor-e-to-me-di-al-y-sis

Cori cy-cle
co-ri-an-der
co-ri-um
corn
cor-ne-a
Cornell—Coxe Per-form-ance A-bil-i-ty Scale
cor-ne-o-bleph-a-ron
cor-ne-o-scle-ra
cor-ne-ous
cor-ne-um
cor-nic-u-late
cor-nic-u-lum
cor-ni-fi-ca-tion
cor-nu
co-ro-na
cor-o-na-le
co-ro-ne
cor-o-ner
cor-o-net
co-ro-ni-on
co-ro-no-bas-i-lar
co-ro-no-fa-cial
cor-o-noid
cor-o-pa-rel-cy-sis
co-ros-co-py
cor-po-ra
corpse
corps ronds
cor-pu-lent
corpus al-bi-cans
cor-pus cal-lo-sum
cor-pus cav-er-no-sum
cor-pus fi-bro-sum
cor-pus hem-or-rhag-ic-um
cor-pus lu-te-um
cor-pus spon-gi-o-sum
cor-pus stri-a-tum
cor-pus u-ter-i
cor-pus-cle

cor-pus-cu-lum
corpus delecti
cor-rec-tion
cor-rec-tive
cor-re-la-tion
cor-re-spond-ence
Corrigan pulse
cor-ro-sion
cor-ro-sive
cor-ru-ga-tor
cor-set
cor-tex
cor-ti-cate
cor-ti-ces
cor-ti-cif-u-gal
cor-ti-cip-e-tal
cor-ti-coid
cor-ti-co-pon-to-cer-e-bel-lar
cor-ti-co-spi-nal
cor-ti-cos-ter-oid
cor-ti-cos-te-rone
cor-ti-co-stri-ate
cor-ti-co-tro-phin
cor-ti-lac-tin
cor-tin
cor-ti-sone
cor-us-ca-tion
cor-ym-bi-form
Co-ry-ne-bac-te-ri-um
Co-ry-ne-bac-te-ri-um diph-the-ri-ae
co-ry-za
cos-met-ic
cos-mo-tron
cos-tal
cos-tal-gi-a
cos-tal-is
cos-tate
cos-tec-to-my
cos-ti-car-ti-lage
cos-ti-form

cos-tive
cos-to-car-ti-lage
cos-to-cer-vi-cal-is
cos-to-chon-dral
cos-to-cla-vic-u-lar
cos-to-cor-a-coid
cos-to-phren-ic
cos-to-scap-u-lar
cos-to-tome
cos-tot-o-my
cos-to-trans-verse
cos-to-trans-ver-sec-to-my
cos-to-ver-te-bral
cos-to-xiph-oid
cot
co-throm-bo-plas-tin
co-trans-am-i-nase
cot-ton
cot-y-le-don
cot-y-loid
cough
cou-lomb
count-er
coun-ter-ac-tion
coun-ter-ex-ten-sion
coun-ter-ir-ri-tant
coun-ter-o-pen-ing
coun-ter-pres-sure
coun-ter-shock
coun-ter-stain
coun-ter-trac-tion
coun-ter-trans-fer-ence
cou-ple
Courvoisier sign
Couvelaire u-ter-us
co-va-lence
cov-er glass
Cowling's rule
Cowper's glands
cow-per-i-tis
cow-pox

cox-a pla-na
cox-a val-ga
cox-a va-ra
cox-al-gi-a
Cox-i-el-la bur-net-i
cox-i-tis
cox-o-dyn-i-a
Cox-sa-ck-ie vi-rus
co-zy-mase
crab yaws
cracked—pot sound
cra-dle
cramp
cra-ni-ec-to-my
cra-ni-o-cer-vi-cal
cra-ni-oc-la-sis
cra-ni-o-clast
cra-ni-o-clei-do-dys-os-
  to-sis
cra-ni-o-fa-cial
cra-ni-o-fe-nes-tri-a
cra-ni-o-graph
cra-ni-og-ra-phy
cra-ni-ol-o-gy
cra-ni-om-e-ter
cra-ni-o-met-ric point
cra-ni-om-e-try
cra-ni-op-a-gus
cra-ni-op-a-thy
cra-ni-o-pha-ryn-ge-al
cra-ni-o-pha-ryn-gi-o-ma
cra-ni-o-plas-ty
cra-ni-o-rha-chis-chi-sis
cra-ni-o-sa-cral
cra-ni-os-chi-sis
cra-ni-o-spi-nal
cra-ni-o-stat
cra-ni-o-ste-no-sis
cra-ni-os-to-sis
cra-ni-o-syn-os-to-sis
cra-ni-o-ta-bes
cra-ni-o-tome

cra-ni-ot-o-my
cra-ni-o-trac-tor
cra-ni-o-trip-so-tome
cra-ni-o-tym-pan-ic
cra-ni-um
cran-ter
cra-quel-é
cra-ter-i-za-tion
cra-vat
craw—craw
cream
crease
cre-a-tine
cre-a-ti-ne-mi-a
cre-at-i-nine
cre-a-ti-nu-ri-a
cre-a-tor-rhe-a
Credé's meth-od
Credé's treat-ment
creek dots
creep-ing e-rup-tion
cre-mas-ter
cre-ma-tion
cre-ma-to-ry
crem-no-pho-bi-a
cre-na
cre-nat-ed
cre-na-tion
Cren-o-thrix pol-y-spor-a
cre-o-sol
cre-o-sote
crep-i-ta-tion
crep-i-tus
cres-cent
cre-sol
crest
cres-yl blue
cres-yl vi-o-let
cre-ta
cre-ta-ce-ous
cre-tin
cre-tin-ism

crev-ice
crib-bing
crib-rate
crib-ri-form
crib-rose
Cri-ce-tus
crick
cri-co-ar-y-te-noid
cri-coid
cri-coi-dec-to-my
cri-co-pha-ryn-ge-al
cri-co-phar-yn-ge-us
cri-co-thy-roid
cri-cot-o-my
cri-co-tra-che-al
cri-co-tra-che-ot-o-my
crim-i-nol-o-gy
crimp-er
crin-o-gen-ic
cri-nose
crise de de-glob-u-
  li-sa-tion
cri-sis
cris-pa-tion
cris-pa-tu-ra
cris-ta
crit
crit-i-cal
Crooke's change
cross
crossed
cross-ing o-ver
cross match-ing
cross sec-tion
Cro-tal-i-dae
crot-a-line
Crot-a-lus
cro-taph-i-on
crotch
crotch-et
cro-ton oil
cro-ton-al-de-hyde

cro-ton-ism
cro-tox-in
croup
croup-ine
croup ket-tle
Crouzon's dis-ease
crown
crown-work
cru-cial
cru-ci-ate
cru-ci-ble
cru-ci-form
crup-per
cru-re-us
crus
crush
crust
crus-ta
Crus-ta-ce-a
crutch
Crutchfield tongs
cry-al-ge-si-a
cry-an-es-the-si-a
cry-es-the-si-a
cry-mo-dyn-i-a
cry-o-cau-ter-y
cry-o-glob-u-lin
cry-o-glob-u-li-ne-mi-a
cry-om-e-ter
cry-o-scope
cry-o-stat
cry-o-ther-a-py
crypt
cryp-tag-glu-tin-oid
crypt-an-am-ne-si-a
cryp-ti-tis
cryp-to-coc-co-sis
Cryp-to-coc-cus his-tol-y-ti-cus
cryp-tog-a-mous
cryp-to-gen-ic
cryp-to-lith

cryp-to-men-or-rhe-a
cryp-tom-ne-si-a
cryp-toph-thal-mos
crypt-or-chid-ec-to-my
crypt-or-chid-ism
crypt-or-chid-o-pex-y
crypt-or-chism
cryp-to-xan-thin
cryp-to-zo-ite
cryp-toz-y-gous
crys-tal
crys-tal-bu-min
crys-tal-fi-brin
crys-tal-lin
crys-tal-line
crys-tal-li-tis
crys-tal-li-za-tion
crys-tal-log-ra-phy
crys-tal-loid
crys-tal-lo-mag-net-ism
crys-tal-lu-ri-a
crys-tal-vi-o-let
Cten-o-ce-phal-i-des
Cten-op-syl-lus seg-nis
cu-bi-form
cu-bi-tus
cu-boid
cu-boi-de-o-na-vic-u-lar
cu-cum-ber shin
cud-bear
cui-rass
cul—de—sac
cul-do-cen-te-sis
cul-do-scope
cul-dos-cop-y
cul-dot-o-my
Cu-lex
Cu-lic-i-dae
cu-li-cide
cu-lic-i-fuge
Cu-li-ci-nae
Cu-li-coi-des

cul-men
cult
cul-ti-va-tion
cul-ture
cu-mu-la-tive
cu-mu-lus
cu-ne-ate
cu-ne-i-form
cu-ne-o-cu-boid
cu-ne-o-na-vic-u-lar
cu-ne-o-scaph-oid
cu-ne-us
cu-nic-u-lar
cu-nic-u-lus
cun-jah
cun-ni-lin-gus
cun-nus
cu-o-rin
cup
cu-po-la
cupped
cup-ping
cu-pram-mo-ni-a
cu-pric
cu-prous
cu-prum
cu-pu-la
cu-pu-lom-e-try
cu-ra-re
cu-ra-rize
cu-ra-ri-mi-met-ic
cu-ra-ri-za-tion
cu-ra-tive
curd
cure
cu-ret
cu-ret-tage
cu-rie
cu-rine
cu-ri-um
curled
Curling's ul-cer

112

cur-rent
Curschmann's spi-rals
cur-va-ture
curve
Cushing's syn-drome
cush-ion
cusp
cus-pid
cu-ta-ne-o-mu-co-sal
cu-ta-ne-ous
cu-ti-cle
cu-ti-col-or
cu-tic-u-lar
cu-tin
cu-tis
cu-ti-sec-tor
cu-ti-za-tion
cu-vette
cy-an-am-ide
cyan—hematin
cy-an-he-mo-glo-bin
cy-an-hi-dro-sis
cy-an-ic ac-id
cy-a-nide
cy-an-met-he-mo-glo-bin
cy-an-o-co-bal-a-min
cy-an-o-gen
cy-an-o-phil
cy-an-o-phose
cy-a-nop-sin
cy-a-nosed
cy-a-no-sis
cy-a-nu-ric ac-id
cy-as-ma
cy-ber-net-ics
cyc-la-mate so-di-um
cy-cle
cy-clec-to-my
cy-clen-ceph-a-lus
cy-clic
cy-cli-cot-o-my
cy-clo-ceph-a-lus

cy-clo-cho-roid-i-tis
cy-clo-di-al-y-sis
cy-clog-e-ny
cy-clo-hex-ane
cy-clo-hex-a-nol
cy-clo-hex-a-none
cy-cloid
cy-clo-pen-tane
cy-clo-pen-te-no-phen-
  an-threne
cy-clo-phor-ase
cy-clo-pho-ri-a
cy-clo-pi-a
cy-clo-ple-gi-a
cy-clo-pro-pane
Cy-clops
cy-clo-scope
cy-clo-ser-ine
cy-clo-sis
cy-clo-stage
cy-clo-thy-mic per-son-
  al-i-ty
cy-clo-tome
cy-clot-o-my
cy-clo-tron
cy-clo-tro-pi-a
cy-e-si-og-no-sis
cy-e-si-ol-o-gy
cy-e-sis
cyl-in-der
cy-lin-dri-form
cyl-in-droid
cyl-in-dro-ma
cyl-in-dro-sis
cyl-in-dru-ri-a
cyl-lo-so-ma
cym-ba
cym-bi-form
cym-bo-ceph-a-ly
cy-nan-thro-py
cyn-i-a-tri-a
cyn-ic

cyn-o-ceph-a-lous
cyn-o-don-tes
cyn-o-pho-bi-a
cy-o-pho-ri-a
cy-oph-o-rin
cy-ot-ro-phy
cyr-to-ceph-a-lus
cyr-toid
cyr-tom-e-ter
cyr-to-me-to-pus
cyr-to-pis-tho-cra-ni-us
cyr-tu-ran-us
cyst
cyst-ad-e-no-car-ci-no-ma
cyst-ad-e-no-ma
cyst-ad-e-no-sar-co-ma
cys-tal-gi-a
cyst-ec-ta-si-a
cys-tec-to-my
cys-te-ic ac-id
cys-te-ine
cyst-ic
cys-ti-cer-coid
cys-ti-cer-co-sis
cys-ti-cer-cus
cys-ti-form
cys-tine
cys-ti-ne-mi-a
cys-ti-no-sis
cys-ti-nu-ri-a
cys-ti-tis
cys-tit-o-my
cys-to-car-ci-no-ma
cys-to-cele
cys-to-gram
cys-tog-ra-phy
cyst-oid
cys-to-li-thi-a-sis
cys-to-li-thot-o-my
cys-to-ma
cys-tom-e-ter
cys-to-met-ro-gram

cys-to-pex-y
cys-to-pho-tog-ra-phy
cys-to-plas-ty
cys-to-pros-ta-tec-to-my
cys-to-py-e-li-tis
cys-to-py-e-lo-ne-phri-tis
cys-tor-rha-phy
cys-to-sar-co-ma
cys-to-scope
cys-tos-co-py
cys-tos-te-a-to-ma
cys-tos-to-my
cys-to-tome
cys-tot-o-my
cys-to-u-re-thro-gram
cys-to-u-re-throg-ra-phy
cys-to-u-re-thro-scope
cy-tas-ter
cyth-e-mo-ly-sis
cyt-i-dine
cyt-i-dyl-ic ac-id
cyt-i-sine
cy-to-ar-chi-tec-ton-ic
cy-to-ar-chi-tec-ture
cy-to-blast
cy-to-blas-te-ma
cy-to-cen-trum
cy-to-chem-ism
cy-to-chem-is-try
cy-to-chrome
cy-to-cide
cy-toc-la-sis
cy-to-crin-i-a
cy-to-derm
cy-to-di-ag-no-sis
cy-to-gene
cy-to-gen-e-sis
cy-tog-e-ny
cy-to-glob-u-lin
cy-toid
cy-to-ki-ne-sis
cy-tol-er-gy

cy-tol-o-gy
cy-to-ly-sin
cy-tol-y-sis
cy-tom-e-ter
cy-to-mi-cro-some
cy-to-mi-tome
cy-to-mor-pho-sis
cy-ton
cy-to-path-o-gen-ic
cy-to-pa-thol-o-gy
cy-to-pe-ni-a
cy-to-phil
cy-to-phys-i-ol-o-gy
cy-to-plasm
cy-to-plas-tin
cy-to-poi-e-sis
cy-to-prox-i-mal
cy-to-re-tic-u-lum
cy-tos-co-py
cy-to-sid-er-in
cy-to-sine
cy-to-skel-e-ton
cy-to-some
cy-to-spon-gi-um
cy-tost
cy-to-stome
cy-to-tax-is
cy-toth-e-sis
cy-to-tox-in
cy-to-troph-o-blast
cy-tot-ro-pism
cy-tot-rop-ic
cy-to-zo-on
cy-to-zyme
Czerny's su-ture

D

dac-ry-ag-o-ga-tre-si-a
dac-ry-a-gogue

dac-ry-o-ad-e-nal-gi-a
dac-ry-o-ad-e-nec-to-my
dac-ry-o-ad-e-ni-tis
dac-ry-o-blen-nor-rhe-a
dac-ry-o-cys-tec-to-my
dac-ry-o-cys-ti-tis
dac-ry-o-cys-to-blen-
  nor-rhe-a
dac-ry-o-cys-to-cele
dac-ry-o-cys-to-rhi-nos-
  to-my
dac-ry-o-cys-tos-to-my
dac-ry-o-cys-to-tome
dac-ry-o-cys-tot-o-my
dac-ry-o-lin
dac-ry-o-lith
dac-ry-o-li-thi-a-sis
dac-ry-o-ma
dac-ry-on
dac-ry-op-to-sis
dac-ry-or-rhe-a
dac-ry-o-so-le-ni-tis
dac-ry-o-ste-no-sis
dac-ry-o-syr-inx
dac-tyl
dac-tyl-ar
dac-ty-lif-er-ous
dac-tyl-i-on
dac-ty-li-tis
dac-ty-lo-meg-a-ly
dac-ty-lo-sym-phy-sis
dac-ty-lus
dahl-ia pa-per
dahl-ia vi-o-let
dahl-lite
Dakin's so-lu-tion
Dalton's laws
dam
D and C
dan-de-li-on
dan-der
dan-druff

114

D'Antoni stain
Darier's dis-ease
dark—field il-lu-mi-na-tion
dar-tos
Darwin's tu-ber-cle
dat-u-rism
dau-er-schlaf
daught-er
Da-vai-ne-a
Davis graft
day rods
de-ac-ti-va-tion
dead
dead-ly night-shade
dead time
deaf-ened
de-af-fer-en-ta-tion
deaf—mu-tism
deaf-ness
de-al-bate
de-al-co-hol-i-za-tion
de-al-ler-gi-za-tion
de-am-i-dase
de-am-i-di-za-tion
de-am-i-nase
de-am-i-na-tion
death
de-bil-i-tant
de-bil-i-ty
de-bride-ment
de-bris
dec-a-gram
de-cal-ci-fi-ca-tion
dec-a-li-ter
dec-a-me-ter
dec-a-me-tho-ni-um
de-can-cel-la-tion
dec-a-nor-mal
de-cant
de-cap-i-ta-tion
de-cap-i-ta-tor

de-cap-su-la-tion
de-car-bon-ate
de-car-bon-i-za-tion
de-car-box-yl-ase
de-car-box-y-la-tion
de-ca-thec-tion
de-cay
de-cen-tered
de-cer-e-bel-la-tion
de-cer-e-brate
de-cer-e-bra-tion
de-chlo-ri-da-tion
de-chlo-ru-ra-tion
dec-i-bel
de-cid-u-a
de-cid-u-ate
de-cid-u-a-tion
de-cid-u-i-tis
de-cid-u-o-ma
de-cid-u-o-sis
de-cid-u-ous
dec-i-gram
dec-i-li-ter
dec-i-me-ter
dec-i-nor-mal
de-clive
de-coc-tion
de-col-la-tor
de-col-or-ant
de-col-or-ize
de-com-pen-sa-tion
de-com-po-si-tion
de-com-pres-sion
de-con-ges-tive
de-con-tam-i-na-tion
de-cor-ti-ca-tion
de-cu-bi-tal
de-cu-bi-tus
de-cus-sate
de-cus-sa-tion
de-den-ti-tion
de-dif-fer-en-ti-a-tion

deer fly
def-e-ca-tion
de-fect
de-fem-i-na-tion
de-fense mech-a-nism
de-fense re-ac-tion
def-er-ent
def-er-en-tial
def-er-en-ti-tis
de-fer-ves-cence
de-fib-ril-la-tion
de-fib-ril—la-tor
de-fi-bri-na-tion
def-i-ni-tion
def-la-gra-tion
de-flec-tion
def-lo-ra-tion
de-flo-res-cence
de-flu-vi-um un-gui-um
de-form-i-ty
de-fuse
de-gen-er-a-cy
de-gen-er-ate
de-gen-er-a-tion
de-gen-i-tal-i-ty
de-glu-ti-tion
deg-ra-da-tion
de-grease
de-gree
de-gus-ta-tion
de-his-cence
de-hy-drase
de-hy-dra-tion
de-hy-dro-cho-lic ac-id
de-hy-dro-cor-ti-cos-te-rone
de-hy-dro-gen-ase
de-hy-dro-gen-ate
de-hy-dro-i-so-an-dros-ter-one
de-hy-dro-stil-bes-trol
de-i-on-iz-er

Deiter's cells
de-jà vu
de-jec-tion
Dejerine—Sottas dis-ease
Delafield's he-ma-
tox-y-lin
de-lam-i-na-tion
Del-hi boil
de-lim-i-ta-tion
de-lim-it-ed
de-lin-quen-cy
de-lip-i-da-tion
del-i-ques-cence
de-lir-i-um
de-lo-mor-phous
de-louse
Del-phin-i-um
del-ta
del-toid
de-lu-sion
de-mar-ca-tion
de-ment-ed
de-men-ti-a
de-men-ti-a pre-cox
de-meth-yl-a-tion
dem-i-fac-et
dem-i-lune
de-min-er-al-i-za-tion
dem-i-pen-ni-form
Dem-o-dex fol-li-cu-
lor-um
de-mog-ra-phy
de-mon-ol-a-try
de-mon-o-ma-ni-a
de-mon-o-pho-bi-a
de-mor-phin-i-za-tion
de-mul-cent
de-my-e-lin-ate
de-nar-co-tized
de-na-tur-ant
de-na-tured
de-na-tur-i-za-tion

Den-dr-as-pis an-gus-
ti-ceps
den-drite
den-drit-ic
den-dron
den-dro-phag-o-cy-to-
sis
de-ner-va-ted
de-ner-va-tion
den-gue
de-ni-al
den-i-da-tion
de-ni-gra-tion
de-ni-tri-fy
de-ni-tro-gen-a-tion
dens
dens in den-te
den-sit-om-e-ter
den-si-ty
den-so-gram
den-tag-ra
den-tal
den-tal floss
den-tal hy-gien-ist
den-tar-y
den-tate
den-ta-tum
den-te-la-tion
den-tes
den-ti-a-pre cox
den-ti-a-ski-a-scope
den-ti-cle
den-tic-u-late
den-ti-fi-ca-tion
den-ti-form
den-ti-frice
den-tig-er-ous
den-tin
den-tin-i-fi-ca-tion
den-ti-no-blas-to-ma
den-ti-no-ce-men-tal

den-ti-no-gen-e-sis im-
per-fec-ta
den-ti-noid
den-ti-no-ma
den-ti-nos-te-oid
den-tip-a-rous
den-tist
den-tis-try
den-ti-tion
den-to-al-ve-o-lar
den-to-fa-cial
den-tog-ra-phy
den-toid
den-to-le-gal
den-ton-o-my
den-ture
de-nu-cle-a-ted
de-nude
de-o-dor-ant
de-o-ral-i-ty
de-or-sum-duc-tion
de-or-sum-ver-gence
de-os-si-fi-ca-tion
de-ox-y-gen-a-tion
de-per-son-al-i-za-tion
de-pig-men-ta-tion
dep-i-late
dep-i-lous
de-ple-tion
de-po-lar-i-za-tion
de-po-lym-er-ase
de-pol-y-mer-i-za-tion
de-pos-it
de-pot
de-pres-sant
de-pres-sion
de-pres-sor
dep-side
depth
de-pu-li-za-tion
de-range-ment
de-re-al-i-za-tion

de-re-is-tic
der-en-ceph-a-ly
der-i-va-tion
de-riv-a-tive
der-ma
Der-ma-cen-tor
  an-der-soni
Der-ma-cen-tor
  va-ri-a-bil-is
Der-ma-cen-trox-e-nus
der-man-a-plas-ty
der-ma-tal-gi-a
der-ma-ta-neu-ri-a
der-mat-he-mi-a
der-ma-therm
der-mat-ic
der-ma-ti-tis
der-ma-ti-tis ex-fol-i-a-
  tiva ne-on-a-to-rum
der-ma-ti-tis fac-ti-tia
der-ma-ti-tis her-pet-i-
  form-is
der-ma-ti-tis med-i-ca-
  men-to-sa
der-ma-ti-tis seb-or-
  rhe-i-ca
der-ma-ti-tis ven-en-at-a
Der-ma-to-bi-a hom-i-nis
der-ma-to-bi-a-sis
der-ma-to-cel-lu-li-tis
der-ma-to-cyst
der-ma-to-fi-bro-ma
der-ma-to-fi-bro-sar-
  co-ma pro-tu-ber-ans
der-ma-to-glyph-ics
der-ma-to-graph-ism
der-ma-tog-ra-phy
der-ma-tol-o-gist
der-ma-tol-o-gy
der-ma-tol-y-sis
der-ma-tome
der-ma-to-my-ces

der-ma-to-my-cete
der-ma-to-my-co-sis
der-ma-to-my-o-ma
der-ma-to-my-o-si-tis
der-ma-to-neu-ro-sis
der-ma-to-pa-thol-o-gy
der-ma-top-a-thy
der-ma-to-phi-li-a-sis
der-ma-to-phy-te
der-ma-to-phy-to-sis
der-ma-to-plas-ty
der-ma-to-scle-ro-sis
der-ma-to-sis
der-ma-to-some
der-ma-to-stom-a-ti-tis
der-ma-to-ther-a-py
der-ma-to-thla-si-a
der-ma-to-zo-on
der-ma-to-zo-on-o-sis
der-mis
der-mo-blast
der-mo-ep-i-der-mal
der-mo-graph-i-a
der-mog-ra-phy
der-moid
der-moid-ec-to-my
der-mo-la-bi-al
der-mo-phle-bi-tis
der-mos-to-sis
der-mo-syn-o-vi-tis
des-am-i-dase
de-sat-u-ra-tion
des-ce-me-ti-tis
des-ce-met-o-cele
de-scend-ens
de-scen-sus
de-scent
de-sen-si-ti-za-tion
de-sen-si-tize
de-sex-u-al-i-ty
de-sex-u-al-i-za-tion
des-ic-cant

des-ic-ca-tion
des-ic-ca-tor
des-mo-cra-ni-um
des-mo-cyte
des-mo-gly-co-gen
des-moid
des-mo-lase
des-mone
des-mo-pla-si-a
des-mo-some
des-mot-o-my
des-o-mor-phine
de-sorp-tion
11—des-ox-o-cor-ti-sone
des-ox-y-cho-lic ac-id
des-ox-y-cor-ti-cos-
  te-rone
des-ox-y-cor-ti-sone
des-ox-y-e-phed-rine
11—des-ox-y—17—hy-
  drox-y-cor-ti-cos-
  ter-one
des-ox-y-ri-bo-nu-cle-ase
des-ox-y-ri-bo-nu-cle-ic
  ac-id
des-ox-y-ri-bose
de-spe-ci-a-tion
des-qua-ma-tion
de-stru-do
de-tach-ment
de-ter-gent
de-ter-mi-nant
de-ter-mi-na-tion
de-tor-sion
de-tox-i-ca-tion
de-tox-i-fy
de-tox-i-fi-ca-tion
de-tri-tion
de-tri-tus
de-trun-ca-tion
de-tru-sion
de-tru-sor

de-tu-mes-cence
deu-ter-a-no-pi-a
deu-ter-a-tion
deu-ter-i-um
deu-ter-on
deu-ter-o-plasm
deu-ter-o-pro-te-ose
deu-ter-os-to-ma
deu-ter-o-tox-in
deu-to-plas-mol-y-sis
deu-to-sco-lex
de-vel-op-ment
de-vi-a-tion
de-vi-om-e-ter
de-vi-tal-ize
dev-o-lu-tion
dew-claw
dew-lap
dex-ter
dex-trad
dex-tral
dex-tral-i-ty
dex-tra-li-za-tion
dex-tran
dex-trau-ral
dex-trin
dex-tri-nu-ri-a
dex-tro-car-di-a
dex-tro-car-di-o-gram
dex-tro-cer-e-bral
dex-tro-com-pound
dex-troc-u-lar
dex-tro-duc-tion
dex-tro-man-u-al
dex-tro-pe-dal
dex-tro-pho-ri-a
dex-tro-ro-ta-to-ry
dex-trose
dex-tro-sin-is-tral
dex-tro-su-ri-a
dex-tro-tor-sion
dex-tro-ver-sion

dho-bie itch
di-a-be-tes
di-a-be-tes in-sip-id-us
di-a-be-tes mel-li-tus
di-a-bet-ic
di-a-be-to-gen-ic
di-a-be-tog-e-nous
di-a-be-to-pho-bi-a
di-ab-o-lep-sy
di-a-ce-tic ac-id
di-ac-e-tin
di-ac-e-tu-ri-a
di-ac-e-tyl-mor-phine
di-ac-la-sis
di-a-clast
di-a-crit-ic
di-ac-tin-ic
di-ad
di-ad-o-cho-ki-ne-si-a
di-ad-o-ko-ki-ne-sis
di-ag-nos-a-ble
di-ag-no-sis
di-ag-nos-tic
di-ag-nos-ti-cian
di-a-ki-ne-sis
di-al-y-sate
di-al-y-sis
di-al-y-zate
di-a-ly-zer
di-a-mag-net-ic
di-am-e-ter
di-am-i-dine
di-a-mine
di-a-mi-no-pu-rine
di-a-pa-son
di-a-pe-de-sis
di-a-phane
di-aph-a-nom-e-ter
di-aph-a-no-scope
di-aph-e-met-ric
di-aph-o-rase
di-a-pho-re-sis

di-a-pho-ret-ic
di-a-phragm
di-a-phrag-mi-tis
di-aph-y-sec-to-my
di-aph-y-sis
di-a-poph-y-sis
di-ar-rhe-a
di-ar-thric
di-ar-thro-sis
di-ar-tic-u-lar
di-as-chi-sis
di-a-schis-tic
di-as-cop-y
di-a-stal-sis
di-a-stase
di-as-ta-sis
di-a-stat-ic
di-a-ste-ma
di-a-stem-a-to-my-e-li-a
di-a-ster-e-o-i-so-mer
di-as-to-le
di-a-tax-i-a
di-a-ther-mic
di-a-ther-mo-co-ag-u-la-
    tion
di-a-ther-mom-e-ter
di-a-ther-my
di-ath-e-sis
di-a-tom
di-a-to-ma-ceous earth
di-a-tom-ic
di-a-zine
di-az-o
di-az-o-ti-za-tion
di-ba-sic
di-ben-zan-thra-cene
di-car-box-yl-ic ac-id
di-ceph-a-lus
di-ceph-a-ly
di-chlor-a-mine—T
di-chlo-ro-a-ce-tic ac-id

118

di-chlo-ro-di-eth-yl-sul-
    fide
di-chlo-ro—di-flu-o-ro-
    meth-ane
di-chlo-ro-di-phen-yl-tri-
    chlo-ro-eth-ane
di-chot-o-mize
di-chot-o-my
di-chro-ic
di-chro-mate
di-chro-mat-ic
di-chro-ma-tism
di-chro-mic
di-chro-mism
di-chro-mo-phil
Dick test
di-cou-ma-rin
di-crot-ic notch
dic-ty-o-cyte
dic-ty-o-cy-to-ma
di-dac-tic
di-dac-tyl-ism
di-del-phic
Didot's op-er-a-tion
did-y-mi-tis
di-el-drin
di-en-ceph-a-lon
di-en-es-trol
Di-en-ta-moe-ba fra-
    gil-is
di-es-trus
di-et
di-e-tar-y
di-e-tet-ics
di-eth-yl e-ther
di-eth-yl-stil-bes-trol
di-e-ti-tian
di-e-to-ther-a-py
dif-fer-en-tial
dif-fer-en-ti-a-tion
dif-flu-ence

dif-frac-tion
dif-fus-ate
dif-fuse
dif-fus-i-bil-i-ty
dif-fu-si-om-e-ter
dif-fu-sion
di-gas-tric
Di-ge-ne-a
di-gen-e-sis
di-ge-net-ic
Di-gen-et-ic-a
di-gen-ic
di-gest-ant
di-gest-er
di-ges-tion
dig-it
dig-i-ta-lin
dig-i-tal-is
dig-i-tal-i-za-tion
dig-i-ta-tion
dig-i-ti-form
dig-i-tox-in
dig-i-tus
di-glos-si-a
di-glos-sus
di-glu-ta-thi-one
di-gnath-us
di-gox-in
di-hy-brid
di-hy-drate
di-hy-dric
di-hy-dro-cho-les-ter-ol
di-hy-dro-co-de-i-none
di-hy-dro-co-en-zyme
di-hy-dro-er-got-a-mine
di-hy-drol
di-hy-dro-mor-phi-none
    hy-dro-chlo-ride
di-hy-dro-strep-to-my-cin
di-hy-dro-the-e-lin
di-hy-drox-y-a-lu-mi-num
    a-mi-no-ac-e-tate

di-hy-drox-y-phen-yl-al-a-
    nine
di-i-o-do-hy-drox-y-quin
di-i-o-do-hy-drox-y-quin-
    o-line
di-i-o-do-ty-ro-sine
di-i-so-pro-pyl flu-o-ro-
    phos-phate
di-kar-y-on
dil-a-ta-tion
di-la-tion
di-la-tor
dil-u-ent
di-lute
di-lu-tion
di-meg-a-ly
di-men-sion
di-mer-cap-to-pro-pan-ol
dim-er-ous
di-meth-yl-a-mi-no—az-
    o-ben-zene
di-meth-yl-ke-tone
di-me-tri-a
di-mor-phous
dim-ple
dimp-ling
di-neu-tron
di-ni-tro-phe-nol
di-ni-tro-phen-yl-hy-
    dra-zine
di-nu-cle-o-tide
di-oc-tyl so-di-um sul-
    fo-suc-ci-nate
di-o-nism
di-op-sim-e-ter
di-op-ter
di-op-tom-e-ter
di-op-tric
di-op-trics
di-or-tho-sis
di-or-thot-ic
di-ose

119

di-o-tic
di-ox-ane
di-ox-ide
di-pep-ti-dase
di-pep-tide
di-phen-yl-a-mine
di-phen-yl-car-ba-zide
di-pho-ni-a
di-phos-pho-gly-cer-ic ac-id
di-phos-pho-pyr-i-dine nu-cle-o-tide
di-phos-pho-thi-a-mine
diph-the-ri-a
diph-the-ri-tis
diph-the-roid
diph-the-ro-tox-in
diph-thon-gi-a
diph-y-gen-ic
di-phyl-lo-both-ri-a-sis
Di-phyl-lo-both-ri-um la-tum
di-phy-o-dont
dip-la-cu-sis
di-plas-tic
di-ple-gi-a
dip-lo-ba-cil-lus
dip-lo-blas-tic
dip-lo-ceph-a-lus
dip-lo-coc-cin
dip-lo-coc-coid
Dip-lo-coc-cus
dip-lo-e
dip-loid
dip-lo-mate
dip-lo-my-cin
di-plop-i-a-gus
di plo pi a
di-plo-sis
dip-lo-some
di-po-lar
di-pole

di-pole mo-ment
dip-ping
di-pro-so-pus
dip-so-ma-ni-a
dip-so-pho-bi-a
dip-sor-rhex-i-a
Dip-ter-a
dip-ter-ous
di-pus
dip-y-lid-i-a-sis
Di-py-lid-i-um can-i-num
di-rec-tor
Di-ro-fi-la-ri-a
dir-rhi-nus
di-sac-cha-ride
dis-ag-gre-ga-tion
dis-ar-tic-u-la-tion
dis-as-so-ci-a-tion
disc
dis-charge
dis-charg-ing
dis-cis-sion
disc-i-tis
disc-o-gram
dis-cog-ra-phy
dis-coid
dis-col-or-a-tion
dis-com-po-si-tion
dis-crete
dis-crim-i-na-tion
dis-cus
dis-cu-tient
dis-ease
dis-en-gage-ment
dis-e-qui-lib-ri-um
dis-in-fect-ant
dis-in-fec-tion
dis-in-fes-ta-tion
dis-in-hi-bi-tion
dis-in-te-grate
dis-in-te-gra-tion
dis-joint

disk
dis-lo-cate
dis-lo-cat-ed
dis-lo-ca-tion
dis-mem-ber
dis-mu-ta-tion
dis-oc-clude
dis-ord-er
dis-or-gan-i-za-tion
dis-o-ri-en-ta-tion
dis-pa-rate
dis-par-i-ty
dis-pen-sa-ry
dis-pen-sa-to-ry
dis-pense
dis-per-sion
dis-pers-oid
dis-place-ment
dis-po-si-tion
dis-rup-tive
dis-sect
dis-sec-tion
dis-sec-tor
dis-sem-i-na-tion
dis-sim-u-la-tion
dis-so-ci-a-tion
dis-so-ci-a-tive-re-ac-tion
dis-sog-e-ny
dis-so-lu-tion
dis-solve
dis-tad
dis-tal
dis-tal-ly
dis-tance
dis-tem-per
dis-ten-tion
dis-tich-i-a
dis-til-land
dis-til-late
dis-til-la-tion
dis-to-buc-cal

dis-to-buc-co-oc-clu-sal
dis-to-oc-clu-sal
dis-to-clu-sion
dis-to-la-bi-al
dis-to-lin-gual
dis-to-lin-guo-oc-clu-sal
Di-sto-ma-ta
dis-to-mi-a-sis
dis-to-mo-lar
dis-tor-tion
dis-to-ver-sion
dis-tri-bu-tion
dis-tri-chi-a-sis
dis-trix
di-sul-fide
di-thi-o-bi-u-ret
di-thi-zone
dit-o-kous
Dittrich's plugs
di-u-re-ide
di-u-re-sis
di-u-ret-ic
di-ur-nule
di-va-ga-tion
di-va-lent
di-var-i-ca-tion
di-ver-gence
di-ver-tic-u-lar
di-ver-tic-u-lec-to-my
di-ver-tic-u-li-tis
di-ver-tic-u-lo-sis
di-ver-tic-u-lum
vi-nyl e-ther
di-vi-sion
di-vul-sion
di-vul-sor
di-zy-got-ic
diz-zi-ness
doc-tor
Doderlein's ba-cil-lus
Doellinger's ring
dol-sy-nol-ic ac-id

dol-i-cho-ceph-a-lus
dol-i-cho-ceph-a-ly
dol-i-cho-cham-ae-
    cra-ni-al
dol-i-choc-ne-mic
dol-i-cho-fa-cial
dol-i-cho-mor-phic
dol-i-cho-pel-vic
dol-i-chor-rhine
dol-i-cho-u-ran-ic
do-lor
do-lo-rim-e-ter
dol-or-o-gen-ic
dom-in-ance
dom-i-nant
dom-i-na-tor
Donders' rings
do-nee
do-nor
Donovan bod-ies
do-pa
dope
Doppler's ef-fect
dor-mant
dor-sa
dor-sad
dor-sal
dor-sa-lis pe-dis
dor-si-flex-ion
dor-si-ven-tral
dor-so-an-te-ri-or
dor-so-ceph-al-ad
dor-so-lat-er-al
dor-so-lum-bar
dor-so-me-di-an
dor-so-na-sal
dor-so-pos-te-ri-or
dor-so-ra-di-al
dor-so-ul-nar
dor-so-ven-tral
dor-sum
do-sage

dose
do-sim-e-ter
do-sim-e-try
doub-let
douche
Dover's pow-der
drachm
dra-cun-cu-lo-sis
Dra-cun-cu-lus
draft
Dragstedt's op-er-a-tion
drain
drain-age
dram
dram-a-tism
drape
draught
draw
draw—sheet
dread
dream
drench
drep-a-no-cyte
drep-a-no-cy-to-sis
dress-er
dress-ing
drib-ble
drierite
drift
drill
Drinker res-pi-ra-tor
Drinker's meth-od
drip
driv-el-ing
dri-ving
drom-o-ma-ni-a
drom-o-pho-bi-a
drop
drop-let
drop-per
drop-sy

Dro-soph-i-la me-lan-o-
gas-ter
drug
drug-gist
drum
drunk-en-ness
drunk-om-e-ter
Duchenne's pa-ral-y-sis
Ducrey's ba-cil-lus
duct
duct-less
duct-ule
duc-tu-lus
duc-tus ar-te-ri-o-sus
Duhrssen's in-ci-sions
dul-cin
dul-ci-tol
dul-cose
dull-ness
dum-my
Duncan's po-si-tion
Dun-ferm-line scale
du-o-crin-in
du-o-de-nec-to-my
du-o-de-ni-tis
du-o-de-no-chol-e-cys-
tos-to-my
du-o-de-no-cho-led-o-
chot-o-my
du-o-de-no-col-ic
du-o-de-no-cys-tos-to-my
du-o-de-no-en-ter-os-
to-my
du-o-de-no-gram
du-o-de-no-he-pat-ic
du-o-de-no-il-e-os-to-my
du-o-de-no-jej-u-nos-
to-my
du-o-de-no-pan-cre-a-
tec-to-my
du-o-de-no-plas-ty

du-o-de-no-py-lo-rec-
to-my
du-o-de-nor-rha-phy
du-o-de-nos-co-py
du-o-de-nos-to-my
du-o-de-not-o-my
du-o-de-num
du-pli-ca-ture
du-pli-ca-tus cru-ci-a-ta
du-plic-i-tas
du-plic-i-ty
Dupuytren's frac-ture
Dupuytren's con-
trac-ture
du-ra
du-ra ma-ter
du-ra-plas-ty
du-ro-ar-ach-ni-tis
Duval's ba-cil-lus
dwarf
dwarf-ism
dy-ad
dye
dy-nam-ic
dy-na-mo
dy-na-mom-e-ter
dyne
dys-a-cou-si-a
dys-a-cou-sis
dys-ad-ap-ta-tion
dys-an-ti-graph-i-a
dys-a-phi-a
dys-ar-thri-a
dys-ar-thro-sis
dys-au-to-no-mi-a
dys-bar-ism
dys-ba-si-a
dys-bu-li-a
dys-chi-ri-a
dys-chi-zi-a
dys-chon-dro-pla-si-a
dys-chro-ma-top-si-a

dys-chro-mi-a
dys-chro-nous
dys-co-ri-a
dys-cra-si-a
dys-cri-nism
dys-di-ad-o-cho-ki-ne-si-a
dys-em-bry-o-ma
dys-em-bry-o-pla-si-a
dys-e-me-si-a
dys-en-doc-rin-ism
dys-en-ter-y
dys-es-the-si-a
dys-func-tion
dys-gen-ic
dys-ger-mi-no-ma
dys-geu-si-a
dys-glan-du-lar
dys-gnath-ic
dys-gno-si-a
dys-gon-ic
dys-gram-ma-tism
dys-graph-i-a
dys-hi-dro-sis
dys-ker-a-to-sis
dys-ki-ne-si-a
dys-la-li-a
dys-lex-i-a
dys-lo-gi-a
dys-ma-se-si-a
dys-men-or-rhe-a
dys-me-tri-a
dys-mim-i-a
dys-mne-si-a
dys-mor-phic
dys-no-mi-a
dys-o-pi-a
dys-o-rex-i-a
dys-os-mi-a
dys-os-to-sis
dys-par-a-thy-roid-ism
dys-pa-reu-ni-a
dys-pep-si-a

dys-pep-tic
dys-pha-gi-a
dys-pha-si-a
dys-phe-mi-a
dys-pho-ni-a
dys-pho-ri-a
dys-phra-si-a
dys-pla-si-a
dysp-ne-a
dysp-ne-ic
dys-prax-i-a
dys-pro-si-um
dys-ra-phism
dys-rhyth-mi-a
dys-se-ba-ci-a
dys-sper-mi-a
dys-sta-si-a
dys-syn-er-gy
dys-tax-i-a
dys-tec-tic
dys-tha-na-si-a
dys-thy-mi-a
dys-to-ci-a
dys-to-ni-a
dys-ton-ic
dys-top-ic
dys-tro-phy
dys-u-ri-a

E

ear-ache
ear-drum
ear-plug
ear-wax
E-ber-thel-la ty-pho-sa
e-bur
e-bur-na-tion
ec-bol-ic
ec-cen-tric

ec-ceph-a-lo-sis
ec-chon-dro-ma
ec-chon-dro-sis
ec-chon-dro-tome
ec-chy-mo-sis
ec-crine
ec-cy-e-sis
ec-dem-ic
e-chid-nase
e-chid-nin
Ech-id-noph-a-ga
e-chid-no-tox-in
ech-i-na-ce-a
e-chi-no-chrome
e-chi-no-coc-ci-a-sis
e-chi-no-coc-co-sis
E-chi-no-coc-cus gran-u-
    lo-sus
E-chi-no-der-ma-ta
E-chi-no-sto-ma
Ech-is ca-ri-na-tus
ech-o
ech-o-a-cou-si-a
ech-o-graph-i-a
ech-o-la-li-a
ech-op-a-thy
ech-oph-o-ny
ech-o-prax-i-a
ec-la-bi-um
ec-lamp-si-a
ec-lamp-tic
ec-lec-tic
ec-ly-sis
ec-mne-si-a
e-col-o-gy
e-co-ma-ni-a
e-co-site
e-cos-tate
ec-pho-ri-a
é-cra-seur
ec-sta-sy
ec-tad

ec-tal
ec-ta-si-a
ec-thy-ma
ec-to-car-di-a
ec-to-cho-roi-de-a
ec-to-cor-ne-a
ec-to-cra-ni-al
ec-to-derm
ec-to-der-mo-sis e-ro-
    siv-a plu-ri-or-i-fi-
    ci-a-lis
ec-to-en-zyme
ec-tog-e-nous
ec-tog-o-ny
ec-to-men-inx
ec-to-mere
ec-to-mes-o-derm
ec-to-morph
ec-to-pa-gi-a
ec-top-a-gus
ec-to-par-a-site
ec-to-phyte
ec-to-phyt-ic
ec-to-pi-a
ec-to-plasm
ec-to-pot-o-my
ec-to-ret-i-na
ec-to-sarc
ec-to-thrix
Ec-to-tri-choph-y-ton
ec-to-zo-on
ec-tro-dac-tyl-i-a
ec-trog-e-ny
ec-tro-me-li-a
ec-trom-e-lus
ec-tro-pi-on
ec-trop-o-dism
ec-tro-syn-dac-ty-ly
ec-trot-ic
ec-ty-lot-ic
ec-ze-ma
ec-zem-a-tid

ec-zem-a-ti-za-tion
ec-zem-a-toid
ec-zem-a-to-sis
ec-zem-a-tous
Eddowes' dis-ease
e-de-ma
e-dem-a-tous
e-den-tate
e-den-tu-lous
e-de-ol-o-gy
e-des-tin
ed-i-ble
Edinger—Westphal nu-
cle-us
ef-fect
ef-fec-tor
ef-fer-ent
ef-fer-ves-cence
ef-fer-ves-cent
ef-fleu-rage
ef-flo-res-cence
ef-flu-ent
ef-flu-vi-um
ef-fuse
ef-fu-sion
e-ga-grop-i-lus
e-ger-sis
e-ges-ta
egg white
e-glan-du-lar
e-go
e-go-bron-choph-o-ny
e-go-cen-tric
e-go i-de-al
e-go-ma-ni-a
e-goph-o-ny
Ehlers—Danlos
syn-drome
Ehrlich's test
ei-det-ic im-age
ei-do-gen
Einstein

Einthoven's tri-an-gle
Eisenmenger's com-plex
e-jac-u-la-tion
e-jec-ta
e-jec-tion
e-jec-tor
e-lab-o-ra-tion
E-lap-i-dae
e-las-tase
e-las-tic
e-las-ti-ca
e-las-tin
e-las-ti-nase
e-las-tom-e-ter
e-las-tose
e-làs-to-sis se-ni-lis
el-bow
Electra com-plex
e-lec-tric
e-lec-tric-i-ty
e-lec-tri-fy
e-lec-tri-za-tion
e-lec-tro-af-fin-i-ty
e-lec-tro-an-es-the-si-a
e-lec-tro-bi-ol-o-gy
e-lec-tro-bi-os-co-py
e-lec-tro-cap-il-lar-i-ty
e-lec-tro-car-di-o-gram
e-lec-tro-car-di-o-graph
e-lec-tro-car-di-og-ra-phy
e-lec-tro-car-di-o-pho-
nog-ra-phy
e-lec-tro-ca-tal-y-sis
e-lec-tro-cau-ter-y
e-lec-tro-chem-is-try
e-lec-tro-chro-ma-tog-ra-
phy
e-lec-tro-co-ag-u-la-tion
e-lec-tro-con-duc-tiv-i-ty
e-lec-tro-con-trac-til-i-ty
e-lec-tro-cor-ti-cog-ra-
phy

e-lec-tro-cu-tion
e-lec-trode
e-lec-tro-dent
e-lec-tro-der-ma-tome
e-lec-tro-des-ic-ca-tion
e-lec-tro-di-al-y-sis
e-lec-tro-di-aph-any
e-lec-tro-dy-nam-ics
e-lec-tro-dy-na-mom-
e-ter
e-lec-tro-en-ceph-a-lo-
gram
e-lec-tro-en-ceph-a-lo-
graph
e-lec-tro-en-ceph-a-log-
ra-phy
e-lec-tro-form
e-lec-tro-gen-e-sis
e-lec-tro-he-mo-sta-sis
e-lec-tro-ki-net-ics
e-lec-tro-ky-mo-graph
e-lec-tro-li-thot-ri-ty
e-lec-trol-o-gy
e-lec-trol-y-sis
e-lec-tro-lyte
e-lec-tro-lyt-ic
e-lec-tro-ly-zer
e-lec-tro-mag-net
e-lec-tro-mag-net-ics
e-lec-tro-mas-sage
e-lec-trom-e-ter
e-lec-tro-mo-tive
e-lec-tro-my-o-gram
e-lec-tro-my-og-ra-phy
e-lec-tron
e-lec-tro-nar-co-sis
e-lec-tro-neg-a-tive
e-lec-tro-neg-a-tiv-i-ty
e-lec-tron lens
e-lec-tron op-tics
e-lec-tron volt
e-lec-tro-os-mo-sis

124

e-lec-tro-pa-thol-o-gy
e-lec-tro-pho-bi-a
e-lec-tro-pho-re-sis
e-lec-tro-phys-i-ol-o-gy
e-lec-tro-pos-i-tive
e-lec-tro-py-rex-i-a
e-lec-tro-re-sec-tion
e-lec-tro-ret-i-no-gram
e-lec-tro-scis-sion
e-lec-tro-scope
e-lec-tro-sec-tion
e-lec-tro-shock
e-lec-tro-sol
e-lec-tro-some
e-lec-tro-stat-ics
e-lec-tro-steth-o-phone
e-lec-tro-stric-tion
e-lec-tro-sur-ger-y
e-lec-tro-syn-the-sis
e-lec-tro-tax-is
e-lec-tro-thal-a-mo-gram
e-lec-tro-tha-na-si-a
e-lec-tro-ther-a-peu-tics
e-lec-tro-ther-a-py
e-lec-tro-ther-mal
e-lec-tro-tome
e-lec-tro-ton-ic ef-fect
e-lec-tro-va-lence
e-le-i-din
el-e-ment
el-e-o-ma
el-e-om-e-ter
el-e-phan-ti-a-sis
el-e-va-tor
Elford mem-brane
e-lim-i-nant
e-lim-i-na-tion
e-lin-gua-tion
e-lix-ir
el-lip-sin
el-lip-soid
el-lip-to-cyte

el-lip-to-cy-to-sis
e-lon-ga-tion
el-u-ant
el-u-ate
e-lu-tion
e-lu-tri-a-tion
Ely's ta-ble
e-ma-ci-a-tion
e-mac-u-la-tion
em-a-na-tion
e-man-ci-pa-tion
e-mas-cu-la-tion
Em-ba-do-mo-nas in-tes-
ti-nal-is
em-balm-ing
em-bed
em-bo-lec-to-my
em-bo-le-mi-a
em-bol-ic
em-bo-lism
em-bo-lo-phra-si-a
em-bo-lus
em-bo-ly
em-bra-sure
em-bro-ca-tion
em-bry-ec-to-my
em-bry-o
em-bry-o-blast
em-bry-o-car-di-a
em-bry-oc-to-ny
em-bry-o-gen-ic
em-bry-oid
em-bry-ol-o-gist
em-bry-ol-o-gy
em-bry-o-ma
em-bry-o-mor-phous
em-bry-o-ni-za-tion
em-bry-o-noid
em-bry-o-tome
em-bry-ot-o-my
em-bry-ul-ci-a
em-bry-ul-cus

e-mer-gen-cy
em-e-sis
e-met-a-tro-phi-a
e-met-ic
em-e-tine
em-e-to-mor-phine
em-e-to-pho-bi-a
e-mic-tion
em-i-gra-tion
em-i-nence
em-i-nen-ti-a
em-is-sar-y
e-mis-sion
em-men-i-a
em-men-i-op-a-thy
em-me-tro-pi-a
e-mol-li-ent
e-mo-tion
em-pa-thy
em-phly-sis
em-phrac-tic
em-phrax-is
em-phy-se-ma
em-pir-ic
em-pir-i-cism
em-pros-thot-o-nos
em-py-e-ma
em-py-e-sis
e-mul-si-fi-er
e-mul-si-fy
e-mul-sion
e-mul-soid
en-am-el
en-am-el-o-ma
en-an-the-ma
en-an-ti-o-morph
en-ar-thro-sis
en-can-this
en-cap-su-la-tion
en-cap-suled
en-ceph-a-lal-gi-a
en-ceph-a-lat-ro-phy

en-ceph-a-li-tis
en-ceph-a-lo-cele
en-ceph-a-lo-dys-pla-si-a
en-ceph-a-lo-gram
en-ceph-a-log-ra-phy
en-ceph-a-loid
en-ceph-a-lol-o-gy
en-ceph-a-lo-ma
en-ceph-a-lo-ma-la-ci-a
en-ceph-a-lo-men-in-gi-tis
en-ceph-a-lo-me-nin-go-cele
en-ceph-a-lo-mere
en-ceph-a-lom-e-ter
en-ceph-a-lo-my-e-li-tis
en-ceph-a-lo-my-e-lop-a-thy
en-ceph-a-lo-my-el-o-sis
en-ceph-a-lo-my-o-car-di-tis
en-ceph-a-lon
en-ceph-a-lop-a-thy
en-ceph-a-lo-punc-ture
en-ceph-a-lo-py-o-sis
en-ceph-a-lor-rha-gi-a
en-ceph-a-los-cop-y
en-ceph-a-lo-sis
en-ceph-a-lo-spi-nal
en-ceph-a-lo-tome
en-ceph-a-lot-o-my
en-chon-dral
en-chon-dro-ma
en-chon-dro-ma-to-sis
en-chon-dro-sar-co-ma
en-chon-dro-sis
en-clit-ic
en-co-pre-sis
en-cyst-ed
en-cyst-ment
en-da-del-phus
En-da-moe-ba co-li

En-da-moe-ba gin-gi-val-is
En-da-moe-ba his-tol-y-ti-ca
en-dan-gi-i-tis
en-da-or-ti-tis
en-dar-ter-ec-to-my
en-dar-te-ri-al
en-dar-te-ri-tis
end-au-ral
end-brain
end—bulb
en-dem-ic
end-er-gon-ic
en-der-mic
en-der-mo-sis
en-do-ab-dom-i-nal
en-do-an-gi-i-tis
en-do-a-or-ti-tis
en-do-ar-te-ri-tis
en-do-bi-ot-ic
en-do-bron-chi-al
en-do-car-di-al
en-do-car-di-tis
en-do-car-di-um
en-do-carp
en-do-cer-vi-cal
en-do-cer-vi-ci-tis
en-do-cer-vix
en-do-chon-dral
en-do-cra-ni-al
en-do-cra-ni-um
en-do-crine
en-do-cri-nol-o-gy
en-do-cri-nop-a-thy
en-do-crin-o-ther-a-py
en-do-cyst
en-do-derm
en-do-der-mo-phy-to-sis
en-do-don-tics
en-do-don-tist
en-do-en-zyme

en-dog-e-nous
en-dog-e-ny
en-do-go-ni-um
en-do-la-ryn-ge-al
En-do-li-max na-na
en-do-lymph
en-do-lymph-at-ic
en-do-men-inx
en-do-mes-o-derm
en-do-me-tri-o-ma
en-do-me-tri-o-sis
en-do-me-tri-tis
en-do-me-tri-um
en-do-mi-to-sis
en-do-morph
en-do-my-o-car-di-tis
en-do-na-sal
en-do-neu-ral
en-do-nu-cle-o-lus
en-do-par-a-site
en-do-per-i-car-di-tis
en-do-per-i-my-o-car-di-tis
en-do-phle-bi-tis
en-doph-thal-mi-tis
en-do-plasm
end or-gan
en-do-scope
en-do-skel-e-ton
en-dos-mo-sis
en-do-sperm
en-do-spore
en-dos-te-o-ma
en-dos-te-um
en-dos-ti-tis
en-dos-to-sis
en-do-the-li-o-an-gi-i-tis
en-do-the-li-o-ma
en-do-the-li-um
en-do-ther-mic
en-do-thrix

en-do-tox-in
end—plate
end prod-uct
en-e-ma
en-er-get-ics
en-er-gom-e-ter
en-er-gy
en-er-va-tion
en-gage-ment
en-gorge-ment
en grappes
en-large-ment
e-nol
e-no-lase
en-oph-thal-mos
en-o-si-ma-ni-a
en-os-to-sis
en-si-form
en-ta-cous-tic
En-ta-moe-ba
en-tel-e-chy
en-ter-ec-to-my
en-ter-e-pip-lo-cele
en-ter-ic
en-ter-i-tis
en-ter-o-a-nas-to-mo-sis
En-ter-o-bac-te-ri-a-ce-ae
en-ter-o-bi-a-sis
En-ter-o-bi-us ver-mic-u-
    lar-is
en-ter-o-cele
en-ter-o-cen-te-sis
en-ter-oc-ly-sis
en-ter-o-coc-cus
en-ter-o-coele
en-ter-o-co-lec-to-my
en-ter-o-co-li-tis
en-ter-o-co-los-to-my
en-ter-o-crin-in
en-ter-o-cyst
en-ter-o-cys-to-cele
en-ter-o-cys-to-plas-ty

en-ter-o-en-ter-ic
en-ter-o-en-ter-os-to-my
en-ter-o-gas-tri-tis
en-ter-o-gas-tro-cele
en-ter-o-gas-trone
en-ter-og-e-nous
en-ter-o-ki-nase
en-ter-ol-y-sis
En-ter-o-mo-nas
    hom-i-nis
en-ter-o-my-co-sis
en-ter-on
en-ter-op-a-thy
en-ter-o-pex-y
en-ter-o-plas-ty
en-ter-o-ple-gi-a
en-ter-op-to-sis
en-ter-or-rha-phy
en-ter-o-scope
en-ter-o-sep-sis
en-ter-o-spasm
en-ter-o-sta-sis
en-ter-o-ste-no-sis
en-ter-os-to-my
en-ter-o-tome
en-ter-ot-o-my
en-ter-o-tox-e-mi-a
en-ter-o-tox-in
en-the-o-ma-ni-a
en-the-sis
en-thet-ic
en-ti-ris
en-to-blast
en-to-derm
en-to-mere
en-to-mi-on
en-to-mol-o-gist
en-to-mol-o-gy
en-to-mo-pho-bi-a
ent-oph-thal-mi-a
ent-op-tic
ent-op-tos-co-py

ent-os-to-sis
en-to-zo-al
en-train-ment
en-tro-pi-on
en-tro-py
en-ty-py
e-nu-cle-ate
en-u-re-sis
en-vi-ron-ment
en-zo-ot-ic
en-zyme
en-zy-mol-o-gy
en-zy-mol-y-sis
e-o-sin
e-o-sin-o-pe-ni-a
e-o-sin-o-phil
e-o-sin-o-phil-i-a
e-o-sin-o-phil-ic
e-pac-tal
ep-ax-i-al
ep-en-dy-ma
ep-en-dy-mi-tis
ep-en-dy-mo-blas-to-ma
ep-en-dy-mo-cyte
ep-en-dy-mo-ma
e-phed-rine
e-phem-er-al
eph-i-dro-sis
ep-i-a-gnath-us
ep-i-can-thus
ep-i-car-di-a
ep-i-car-di-um
ep-i-carp
ep-i-cho-ri-on
ep-i-con-dy-lar
ep-i-con-dy-le
ep-i-con-dy-li-tis
ep-i-cra-ni-um
ep-i-cra-ni-us
ep-i-cri-sis
ep-i-crit-ic
ep-i-cys-ti-tis

ep-i-dem-ic
ep-i-de-mi-ol-o-gist
ep-i-de-mi-ol-o-gy
ep-i-der-ma-to-plas-ty
ep-i-der-mi-dal-i-za-tion
ep-i-der-mis
ep-i-der-mi-tis
ep-i-der-mi-za-tion
ep-i-der-moid
ep-i-der-mol-y-sis
ep-i-der-mol-y-sis bul-lo-sa
ep-i-der-mo-my-co-sis
ep-i-der-moph-y-tid
Ep-i-der-moph-y-ton
ep-i-der-mo-phy-to-sis
ep-i-did-y-mis
ep-i-did-y-mi-tis
ep-i-did-y-mo—or-chi-tis
ep-i-did-y-mo-vas-os-to-my
ep-i-du-ral
ep-i-fas-ci-al
ep-i-gas-tric
ep-i-gas-tri-um
ep-i-gas-tri-us
ep-i-gen-e-sis
ep-i-glot-ti-dec-to-my
ep-i-glot-tis
ep-i-glot-ti-tis
ep-i-gua-nine
ep-i-hy-oid
ep-i-la-mel-lar
ep-i-la-tion
ep-i-lem-ma
ep-i-lep-sy
ep-i-lep-to-gen-ic
ep-i-lep-toid
ep-i-mere
ep-i-my-o-car-di-um
Ep-i-mys rat-tus

ep-i-neph-rine
ep-i-ne-phri-tis
ep-i-neu-ral
ep-i-neu-ri-um
ep-i-ot-ic
ep-i-phar-ynx
ep-i-phe-nom-e-non
e-piph-o-ra
ep-i-phys-i-o-de-sis
ep-i-phys-i-ol-is-the-sis
e-piph-y-sis
e-piph-y-si-tis
ep-i-phyte
ep-i-pleu-ral
e-pip-lo-cele
ep-i-plo-ec-to-my
e-pip-lo-en-ter-o-cele
e-pip-lo-ic
e-pip-lom-phal-o-cele
e-pip-lo-on
e-pip-lo-pex-y
ep-i-plor-rha-phy
ep-i-scle-ra
ep-i-scle-ral
ep-i-scle-ri-tis
e-pi-si-ot-o-my
ep-i-sode
ep-i-spa-di-as
ep-i-spas-tic
ep-i-spi-nal
ep-i-sta-sis
ep-i-stax-is
ep-i-ten-din-e-um
ep-i-thal-a-mus
ep-i-the-li-a
ep-i-the-li-o-cho-ri-al
ep-i-the-li-oid
ep-i-the-li-o-ma
ep-i-the-li-tis
ep-i-the-li-um
ep-i-the-li-za-tion
ep-i-ton-ic

ep-i-to-nos
ep-i-troch-le-ar
ep-i-troch-le-ar-is
ep-i-tu-ber-cu-lo-sis
ep-i-tym-pa-num
ep-i-zo-ic
ep-i-zo-i-cide
ep-i-zo-on
ep-i-zo-ot-ic
ep-o-nym
ep-o-oph-o-ron
Ep-som salt
ep-u-lis
ep-u-lo-fi-bro-ma
e-qua-tion
e-qua-tor
Eq-ui-dae
e-qui-li-bra-tion
e-qui-lib-ri-um
e-qui-mo-lec-u-lar
eq-uine
eq-ui-no-ca-vus
eq-ui-no-va-rus
e-qui-nus
e-quiv-a-lent
Erb's pal-sy
Erben's phe-nom-e-non
er-bi-um
e-rec-tile
e-rec-tion
e-rec-tor
er-e-mo-pho-bi-a
e-rep-sin
er-e-this-tic
erg
er-ga-si-a
er-gas-the-ni-a
er-go-cal-cif-er-ol
er-go-cor-nine
er-go-cris-tine
er-go-cryp-tine

er-go-graph
er-gom-e-ter
er-go-no-vine
er-go-phore group
er-go-sine
er-gos-ter-ol
er-got
er-got-a-mine
er-got-ism
er-got-ized
er-i-gens
Erienmeyer flask
e-rog-e-nous
eros
e-rose
e-ro-si-o in-ter-dig-i-ta-lis blas-to-my-ce-ti-ca
e-ro-sion
e-rot-ic
e-rot-i-ca
er-o-tism
er-o-to-gen-ic
er-o-to-ma-ni-a
er-o-to-pho-bi-a
e-ruc-ta-tion
e-ru-ga-to-ry
e-rup-tion
e-rup-tive
er-y-sip-e-las
er-y-sip-e-loid
Er-y-si-pel-o-thrix
e-rys-i-phake
er-y-the-ma
er-y-the-ma bul-lo-sum
er-y-the-ma mul-ti-forme
er-y-the-ma no-dos-um
er-y-the-ma per-nio
er-y-the-ma per-stans
er-y-the-ma scar-la-ti-ni-forme
er-y-the-ma so-lare
er-y-the-ma-toid

er-y-thras-ma
e-ryth-re-de-ma pol-y-neu-rop-a-thy
er-y-thre-mi-a
e-ryth-ro-blast
e-ryth-ro-blas-to-ma
e-ryth-ro-blas-to-pe-ni-a
e-ryth-ro-blas-to-sis foe-tal-is
e-ryth-ro-chlo-ro-pi-a
e-ryth-ro-conte
e-ryth-ro-cru-or-in
e-ryth-ro-cy-a-no-sis
e-ryth-ro-cyte
e-ryth-ro-cy-the-mi-a
e-ryth-ro-cy-to-ly-sin
e-ryth-ro-cy-tol-y-sis
e-ryth-ro-cy-tom-e-ter
e-ryth-ro-cy-to—op-so-nin
e-ryth-ro-cy-to-poi-e-sis
e-ryth-ro-cy-to-sis
e-ryth-ro-de-gen-er-a-tive
e-ryth-ro-der-ma
e-ryth-ro-gen-e-sis
er-y-throid
e-ryth-ro-leu-ko-blas-to-sis
e-ryth-ro-leu-ko-sis
er-y-throl-y-sin
er-y-throl-y-sis
e-ryth-ro-my-cin
er-y-thron
e-ryth-ro-ne-o-cy-to-sis
er-y-thro-pe-ni-a
e-ryth-ro-pha-go-cy-to-sis
e-ryth-ro-phil
e-ryth-ro-pla-si-a of Quey-rat
e-ryth-ro-poi-e-sis

er-y-thro-psi-a
er-y-throp-sin
e-ryth-ro-sar-co-ma
e-ryth-ro-sine
e-ryth-ro-sin B
e-ryth-ro-sis
Esbach's meth-od
es-cape
es-char
es-cha-rot-ic
Esch-er-ich-i-a co-li
es-cu-lin
es-cutch-eon
Esmarch band-age
e-soph-a-gec-ta-si-a
e-soph-a-gec-to-my
e-soph-a-gi-tis
e-soph-a-go-du-o-de-nos-to-my
e-soph-a-go-en-ter-os-to-my
e-soph-a-go-gas-trec-to-my
e-soph-a-go-gas-tro-scope
e-soph-a-go-gas-tros-co-py
e-soph-a-go-gas-tros-to-my
e-soph-a-go-je-ju-nos-to-my
e-soph-a-go-scope
e-soph-a-go-spasm
e-soph-a-go-ste-no-sis
e-soph-a-gos-to-my
e-soph-a-got-o-my
e-soph-a-gus
e-soph-o-gram
es-o-pho-ri-a
es-o-tro-pi-a
es-sence
es-sential
Esser in-lay graft

129

es-ter
es-ter-ase
es-ter-i-fi-ca-tion
es-the-si-a
es-the-si-om-e-ter
es-the-si-o-phys-i-ol-o-
   gy
es-thet-ic
es-ti-val
es-ti-va-tion
es-tra-di-ol
es-trane
es-tri-ol
es-tro-gen
es-trone
es-trum
es-trus
es-tu-a-ri-um
eth-ane
eth-a-nol
e-ther
e-ther-ide
e-ther-i-fi-ca-tion
e-ther-i-za-tion
eth-ics
e-thi-o-nine
e-this-ter-one
eth-mo-fron-tal
eth-moid
eth-moid-ec-to-my
eth-moid-i-tis
eth-moid-ot-o-my
eth-mo-lac-ri-mal
eth-mo-max-il-lar-y
eth-mo-na-sal
eth-mo-tur-bi-nal
eth-nic
eth-nog-ra-phy
eth-nol-o-gy
eth-yl
eth-yl ac-e-tate
eth-yl al-co-hol

eth-yl-ate
eth-yl-a-tion
eth-yl cel-lu-lose
eth-yl chlo-ride
eth-yl-ene
eth-yl-ene-di-a-mine
eth-yl-ene ox-ide
eth-y-nyl es-tra-di-ol
e-ti-ol-o-gy
e-ti-o-path-o-gen-e-sis
Eu-bac-te-ri-a-les
eu-ca-lyp-tol
eu-ca-lyp-tus
eu-cat-ro-pine hy-dro-
   chlo-ride
eu-chlor-hy-dri-a
eu-chol-i-a
eu-chro-ma-tin
eu-chro-ma-top-si-a
eu-di-om-e-ter
eu-es-the-si-a
eu-gen-ics
eu-ge-nol
eu-glob-u-lin
eu-gon-ic
eu-ker-a-tin
eu-mor-phic
Eu-my-ce-tes
eu-nuch
eu-nuch-ism
eu-nuch-oid
eu-pa-ral
eu-pho-ni-a
Eu-phor-bi-a-ce-ae
eu-phor-bi-um
eu-pho-ri-a
eu-ploid
eu-prax-i-a
eu-ro-pis-o-ceph-a-lus
eu-ro-pi-um
eu-ro-pro-ceph-a-lus
eu-ry-ce-phal-ic

eu-ryc-ne-mic
eu-ry-on
eu-ry-ther-mal
eu-sta-chi-an
eu-sys-to-le
eu-tec-tic
eu-tha-na-si-a
eu-then-ics
Eu-the-ri-a
eu-thy-roid-ism
eu-to-ci-a
Eu-tri-at-o-ma
e-vac-u-ant
e-vac-u-a-tion
e-vag-i-na-tion
ev-a-nes-cent
Evans blue
e-ven-tra-tion
e-ver-sion
ev-i-dence
ev-i-ra-tion
e-vis-cer-a-tion
e-vis-cer-o-neu-rot-o-my
ev-o-ca-tion
ev-o-ca-tor
ev-o-lu-tion
e-vul-sion
Ewald tube
Ewing's sar-co-ma
ex-ac-er-ba-tion
ex-al-ta-tion
ex-am-i-na-tion
ex-an-the-ma
ex-an-them-at-ous
ex-ca-va-tion
ex-ca-va-tor
ex-ce-men-to-sis
ex-cip-i-ent
ex-ci-sion
ex-cit-a-bil-i-ty
ex-ci-tant
ex-ci-ta-tion

ex-clu-sion
ex-co-ri-a-tion
ex-cre-ment
ex-cres-cence
ex-cre-ta
ex-cre-tin
ex-cre-tion
ex-cur-sion
ex-cur-va-ture
ex-cy-clo-pho-ri-a
ex-cy-clo-tro-pi-a
ex-cys-ta-tion
ex-en-ce-phal-ic
ex-en-ter-a-tion
ex-er-cise
ex-er-gon-ic
ex-fe-ta-tion
ex-flag-el-la-tion
ex-fo-li-a-tion
ex-ha-la-tion
ex-haust-er
ex-haus-tion
ex-hi-bi-tion
ex-hi-bi-tion-ism
ex-hil-a-rant
ex-hu-ma-tion
ex-hume
ex-i-tus
Exner's plex-us
ex-o-car-di-a
ex-o-cat-a-pho-ri-a
ex-oc-cip-i-tal
ex-o-crine
ex-o-don-tics
ex-o-don-tist
ex-o-e-ryth-ro-cyt-ic
ex-og-a-my
ex-og-e-nous
ex-om-pha-los
ex-o-pep-ti-dase
ex-o-pho-ri-a
ex-oph-thal-mos

ex-oph-thal-mos—pro-
    duc-ing sub-stance
ex-o-skel-e-ton
ex-os-mo-sis
ex-os-to-sis
ex-o-ther-mic
ex-o-tox-in
ex-o-tro-pi-a
ex-pan-sive
ex-pec-ta-tion
ex-pec-to-rant
ex-pec-to-ra-tion
ex-pel
ex-per-i-ment
ex-per-i-men-tal
ex-per-i-men-ta-tion
ex-pert
ex-pi-ra-tion
ex-pi-ra-tor-y
ex-pire
ex-plant
ex-plode
ex-plo-ra-tion
ex-plor-a-tor-y
ex-plor-er
ex-po-sure
ex-pres-sion
ex-pres-siv-i-ty
ex-pul-sion
ex-san-gui-nate
ex-sic-cant
ex-sic-ca-tion
ex-stro-phy
ex-ten-sion
ex-ten-sor
ex-ten-sor car-pi ra-di-
    a-lis brev-is
ex-ten-sor car-pi ra-di-
    a-lis lon-gus
ex-ten-sor car-pi ul-nar-is
ex-ten-sor dig-i-ti quin-
    ti pro-pri-us

ex-ten-sor dig-i-tor-um
    brev-is ped-is
ex-ten-sor dig-i-tor-um
    com-mun-is
ex-ten-sor dig-i-tor-um
    lon-gus
ex-ten-sor hal-lu-cis
    brev-is
ex-ten-sor hal-lu-cis lon-
    gus
ex-ten-sor in-di-cis pro-
    pri-us
ex-ten-sor pol-li-cis
    brev-is
ex-ten-sor pol-li-cis lon-
    gus
ex-te-ri-or-i-za-tion
ex-tern
ex-ter-nal
ex-ter-nal-ize
ex-ter-o-cep-tor
ex-ter-o-fec-tive
ex-tinc-tion
ex-tir-pa-tion
ex-tor-sion
ex-tra-ar-tic-u-lar
ex-tra-buc-cal
ex-tra-bulb-ar
ex-tra-cap-su-lar
ex-tra-car-pal
ex-tra-cel-lu-lar
ex-tra-cer-e-bral
ex-tra-cor-po-re-al
ex-tra-cor-pus-cu-lar
ex-tra-cra-ni-al
ex-tract
ex-trac-tion
ex-trac-tive
ex-trac-tor
ex-tra-cyst-ic
ex-tra-du-ral
ex-tra-em-bry-on-ic

ex-tra-e-so-phag-e-al
ex-tra-gen-i-tal
ex-tra-he-pat-ic
ex-tra-med-ul-lar-y
ex-tra-mu-ral
ex-tra-nu-cle-ar
ex-tra-pa-ren-chy-mal
ex-tra-pel-vic
ex-tra-per-i-ne-al
ex-tra-per-i-to-ne-al
ex-tra-pla-cen-tal
ex-tra-pros-tat-ic
ex-tra-py-ram-i-dal
ex-tra-sen-sor-y
ex-tra-sys-to-le
ex-tra-tu-bal
ex-tra-u-ter-ine
ex-tra-vag-i-nal
ex-trav-a-sa-tion
ex-tra-vas-cu-lar
ex-tra-ven-tric-u-lar
ex-tra-vis-u-al
ex-trem-i-ty
ex-trin-sic
ex-tro-phy
ex-tro-vert
ex-tru-sion
ex-tu-ba-tion
ex-u-date
ex-u-da-tion
ex-u-vi-a-tion
eye-ball
eye-brow
eye-cup
eye ground
eye-lash
eye-lid
eye-piece
eye-point
eye-spot
sye-strain
eye-tooth
eye-wash

F

fa-bel-la
fab-ri-ca-tion
face bow
fac-et
fa-cial ar-ter-y
fa-ci-es
fa-cil-i-ta-tion
fac-ti-tious
fac-tor
fac-ul-ta-tive
fa-gar-ine
fag-o-py-rism
Fahrenheit
fail-ure
faint
fal-ci-form
fal-cu-la
Fal-lo-pi-an tube
false
falx
fa-mes
fa-mil-ial
fam-i-ly
fa-nat-i-cism
Fanconi's dis-ease
Fan-ni-a ca-nic-u-lar-is
fan-ta-sy
far-ad
far-a-day
fa-rad-ic
far-a-di-za-tion
far-a-do-con-trac-til-i-ty
far-a-do-mus-cu-lar
far-a-do-ther-a-py
far-i-na-ceous
far—point
far-sight-ed-ness
fas-ci-a
fas-ci-cle

fas-cic-u-la-ted
fac-cic-u-la-tion
fas-cic-u-lus
fas-ci-ec-to-my
Fas-ci-o-la gi-gan-ti-ca
Fas-ci-o-la he-pat-i-ca
fas-ci-o-la ci-ne-re-a
Fas-ci-o-loi-des
fas-ci-o-lop-si-a-sis
Fas-ci-o-lop-sis bus-ki
fas-ci-or-rha-phy
fas-ci-ot-o-my
fas-ci-tis
fast green FCF
fas-tig-i-um
fat-i-ga-bil-i-ty
fa-tigue
fat—sol-u-ble
fat-ty ac-id
fau-ces
Fauchard's dis-ease
fau-na
fa-ve-o-late
fa-ve-o-lus
fa-vism
fa-vus
fea-ture
feb-ri-cant
feb-ri-fa-cient
feb-ri-fuge
fe-brile
fe-ca-lith
fe-cal-oid
fe-ces
fec-u-la
fec-u-lent
fe-cun-da-tion
fe-cun-di-ty
fee-ble-mind-ed-ness
feed-ing
feel-ing
Fehling's re-a-gent

fel
fe-line
fel-la-ti-o
fel-la-tor
fel-la-trice
fel-on
Felty's syn-drome
fe-male
fem-i-nism
fem-or-al
fe-mur
fe-nes-tra
fen-es-tra-tion
fen-nel
fer—de—lance
Ferguson's tech-nique
fer-ment
fer-men-ta-tion
fer-ra-ted
fer-ric
fer-ri-cy-a-nide
fer-ri-heme
fer-ri-he-mo-glo-bin
fer-ri-tin
fer-ro-cy-a-nide
fer-ro-heme
fer-ro-he-mo-glo-bin
fer-rous
fer-ru-gi-na-tion
fer-ru-gi-nous
fer-tile
fer-til-i-ty
fer-ti-li-za-tion
fer-ti-li-zin
fes-ter
fes-ti-na-tion
fes-toon
fe-tal-ism
fe-ta-tion
fe-ti-cide
fet-id
fe-tish

fet-lock
fe-tom-e-try
fe-tor
fe-tus
fe-ver
fi-at
fi-ber
fi-bra
fi-bre-mi-a
fi-bri-form
fi-bril
fi-bril-la-tion
fi-brin
fi-bri-ne-mi-a
fi-brin-o-gen
fi-brin-o-gen-o-pe-ni-a
fi-bri-noid
fi-brin-o-kin-ase
fi-bri-no-ly-sin
fi-brin-ol-y-sis
fi-brin-o-pe-ni-a
fi-bro-ad-e-no-ma
fi-bro-ad-i-pose
fi-bro-an-gi-o-ma
fi-bro-blast
fi-bro-blas-tic
fi-bro-blas-to-ma
fi-bro-bron-chi-tis
fi-bro-cal-car-e-ous
fi-bro-car-ci-no-ma
fi-bro-car-ti-lage
fi-bro-cel-lu-lar
fi-bro-chon-dro-ma
fi-bro-cys-to-ma
fi-bro-cyte
fi-bro-dys-pla-si-a
fi-bro-e-las-tic
fi-bro-e-las-to-sis
fi-bro-en-chon-dro-ma
fi-bro-gli-o-ma
fi-broid
fi-broid-ec-to-my

fi-bro-lei-o-my-o-ma
fi-bro-li-po-ma
fi-bro-li-po-sar-co-ma
fi-bro-ma
fi-bro-ma-toid
fi-bro-ma-to-sis
fi-bro-mus-cu-lar
fi-bro-my-o-ma
fi-bro-my-o-mec-to-my
fi-bro-my-o-si-tis
fi-bro-myx-o-li-po-ma
fi-bro-myx-o-ma
fi-bro-myx-o-sar-co-ma
fi-bro-neu-ro-ma
fi-bro—os-te-o-chon-dro-
    ma
fi-bro—os-te-o-ma
fi-bro—os-te-o-sar-co-ma
fi-bro-pla-si-a
fi-bro-plate
fi-bro-sar-co-ma
fi-bro-se-rous
fi-bro-sis
fi-bro-si-tis
fi-brous
fib-u-la
fib-u-lo-cal-ca-ne-al
Fick's prin-ci-ple
Fiedler's my-o-car-di-tis
fig-ure
fig-wort
fi-la
fi-la-ceous
fil-a-ment
fil-a-men-ta-tion
fil-a-ri-a
fil-a-ri-a-sis
fi-lar-i-cide
fi-lar-i-form
fil-i-form
fil-let
fill-ing

133

film badge
fil-ter
fil-trate
fil-tra-tion
fil-trum
fim-bri-a
fim-bri-a-ted
fin-ger
fin-ger cot
fin-ger-print
fin-ger stall
Finney's op-er-a-tion
Finochetti's stir-rup
fire-damp
first aid
first in-ten-tion
fis-sile
fis-sion
fis-sip-a-rous
fis-su-la
fis-sure
fis-tu-la
fis-tu-lec-to-my
fis-tu-li-za-tion
fis-tu-lot-o-my
fix-a-tion
fix-a-tive
fixed
fix-ing flu-id
flac-cid
Flag-el-la-ta
flag-el-late
flag-el-la-tion
fla-gel-li-form
flag-el-lo-sis
fla-gel-lum
flank
flap
flare
flask
flat-foot
flat-u-lence

fla-tus
flat-worm
flav-i-cin
fla-vin
Fla-vo-bac-te-ri-um
fla-vo-ki-nase
fla-vone
fla-vo-noid
flav-o-nol
fla-vo-none
fla-vo-pro-te-in
fla-vo-xan-thin
flax-seed
flesh
flex-i-ble
flex-ile
flex-im-e-ter
flex-ion
Flexner re-port
flex-or
flex-or car-pi ra-di-a-lis
flex-or car-pi ul-nar-is
flex-or dig-i-ti quin-ti
    ped-is
flex-or dig-i-tor-um
    brev-is
flex-or dig-i-tor-um
    lon-gus
flex-or dig-i-tor-um pro-
    fun-dus
flex-or dig-i-tor-um
    sub-lim-is
flex-or hal-lu-cis brev-is
flex-or hal-lu-cis lon-gus
flex-or pol-li-cis brev-is
flex-or pol-li-cis lon-
    gus
flex-ure
flick-er
Flint's mur-mur
float-ing
floc-cu-la-tion

floc-cu-lent
floc-cu-lus
floor
flo-ra
flo-res
flor-id
flo-ta-tion
flow
flow-ers
flow-me-ter
fluc-tu-a-tion
flu-id
flu-id-ex-tract
flu-id lev-el
flu-id line
flu-id-ounce
fluke
flu-or-chrome
flu-o-rene
flu-o-res-ce-in
flu-o-res-cence
flu-or-i-date
flu-o-ride
flu-o-ri-dize
flu-o-ri-na-tion
flu-o-rine
flu-o-rite
flu-o-ro-a-ce-tic ac-id
flu-o-ro-car-bon
flu-or-o-chrome
flu-or-o-gen
flu-or-og-ra-phy
flu-o-ro-pho-tom-e-try
flu-o-ro-scope
flu-or-os-co-py
flu-o-ro-sis
flush
flut-ter
flux
foam
fo-cal length
fo-cus

fog-ging
foil
fold
Foley bal-loon cath-e-ter
fo-li-a-ceous
fo-lic ac-id
fo-lie à deux
fo-li-um ca-cum-in-is
fo-li-um ver-mis
fol-li-cle
fol-lic-u-lar
fol-lic-u-li-tis
fo-men-ta-tion
fo-mi-tes
fon-tac-to-scope
fon-ta-nel
foot—can-dle
foot drop
foot—pound
foot-print
fo-ra-men
fo-ra-men mag-num
fo-ra-men of Magendie
fo-ra-men of Monro
fo-ra-men of Winslow
fo-ra-men o-vale
fo-ra-men of Luschka
fo-ra-mi-na
force
for-ceps
fore-arm
fore-brain
fore-con-scious
fore-fin-ger
fore-foot
fore-gut
fore-head
fo-ren-sic
fore-pleas-ure
fore-skin
form
form-al-de-hyde

for-mate
for-ma-tion
form-a-tive
for-mic ac-id
for-mic al-de-hyde
for-mi-ca-tion
for-mo-cre-sol
for-mol
for-mose
for-mu-la
for-mu-lar-y
for-myl
for-ni-cate
for-ni-ca-tion
for-nix
Foshay's test
fos-sa
fos-sette
fos-su-la
foun-der
found-ling
four-chette
fo-ve-a
fo-ve-o-la
Fowler's po-si-tion
Fox—Fordyce dis-ease
fox-glove
frac-tion-al
frac-tion-a-tion
fract-ure
frac-ture—dis-lo-ca-tion
fra-gil-i-tas
fra-gil-i-ty
frag-men-ta-tion
fram-be-si-a
fram-be-si-form
fran-ci-um
frank
frank-in-cense
Fraunhofer's lines
free-mar-tin
free rad-i-cal

Frei test
frem-i-tus
fre-not-o-my
fren-u-lum
fre-num
fren-zy
fre-quen-cy
Freud-i-an
fri-a-ble
fric-tion
Friedlander's ba-cil-lus
Friedman test
Friedreich's a-tax-i-a
fright
fri-gid-i-ty
fringe
Froehlich's syn-drome
front-ad
fron-tal
fron-ta-lis
fron-to-max-il-lar-y
fron-to-men-tal
fron-to-na-sal
fron-to—oc-cip-i-tal
fron-to—tem-po-ra-le
frost-bite
fro-zen sec-tions
fruc-to-fu-ran-ose
fruc-to-py-ran-ose
fruc-tose
fruc-tose—1, 6—di-phos-
    phate
fruc-tose—1—phos-phate
fruc-tose—6—phos-phate
fruc-to-side
fruc-to-su-ri-a
fru-men-tum
frus-trane
frus-tra-tion
frus-tule
Fuchs—Rosenthal count-
    ing cham-ber

fuch-sin
fuch-sin-o-phil
fu-ga-cious
fu-gi-tive
fugue
ful-gu-ra-ting
ful-gu-ra-tion
fu-lig-i-nous
ful-mi-nant
ful-mi-na-ting
fu-ma-rase
fu-mar-ate
Fu-ma-ri-a-ce-ae
fu-mar-ic ac-id
fu-mi-ga-tion
fu-ming
func-tion
func-tion-al
fun-da-ment
fun-dec-to-my
fun-di-form
fun-dus
fun-du-scope
fun-du-sec-to-my
fun-gate
fun-gi
fun-gi-ci-dal
fun-gi-form
fun-gi-stat-ic
fun-goid
fun-gos-i-ty
fun-gus
fu-nic-u-li-tis
fu-nic-u-lus
fu-nis
fun-nel
fun-ny bone
fur-al-de-hyde
fu-ran
fu-ran-ose
fur-cu-la
fur-cu-lum

fur-fur
fur-fur-al
fur-fur-an
fu-ror
fur-row
fu-run-cle
fu-run-cu-lo-sis
Fu-sa-ri-um
fus-cin
fu-sel oil
fu-si-ble
fu-si-form
Fu-si-for-mis
fu-sion
Fu-so-bac-te-ri-um
fu-so-spi-ro-che-tal

G

gad-o-lin-i-um
Ga-dus mor-rhu-a
Gaffky scale
Gaff-ky-a
gag
gage
gait
ga-lac-ta-gogue
ga-lac-tan
ga-lac-tase
gal-ac-te-mi-a
ga-lac-tic
ga-lac-tin
ga-lac-to-cele
ga-lac-to-gen
ga-lac-toid
ga-lac-to-lip-id
gal-ac-tom-e-ter
gal-ac-toph-a-gous
gal-ac-toph-o-ri-tis
gal-ac-toph-y-gous

ga-lac-to-py-ra-nose
ga-lac-tor-rhe-a
ga-lac-tos-a-mine
gal-ac-tos-che-sis
ga-lac-tose
gal-ac-to-se-mi-a
ga-lac-to-side
gal-ac-to-sis
gal-ac-tos-ta-sis
ga-lac-to-su-ri-a
ga-lac-to-tox-in
ga-lac-to-zy-mase
gal-ac-tu-ri-a
ga-lac-tu-ron-ic ac-id
gal-a-lith
ga-le-a a-pon-eu-ro-
ti-ca
ga-le-na
Ga-len-i-cal
gal-e-o-phil-i-a
gal-e-o-pho-bi-a
gall
gall-blad-der
gal-lic ac-id
Gallie's op-er-a-tion
gal-li-um
gal-lon
gall-stone
gal-van-ic
gal-va-nism
gal-va-ni-za-tion
gal-va-nom-e-ter
gal-va-not-ro-pism
Gam-bu-si-a
gam-ete
ga-me-to-cyte
gam-e-to-gen-e-sis
gam-e-tog-o-ny
ga-me-to-phyte
gam-ic
gam-ma
gam-ma-cism

Gamna nod-ules
gam-o-pho-bi-a
gan-gli-a-ted
gan-gli-ec-to-my
gan-gli-o-blas-to-ma
gan-gli-o-cy-to-ma
gan-gli-o-gli-o-ma
gan-gli-oid
gan-gli-o-ma
gan-gli-on
gan-gli-on-ec-to-my
gan-gli-o-neu-ro-blas-
to-ma
gan-gli-o-neu-ro-cy-
to-ma
gan-gli-o-neu-ro-ma
gan-gli-o-ni-tis
gan-gli-o-sides
gan-go-sa
gan-grene
gangue
gan-ja
gan-o-blast
gape-worm
gar-get
gar-gle
gar-goyl-ism
gar-lic
gar-rot-ing
Gartner's duct
gas-om-e-ter
gasp
Gas-ser-i-an gan-gli-
on
gas-sing
Gas-ter-oph-i-lus
gas-tral-gi-a
gas-trec-to-my
gas-tric
gas-trin
gas-tri-tis
gas-tro-an-as-to-mo-sis

gas-tro-cele
gas-troc-ne-mi-us
gas-tro-col-ic
gas-tro-col-pot-o-my
Gas-tro-dis-coid-es
hom-i-nis
gas-tro-disk
gas-tro-du-o-de-nal
gas-tro-du-o-de-ni-tis
gas-tro-du-o-de-nos-
to-my
gas-tro-en-ter-al-gi-a
gas-tro-en-ter-ic
gas-tro-en-ter-i-tis
gas-tro-en-ter-o-a-
nas-to-mo-sis
gas-tro-en-ter-ol-o-gist
gas-tro-en-ter-ol-o-gy
gas-tro-en-ter-os-to-my
gas-tro-ep-i-plo-ic
gas-tro-e-soph-a-gi-tis
gas-tro-gas-tros-to-my
gas-tro-ga-vage
gas-tro-he-pat-ic
gas-tro-in-tes-ti-nal
gas-tro-je-ju-nal
gas-tro-je-ju-ni-tis
gas-tro-je-ju-nos-to-my
gas-tro-lav-age
gas-tro-lith
gas-trol-o-gy
gas-trol-y-sis
gas-tro-meg-a-ly
gas-tro-my-ot-o-my
gas-trop-a-thy
gas-tro-pex-y
gas-tro-phren-ic
gas-tro-plas-ty
gas-trop-to-sis
gas-tro-py-lo-rec-to-my
gas-tror-rha-gi-a
gas-tror-rha-phy

gas-tro-scope
gas-tros-cop-y
gas-tro-spasm
gas-tro-splen-ic
gas-tros-to-my
gas-tro-tho-ra-cop-a-gus
gas-trot-o-my
gas-tro-tym-pa-ni-tes
gas-tru-la
Gatch bed
Gaucher's dis-ease
gauge
gaul-the-ri-a oil
gaul-ther-o-lin
gaunt-let
gauze
ga-vage
Gay—Lussac's law
Gei-ger—Mul-ler count-er
gei-so-ma
gel
ge-lat-i-fi-ca-tion
gel-a-tin
ge-lat-i-nase
ge-lat-i-nize
ge-lat-i-no-lyt-ic
ge-lat-i-nous
gel-a-tion
geld
geld-ing
gel-ose
ge-lot-o-lep-sy
gel-se-mi-um
ge-mel-lus
gem-i-nate
ge-mis-to-cyte
gem-ma
gem-ma-tion
gem-mule
ge-na
gene
gen-er-a

gen-er-al
gen-er-a-tion
gen-er-a-tor
ge-ner-ic
ge-ne-si-ol-o-gy
gen-e-sis
ge-net-ic
ge-net-i-cist
ge-net-ics
ge-net-o-troph-ic
ge-ni-al
ge-nic-u-lar
ge-nic-u-late
ge-nic-u-lum
ge-ni-o-glos-sus
ge-ni-o-hy-oid
ge-ni-o-plas-ty
gen-i-tal
gen-i-ta-li-a
gen-i-tals
gen-i-to-cru-ral
gen-i-to-fem-o-ral
gen-i-to-u-ri-nar-y
gen-i-us
gen-o-cide
ge-nome
gen-o-pho-bi-a
gen-o-type
gen-tian
gen-tian vi-o-let
gen-tis-ic ac-id
ge-nu
ge-nus
gen-y-chei-lo-plas-ty
gen-y-plas-ty
ge-o-med-i-cine
ge-o-met-ric mean
ge-oph-a-gy
ge-o-tri-cho-sis
Ge-ot-ri-chum
ge-ot-ro-pism
ge-ra-ni-um

ger-a-tol-o-gy
Gerhardt's sign
ger-i-a-tri-cian
ger-i-at-rics
ger-mi-nal
ger-ma-ni-um
ger-mi-ci-dal
ger-mi-cide
ger-mi-na-tion
ger-mi-na-tive
ger-mine
ger-mi-no-ma
ger-o-der-ma
ger-o-mor-phism
ge-ron-tic
ger-on-tol-o-gy
ge-ron-to-ther-a-py
ger-on-tox-on
Gesell chart
ge-stalt
ges-ta-tion
ghat-ti gum
Ghon tu-ber-cle
gi-ant
gi-ant-ism
Gi-ar-di-a lam-bli-a
gi-ar-di-a-sis
gib-bos-i-ty
gib-bous
Gibbs—Helmholtz e-qua-tion
gib-bus
gid-di-ness
Giemsa stain
Gifford's sign
gi-gan-tic ac-id
gi-gan-tism
gi-gan-to-blast
gi-gan-to-cyte
Gigli's saw
Gi-la mon-ster
Gilchrist's dis-ease

gill
Gimbernat's lig-a-ment
gin-ger
gin-gi-va
gin-gi-vec-to-my
gin-gi-vi-tis
gin-gi-vo-glos-si-tis
gin-gi-vo-sis
gin-gi-vo-sto-ma-ti-tis
gin-gly-mus
gin-seng
gir-dle
git-a-lin
gi-tox-in
giz-zard
gla-bel-la
gla-brous
gla-cial
glad-i-o-lus
glair-y
gland
glan-ders
glans
glass-es
glass wool
glass-y
Glauber's salt
glau-co-ma
gleet
gle-no-hu-mer-al
gle-noid
gli-a
gli-o-blas-to-ma mul-ti-for-me
gli-o-ma
gli-o-ma-to-sis
gli-o-sar-co-ma
gli-o-sis
gli-o-some
Glisson's cap-sule
globe
glo-bin

glob-ule
glob-u-lin
glob-u-li-nu-ri-a
glob-u-lus
glo-bus hys-ter-i-cus
glo-bus pal-li-dus
glome
glom-er-ate
glo-mer-u-lo-ne-phri-tis
glo-mer-u-lo-scle-ro-sis
glo-mer-u-lus
glo-mus
glos-sa
glos-sal
glos-sal-gi-a
glos-sec-to-my
Glos-si-na
glos-si-tis
glos-so-dyn-i-a
glos-so-ep-i-glot-tic
glos-so-hy-al
glos-so-la-bi-al
glos-so-la-li-a
glos-so-pal-a-tine
glos-so-pal-a-ti-nus
glos-so-pha-ryn-ge-al
glos-so-pha-ryn-ge-us
glos-so-plas-ty
glos-so-ple-gi-a
glos-so-py-ro-sis
glos-so-spasm
glos-so-trich-i-a
glot-tal
glot-tic
glot-tis
glu-ca-gon
glu-co-a-scor-bic ac-id
glu-co-cor-ti-coid
glu-co-fu-ran-ose
glu-co-gen
glu-co-ki-nase
glu-co-kin-in

glu-col-y-sis
glu-co-ne-o-gen-e-sis
glu-con-ic ac-id
glu-co-no-ki-nase
glu-co-no-lac-tone
glu-co-py-ran-ose
glu-cos-a-mine
glu-co-san
glu-co-sa-zone
glu-cose
glu-cose—1—phos-phate
glu-cose—6—phos-phate
glu-co-si-dase
glu-co-side
glu-co-sone
glu-co-su-ri-a
glu-cu-ron-ic ac-id
glu-cu-ron-i-dase
glu-cu-ron-ide
glu-tam-ic ac-id
glu-tam-i-nase
glu-ta-mine
glu-tar-ic ac-id
glu-ta-thi-one
glu-te-al
glu-te-lin
glu-ten
glu-ten bread
glu-te-nin
glu-ten sul-fate
glu-te-us max-i-mus
glu-te-us me-di-us
glu-te-us min-i-mus
glu-tin
glu-ti-nous
glut-ton-y
gly-ce-mi-a
glyc-er-al-de-hyde
gly-cer-ic ac-id
glyc-er-i-dase
glyc-er-ide
glyc-er-in

glyc-er-o-gel-a-tin
glyc-er-ol
glyc-er-o-phos-pha-tase
glyc-er-o-phos-phate
glyc-er-o-phos-phor-ic
   ac-id
glyc-er-ose
glyc-er-ose—3—phos-
   phate
glyc-er-yl
gly-cin
gly-cine ox-i-dase
gly-ci-nin
gly-co-cho-late
gly-co-chol-ic ac-id
gly-co-cy-a-mine
gly-co-gen
gly-co-ge-nase
gly-co-gen-e-sis
gly-co-gen-ic
gly-co-ge-nol-y-sis
gly-co-ge-no-sis
gly-col
gly-col al-de-hyde
gly-col-ic ac-id
gly-co-lip-id
gly-col-y-sis
gly-colyt-ic
gly-co-me-tab-o-lism
gly-co-ne-o-gen-e-sis
gly-co-pe-ni-a
gly-co-phil-i-a
gly-co-phos-pho-mu-tase
gly-co-pro-te-in
gly-co-side
gly-co-su-ri-a
gly-co-su-ric ac-id
glyc-yr-rhi-za
gly-ox-al
gly-ox-a-lase
gly-ox-yl-ic ac-id
gnat

gnath-ic
gna-thi-on
gnath-i-tis
gnath-o-dyn-i-a
gnath-o-plas-ty
gnath-os-chi-sis
Gnath-os-to-ma
gnath-o-sto-mi-a-sis
gno-sis
gnos-tic
gob-let cell
goi-ter
goi-tro-gen-ic
Goldblatt kid-ney
gold-en-rod
Golgi net-work
Golgi's cor-pus-cle
gon-ad
gon-a-dec-to-my
gon-a-do-tro-pin
go-nal-gi-a
gon-ar-thri-tis
go-ni-om-e-ter
go-ni-on
go-ni-o-scope
go-ni-ot-o-my
gon-o-coc-ci
gon-o-coc-cus
gon-o-cyte
gon-or-rhe-a
gon-y-on-cus
goose flesh
Gordon's re-flex
gouge
gout
gout-y
Graaf-i-an fol-li-cle
grac-i-lis
gra-di-ent
grad-u-ate
grad-u-a-ted
graft

Graham—Cole test
Graham's law
Graham Steell mur-mur
grain
gram
gram ion
gram—me-ter
gram-mole
Gram—neg-a-tive
Gram—pos-i-tive
gra-na
gran-di-ose
grand mal
gran-u-la-ted lids
gran-u-la-tion
gran-u-la-tion tis-sue
gran-ule
gran-u-lo-cyte
gran-u-lo-cyt-ic se-ries
gran-u-lo-cy-to-pe-ni-a
gran-u-lo-cy-to-poi-e-sis
gran-u-lo-ma
gran-u-lo-ma an-nu-lare
gran-u-lo-ma in-gui-nale
gran-u-lo-ma py-o-
    gen-i-cum
gran-u-lo-ma-to-sis
gran-u-lo-poi-e-sis
graph
graph-es-the-si-a
graph-ite
graph-ol-o-gy
graph-or-rhe-a
grat-tage
grav-el
Graves's dis-ease
grav-id
gra-vi-da
gra-vim-e-ter
gra-vi-met-ric
grav-i-ta-tion
grav-i-ty

green blind-ness
gre-ga-ri-ous-ness
grippe
gris-e-o-ful-vin
Gritti—Stokes am-pu-ta-
    tion
groin
groove
ground sub-stance
group-ing
growth
Grynfeltt's tri-an-gle
gry-po-sis
g suit
guai-ac
guai-a-col
gua-nase
gua-na-zo-lo
guan-i-dine
gua-nine
gua-no
gua-nyl-ic ac-id
guard
gua-za
gu-ber-nac-u-lum tes-tis
Guillain—Barré syn-
    drome
guil-lo-tine
guin-ea pig
Guin-ea worm
gul-let
gum ar-a-bic
gum trag-a-canth
gum-boil
gum-ma
gum-ma-tous
gun-jah
gur-ney
gus-ta-tion
gus-ta-to-ry
gut
gut-ta

gut-tae
gut-ta—per-cha
gut-tate
gut-ter
gut-ti-form
Guttmann's sign
gym-nas-tics
gym-no-spore
gy-nan-der
gy-nan-dri-a
gy-nan-drism
gy-nan-dro-blas-to-ma
gy-nan-dro-mor-phism
gy-nan-dro-mor-phy
gy-nan-drous
gy-nan-dry
gyn-a-tre-si-a
gyn-e-co-gen-ic
gyn-e-cog-ra-phy
gyn-e-coid
gyn-e-col-o-gist
gyn-e-col-o-gy
gyn-e-col-og-i-cal
gyn-e-co-mas-ti-a
gyn-e-pho-bi-a
gyn-e-phor-ic
gyn-o-gen-e-sis
gyn-o-plas-ty
gyp-sum
gy-ra-tion
Gy-rau-lus
gy-rec-to-my
gyr-en-ceph-a-late
gyr-en-ceph-a-lous
gy-rose
gy-rus

H

ha-ben-u-la
hab-it
hab-i-tat
ha-bit-u-a-tion
hab-i-tus
hack-ing
Hae-ma-dip-sa
Hae-ma-gog-us
Hae-ma-phy-sa-lis
haem-a-tin
Haem-a-to-bi-a
Haem-a-to-ther-ma
Hae-mon-chus
Hae-mo-pro-teus
Hae-mo-spo-rid-i-a
Haff dis-ease
haf-ni-um
Hagedorn nee-dle
Hagner bag
Haines's re-a-gent
hair fol-li-cle
Haldane scale
half—life
half—val-ue lay-er
hal-i-but—liv-er oil
hal-ide
ha-lis-ter-e-sis
hal-ite
hal-i-to-sis
hal-la-chrome
hal-lu-ci-na-tion
hal-lu-ci-no-sis
hal-lux val-gus
hal-lux va-rus
hal-o-gen
Halsted's op-er-a-tion
ham-ar-to-blas-to-ma
ham-ar-to-ma
ha-mate bone

ham-mer
ham-mer-toe
ham-ster
ham-string
ham-u-lus
Hand—Schuller—Christian dis-ease
hand-ed-ness
hang-nail
Hansen's dis-ease
hap-a-lo-nych-i-a
hap-lo-dont
hap-loid
ha-plo-pi-a
hap-ten
hap-te-pho-bi-a
hap-to-glo-bin
hard-ness
hare-lip
Harkins' meth-od
Harris' he-ma-tox-y-lin
Harrison Act
Hartmann's fos-sa
Hartmann's pouch
harts-horn
Hashimoto's dis-ease
hash-ish
haunch
haus-trum
Haverhill fe-ver
Haversian ca-nals
hawk
Hayem's so-lu-tion
hay fe-ver
Haygarth's nodes
head-ache
head-band
heal-er
heal-ing
health
hear
hear-ing aid

heart
heart block
heart-burn
heart fail-ure
heart mur-mur
heart rate
heart sounds
heart-worm
heat pros-tra-tion
heat stroke
heaves
he-be-phre-ni-a
Heberden's nodes
he-bet-ic
hec-a-ter-o-mer-ic
Hecht—Schlaer night vi-sion test
hec-tic
hec-to-gram
hec-to-li-ter
hec-to-me-ter
he-don-ism
he-do-no-pho-bi-a
heel
Hegar's di-la-tors
he-gem-o-ny
Heidenhain's stain
hel-coid
he-lic-i-form
hel-i-coid
hel-i-co-pod
hel-i-co-pro-te-in
hel-i-co-ru-bin
he-li-o-phobe
he-li-o-tax-is
he-li-o-ther-a-py
he-li-ot-ro-pism
he-li-um
he-lix
Hel-ke-si-mas-tix
Hellin's law
Helmholtz the-o-ry

hel-minth
hel-min-thi-a-sis
hel-min-thol-o-gist
hel-min-thol-o-gy
He-lo-der-ma
he-lot-o-my
He-ma-cha-tus hae-ma-cha-tus
he-ma-chrome
he-mag-glu-ti-na-tion
he-mag-glu-ti-nin
he-mal
he-ma-nal-y-sis
he-man-gi-ec-ta-sis
he-man-gi-o-blas-to-ma
he-man-gi-o-en-do-the-li-o-ma
he-man-gi-o-en-do-the-li-o-sar-co-ma
he-man-gi-o-ma
he-man-gi-o-sar-co-ma
he-mar-thro-sis
he-ma-tem-e-sis
he-mat-hi-dro-sis
he-mat-ic
he-ma-tim-e-ter
hem-a-tin
hem-a-tin-ic
hem-a-tin-om-e-ter
hem-a-ti-nu-ri-a
hem-a-tite
hem-a-to-blast
hem-a-to-cele
hem-a-to-col-pos
hem-a-to-crit
hem-a-to-cyst
hem-a-to-cyte
hem-a-to-gen-e-sis
he-ma-toi-din
he-ma-tol-o-gist
he-ma-tol-o-gy

hem-a-to-lym-phan-gi-o-ma
he-ma-tol-y-sis
he-ma-to-ma
hem-a-to-me-di-as-ti-num
he-ma-tom-e-ter
hem-a-to-me-tra
he-ma-to-my-e-li-a
hem-a-to-my-e-li-tis
he-ma-ton-ic
hem-a-to-per-i-car-di-um
hem-a-to-per-i-to-ne-um
hem-a-to-poi-e-sis
hem-a-to-por-phy-rin
hem-a-to-por-phy-ri-ne-mi-a
hem-a-to-por-phy-ri-nu-ri-a
hem-a-to-sal-pinx
hem-a-tose
hem-a-to-sper-ma-to-cele
hem-a-to-sper-mi-a
hem-a-to-tym-pa-num
he-ma-tox-y-lin
hem-a-tu-ri-a
heme
hem-i-a-blep-si-a
hem-i-a-geu-si-a
hem-i-al-bu-mo-su-ri-a
hem-i-an-al-ge-si-a
hem-i-an-es-the-si-a
hem-i-an-op-si-a
hem-i-a-tax-i-a
hem-i-at-ro-phy
Hem-i-bi-a
he-mic
hem-i-cel-lu-lose
hem-i-ceph-a-ly
hem-i-cho-re-a

hem-i-co-lec-to-my
hem-i-cra-ni-a
hem-i-de-cor-ti-ca-tion
hem-i-di-a-phragm
hem-i-fa-cial
hem-i-glos-sec-to-my
hem-i-glos-so-ple-gi-a
hem-i-hy-per-tro-phy
hem-i-hy-pes-the-si-a
hem-i-lam-i-nec-to-my
hem-i-lar-yn-gec-to-my
hem-i-man-di-bu-lec-to-my
hem-i-me-tab-o-lous
he-min
hem-i-ne-phrec-to-my
hem-i-pa-re-sis
hem-i-pel-vect-o-my
hem-i-ple-gi-a
He-mip-ter-a
hem-i-ra-chis-chi-sis
hem-i-sec-tion
hem-i-sphere
hem-i-spher-ec-to-my
He-mis-po-ra
hem-i-spo-ro-sis
hem-i-sys-to-le
hem-i-thy-roid-ec-to-my
hem-i-ver-te-bra
hem-i-zy-gote
hem-lock
he-mo-bil-i-ru-bin
he-mo-blast
he-mo-chro-ma-to-sis
he-mo-con-cen-tra-tion
he-mo-co-ni-o-sis
he-mo-cu-pre-in
he-mo-cy-a-nin
he-mo-cyte
he-mo-cy-to-blast
he-mo-cy-to-gen-e-sis

he-mo-cy-tol-y-sis
he-mo-cy-tom-e-ter
he-mo-di-al-y-sis
he-mo-di-lu-tion
he-mo-dy-nam-ics
he-mo-e-ryth-rin
he-mo-fo-lin
he-mo-fus-cin
he-mo-glo-bin
he-mo-glo-bi-ne-mi-a
he-mo-glo-bi-nom-e-ter
he-mo-glo-bi-nu-ri-a
he-mo-gram
he-mo-his-ti-o-blast
he-mo-lith
he-mo-lymph
he-mol-y-sin
he-mol-y-sis
he-mo-lyze
he-mom-e-ter
he-mo-my-e-lo-gram
he-mo-pa-thol-o-gy
he-mo-per-i-car-di-um
he-mo-per-i-to-ne-um
he-mo-pha-gi-a
he-mo-phil
he-mo-phil-i-a
he-mo-phil-i-ac
he-mo-phil-ic
He-moph-i-lus in-flu-en-zae
He-moph-i-lus per-tus-sis
He-moph-i-lus su-is
he-moph-thal-mi-a
he-mo-pneu-mo-tho-rax
he-mo-poi-e-sis
he-mo-poi-e-tin
he-mop-ty-sis
hem-or-rhage
hem-or-rhoi-dal
hem-or-rhoid-ec-to-my

hem-or-rhoids
he-mo-sid-er-in
he-mo-sid-er-o-sis
he-mo-sta-tis
he-mo-stat
he-mo-stat-ic
he-mo-ther-a-py
he-mo-tho-rax
he-mo-tox-in
he-mo-troph-ic
he-mo-tym-pa-num
hemp
Henderson—Hasselbalch e-qua-tion
Henle's loop
hen-ry
Henry's law
Hensen's duct
he-par
hep-a-rin
hep-a-tec-to-my
he-pat-ic
he-pat-i-co-du-o-de-nos-to-my
he-pat-i-co-li-thot-o-my
he-pat-i-co-pan-cre-at-ic
hep-a-ti-tis
hep-a-ti-za-tion
hep-a-to-cyst-ic
hep-a-to-du-o-de-nal
hep-a-to-gen-ic
hep-a-to-li-e-nal
hep-a-to-lith
hep-a-to-li-thi-a-sis
hep-a-to-ma
hep-a-to-meg-a-ly
hep-a-to-pex-y
hep-a-to-re-nal
hep-a-tor-rha-phy
hep-a-tor-rhex-is
hep-a-to-sple-no-meg-a-ly
hep-a-to-tox-in

hep-tal-de-hyde
hep-tane
hep-tyl-res-or-ci-nol
herb
her-ba-ceous
herb-al
her-biv-o-rous
herd in-stinct
he-red-i-ty
her-e-do-fa-mil-i-al
Hering—Breuer re-flex
her-it-age
her-maph-ro-dite
her-maph-ro-dism
her-met-ic
her-ni-a
her-ni-ated
her-ni-o-plas-ty
her-ni-or-rha-phy
her-ni-ot-o-my
her-o-in
her-o-in-ism
her-pan-gin-a
her-pes
her-pes oph-thal-mi-cus
her-pes pro-gen-i-tal-is
her-pes sim-plex
her-pes zos-ter
her-pet-ic neu-ral-gi-a
her-pet-i-form
her-pe-tol-o-gy
Hertzian rays
Hesselbach's tri-an-gle
het-er-es-the-si-a
het-er-o-ag-glu-ti-nin
het-er-o-blas-tic
het-er-o-cel-lu-lar
het-er-o-chro-ma-tin
het-er-o-chro-mat-ic
het-er-o-chro-mo-some
het-er-o-cy-clic
het-er-o-dont

het-er-o-ga-met-ic
het-er-o-ge-ne-ous
het-er-o-gen-e-sis
het-er-og-e-nous
het-er-og-o-ny
het-er-o-graft
het-er-o-he-mol-y-sin
het-er-oid
het-er-o-ki-ne-si-a
het-er-o-ki-ne-sis
het-er-o-lac-tic
het-er-o-lat-er-al
het-er-ol-o-gous
het-er-o-mer-ic
het-er-om-er-ous
het-er-o-met-a-pla-si-a
het-er-o-me-tro-pi-a
het-er-o-mor-phic
het-er-o-mor-phous
het-er-on-y-mous
het-er-op-a-gus
het-er-o-path-ic
het-er-o-pha-si-a
het-er-o-phil
het-er-o-pho-ni-a
het-er-o-pho-ri-a
Het-er-oph-y-es het-er-
oph-y-es
het-er-o-pla-si-a
het-er-o-plas-tic
het-er-o-pro-te-ose
het-er-op-si-a
Het-er-op-ter-a
het-er-o-pyk-no-sis
het-er-o-sac-cha-ride
het-er-o-scope
het-er-o-sex-u-al-i-ty
het-er-o-sis
het-er-o-sug-ges-ti-bil-i-ty
het-er-o-sug-ges-tion
het-er-o-tax-is
het-er-o-to-ni-a

het-er-o-top-ic
het-er-o-tox-in
het-er-o-trans-plan-ta-
tion
het-er-o-troph-ic
het-er-o-tro-pi-a
het-er-o-typ-ic
het-er-o-ox-e-nous
het-er-o-zy-go-sis
het-er-o-zy-gote
hex-a-chlo-ro-phene
hex-a-chro-mic
hex-a-dac-ty-lism
hex-a-eth-yl-tet-ra-phos-
phate
hex-a-hy-dric
hex-a-me-tho-ni-um
hex-a-meth-yl-en-a-mine
hex-ane
hex-a-va-lent
hex-o-bar-bi-tal
hex-o-ki-nase
hex-os-a-mine
hex-o-san
hex-ose
hex-ose-di-phos-phate
hex-ose-mon-o-phos-
phate
hex-ose-phos-phates
hex-yl-res-or-cin-ol
hi-a-tal
hi-a-tus
hi-ber-na-tion
hic-cup
Hicks's sign
Hicks ver-sion
hid-rad-e-ni-tis
hid-rad-e-no-car-ci-no-ma
hid-rad-e-no-ma
hid-ro-cys-ta-de-no-ma
hid-ro-cys-to-ma
hid-ro-poi-e-sis

144

hi-dros-ad-e-ni-tis
hid-ros-che-sis
hi-dro-sis
hi-drot-ic
hi-lar dance
hi-li
Hilliard's lu-pus
hill-ock
hi-lum
hi-lus
hind-brain
hind-gut
hip-bone
Hip-pe-la-tes
Hip-po-bos-ci-dae
hip-po-cam-pus
Hippocrates
hip-pu-ri-a
hip-pu-ric ac-id
Hirschsprung's dis-ease
hir-sute
hir-sut-ism
hir-u-din
Hir-u-din-e-a
Hi-ru-do
his-tam-i-nase
his-ta-mine
his-ti-dase
his-ti-dine
his-ti-di-nu-ri-a
his-ti-dyl
his-ti-o-cyte
his-ti-o-cy-to-ma
his-ti-o-cy-to-sar-co-ma
his-ti-o-cy-to-sis
his-ti-o-troph-ic
his-to-chem-i-cal
his-to-flu-o-res-cence
his-to-gen-e-sis
his-tol-o-gist
his-tol-o-gy
his-tol-y-sis

his-to-ma
his-to-mor-phol-o-gy
his-tone
his-to-pa-thol-o-gy
his-to-phys-i-ol-o-gy
His-to-plas-ma cap-su-
    la-tum
his-to-plas-min
his-to-plas-mo-sis
his-to-ry
his-to-spec-tros-co-py
his-to-throm-bin
his-tot-o-my
his-to-tox-ic
his-to-troph-ic
his-tri-on-ic
hives
hoar-hound
hoarse
hoar-y
hob-ble
hob-nail liv-er
hock
Hodgkin's dis-ease
hoe
hof
Hofbauer cell
Hoffmann's at-ro-phy
Hoffmann's ba-cil-lus
ho-lan-dric
hol-ism
hol-is-tic
hol-mi-um
hol-o-blas-tic
hol-o-crine
hol-o-en-zyme
hol-o-gyn-ic
hol-o-met-a-bol-ic
hol-o-sac-cha-ride
hol-o-zo-ic
hom-a-lo-ceph-a-lus
hom-a-lo-cor-y-phus

hom-a-lo-me-to-pus
hom-a-lo-pis-tho-cra-
    ni-us
hom-a-lu-ra-nus
Homans' sign
hom-at-ro-pine
ho-me-o-ki-ne-sis
ho-me-o-mor-phous
ho-me-o-path-ic
ho-me-op-a-thy
ho-me-o-plas-tic
ho-me-os-ta-sis
ho-me-os-tat-ic
ho-me-o-ther-mal
home-sick-ness
hom-i-cide
Ho-mo
ho-mo-cen-tric
ho-mo-chro-mo-i-som-er-
    ism
ho-mo-cy-clic
ho-mo-cys-te-ine
ho-mo-cys-tine
ho-mo-dont
ho-mo-dy-na-my
ho-mo-er-o-tism
ho-mo-fer-men-ta-tive
ho-mo-ga-met-ic
ho-mog-e-nate
ho-mo-ge-ne-ous
ho-mo-gen-ic
ho-mo-ge-ni-za-tion
ho-mog-e-nous
ho-mo-gen-tis-ic ac-id
ho-mo-glan-du-lar
ho-mo-graft
ho-mo-i-o-ther-mic
ho-mo-lat-er-al
ho-mol-o-gous
ho-mon-o-mous
ho-mon-y-mous
ho-mo-plas-tic

Ho-mop-ter-a
ho-mo-ser-ine
ho-mo-sex-ual
ho-mo-ther-mic
hom-o-tope
ho-mo-trans-plan-ta-tion
ho-mo-type
ho-mo-zy-gote
hon-ey
hook-worm
hora
hor-de-o-lum
hor-mi-on
Hor-mo-den-drum
hor-mone
hor-mo-no-poi-et-ic
horn
Horner's syn-drome
horn-i-fi-ca-tion
ho-rop-ter
horse-shoe
Horsley's wax
hos-pi-tal
hos-pit-al-i-za-tion
host
hot lab-or-a-tor-y
house-maid's knee
house phy-si-cian
house staff
Houston's valves
Howard's meth-od
Howell—Jolly bod-ies
H—sub-stance
Hudson's bone drill
hue
hum
hu-man
hu-mer-o-ra-di-al
hu-mer-o-scap-u-lar
hu-mer-o-ul-nar
hu-mer-us
hu-mid-i-fi-ca-tion

hu-mid-i-ty
hu-mor
hu-mor-al
hump-back
hu-mu-lus
hu-mus
hunch-back
hun-ger
Hunter's ca-nal
Huntington's cho-re-a
Hurler's dis-ease
Hutchinson's teeth
hy-a-lin
hy-a-lin-i-za-tion
hy-a-lin-o-sis
hy-a-li-nu-ri-a
hy-a-li-tis
hy-al-o-gen
hy-a-loid
Hy-a-lom-ma
hy-a-lo-mu-coid
hy-a-lo-plasm
hy-a-lu-ron-ic ac-id
hy-a-lu-ron-i-dase
hy-brid
hy-brid-i-za-tion
hy-dan-to-ic ac-id
hy-dan-to-in
hy-dat-id
hy-dat-id-i-form mole
hy-dat-i-do-sis
hy-dra-gog
hy-dram-ni-os
hy-drar-gyr-i-a
hy-drar-thro-sis
hy-drase
hy-dra-tion
hy-drate
hy-drau-lics
hy-dra-zine
hy-dre-mi-a
hy-dren-ceph-a-lo-cele

hy-dren-ceph-a-lo-me-
    nin-go-cele
hy-dride
hy-dri-od-ic ac-id
hy-dri-on
hy-dro-bro-mic ac-id
hy-dro-bro-mide
hy-dro-ca-lix
hy-dro-car-bon
hy-dro-cele
hy-dro-ce-lec-to-my
hy-dro-ceph-al-ic
hy-dro-ceph-a-lus
hy-dro-ceph-a-ly
hy-dro-chlo-ric ac-id
hy-dro-chlo-ride
hy-dro-chol-er-et-ic
hy-dro-col-loid
hy-dro-col-pos
hy-dro-cor-ti-sone
hy-dro-cy-an-ic ac-id
hy-dro-dex-tran
hy-dro-dy-nam-ics
hy-dro-flu-or-ic ac-id
hy-dro-gen
hy-dro-gen-a-tion
hy-dro-gen i-on
hy-dro-gen per-ox-ide
hy-dro-gen sul-fide
hy-dro-ki-net-ics
hy-drol
hy-dro-lac-tom-e-ter
hy-dro-lase
hy-drol-o-gy
hy-drol-y-sate
hy-drol-y-sis
hy-dro-lyst
hy-dro-lyte
hy-dro-lyt-ic
hy-dro-lyze
hy-drol-y-zate
hy-dro-ma

hy-dro-mas-sage
hy-dro-me-nin-go-cele
hy-drom-e-ter
hy-dro-met-ric
hy-dro-mi-cro-ceph-a-ly
hy-dro-my-e-li-a
hy-dro-my-e-lo-cele
hy-dro-my-rinx
hy-dro-ne-phro-sis
hy-dro-ni-um
hy-dro-nol
hy-dro-per-i-car-di-tis
hy-dro-per-i-car-di-um
hy-dro-per-i-on
hy-dro-per-i-to-ne-um
Hy-droph-i-dae
hy-dro-phil
hy-dro-phil-ic
hy-droph-i-lism
hy-droph-i-lous
hy-dro-pho-bi-a
hy-dro-pho-bic
hy-dro-phone
hy-droph-thal-mos
hy-dro-pneu-ma-to-sis
hy-dro-pneu-mo-per-i-car-di-um
hy-dro-pneu-mo-per-i-to-ne-um
hy-dro-pneu-mo-tho-rax
hy-drops
hy-dro-quin-ol
hy-dro-qui-none
hy-dror-rhe-a grav-i-dar-um
hy-dro-sal-pinx
hy-dro-sol
hy-dro-sol-u-ble
hy-dro-spi-rom-e-ter
hy-dro-stat
hy-dro-stat-ics
hy-dro-sul-fu-ric ac-id

hy-dro-sy-rin-go-my-e-li-a
hy-dro-tax-is
hy-dro-ther-a-peu-tics
hy-dro-ther-a-py
hy-dro-ther-mal
hy-dro-tho-rax
hy-dro-trop-ic
hy-drot-ro-pism
hy-dro-tym-pa-num
hy-dro—u-re-ter
hy-drous
hy-drcx-ide
hy-drox-y-ap-a-tite
hy-drox-y-ben-zo-ic ac-id
β—hy-drox-y-bu-try-ic ac-id
17—hy-drox-y-cor-ti-cos-te-rone
17—hy-drox-y—11—de-hy-dro-cor-ti-cos-ter-one
17—hy-drox-y—11—des-ox-y-cor-ti-cos-te-rone
hy-drox-yl
hy-drox-yl-a-mine
hy-drox-y-ly-sine
hy-drox-y-man-del-ic ac-id
hy-drox-y-pro-line
hy-drox-y-quin-o-line
hy-dru-ri-a
Hygeia
hy-giene
hy-gi-en-ist
hy-gric
hy-gro-ma
hy-grom-e-ter
hy-gro-met-ric
hy-gro-scope

hy-gro-scop-ic
hy-lo-trop-ic
hy-men
hy-me-nec-to-my
Hy-me-nol-e-pid-i-dae
Hy-me-nol-e-pis di-mi-nu-ta
Hy-me-nol-e-pis na-na
Hy-me-nop-ter-a
hy-me-not-o-my
hy-o-ep-i-glot-tic
hy-o-glos-sal
hy-o-glos-sus
hy-oid
hy-o-man-dib-u-lar
hy-os-cine
hy-os-cy-a-mine
hy-os-cy-a-mus
hy-o-thy-roid
hyp-a-cu-si-a
hyp-a-cu-sis
hyp-al-bu-min-o-sis
hyp-al-ge-si-a
hyp-am-ni-on
hy-pas-the-ni-a
hy-per-ab-duc-tion
hy-per-a-cid-i-ty
hy-per-ac-tiv-i-ty
hy-per-a-cu-i-ty
hy-per-a-cu-si-a
hy-per-a-dre-nal-cor-ti-cal-ism
hy-per-ad-re-nal-ism
hy-per-ad-re-no-cor-ti-cism
hy-per-al-ge-si-a
hy-per-al-i-men-ta-tion
hy-per-am-in-o-ac-id-u-ri-a
hy-per-am-ne-si-a
hy-per-az-o-te-mi-a
hy-per-az-o-tu-ri-a

147

hy-per-bar-ic
hy-per-bar-ism
hy-per-bil-i-ru-bi-ne-mi-a
hy-per-cal-ce-mi-a
hy-per-cal-ci-nu-ri-a
hy-per-cap-ni-a
hy-per-ca-thar-sis
hy-per-ca-thex-is
hy-per-ce-men-to-sis
hy-per-cham-aer-rhine
hy-per-chlo-re-mi-a
hy-per-chlor-hy-dri-a
hy-per-cho-les-ter-e-mi-a
hy-per-cho-les-ter-o-le-mi-a
hy-per-cho-li-a
hy-per-chro-mat-ic
hy-per-chro-ma-tism
hy-per-chro-ma-to-sis
hy-per-chro-mi-a
hy-per-chy-li-a
hy-per-cor-ti-cism
hy-per-dis-ten-tion
hy-per-dy-nam-ic
hy-per-em-e-sis
hy-per-em-e-sis grav-i-dar-um
hy-per-e-qui-lib-ri-um
hy-per-er-gi-a
hy-per-er-gy
hy-per-es-o-pho-ri-a
hy-per-es-the-si-a
hy-per-es-trin-ism
hy-per-es-tro-ge-ne-mi-a
hy-per-ex-o-pho-ri-a
hy-per-ex-ten-sion
hy-per-flex-ion
hy-per-func-tion
hy-per-gen-e-sis
hy-per-geu-si-a
hy-per-glob-u-li-ne-mi-a
hy-per-gly-ce-mi-a

hy-per-gly-co-ge-nol-y-sis
hy-per-gly-co-su-ri-a
hy-per-gon-ad-ism
hy-per-go-ni-a
hy-per-he-don-ism
hy-per-hi-dro-sis
hy-per-his-ta-mi-ne-mi-a
hy-per-hor-mo-nal
hy-per-i-no-sis
hy-per-in-su-lin-ism
hy-per-in-vo-lu-tion
hy-per-ka-le-mi-a
hy-per-ker-a-tin-i-za-tion
hy-per-ker-a-to-sis
hy-per-ke-to-nu-ri-a
hy-per-ki-ne-mi-a
hy-per-ki-ne-si-a
hy-per-ki-net-ic
hy-per-lac-ta-tion
hy-per-li-pe-mi-a
hy-per-lo-gi-a
hy-per-ma-ni-a
hy-per-man-ic
hy-per-mas-ti-a
hy-per-ma-ture
hy-per-men-or-rhe-a
hy-per-me-tro-pi-a
hy-per-mim-i-a
hy-per-mo-til-i-ty
hy-per-na-tre-mi-a
hy-per-ne-phro-ma
hy-per-nu-tri-tion
hy-per-o-nych-i-a
hy-per-or-tho-gna-thy
hy-per-os-mi-a
hy-per-os-mo-lar-i-ty
hy-per-os-te-og-e-ny
hy-per-os-to-sis
hy-per-ox-e-mi-a
hy-per-ox-y-gen-a-tion

hy-per-par-a-thy-roid-ism
hy-per-path-i-a
hy-per-per-i-stal-sis
hy-per-pha-gi-a
hy-per-pha-lan-gism
hy-per-pho-ne-sis
hy-per-pho-ni-a
hy-per-pho-ri-a
hy-per-phos-pha-te-mi-a
hy-per-phos-pha-tu-ri-a
hy-per-pig-men-ta-tion
hy-per-pi-tu-i-ta-rism
hy-per-pla-si-a
hy-per-plas-tic
hy-perp-ne-a
hy-per-po-ro-sis
hy-per-pot-as-se-mi-a
hy-per-pra-gi-a
hy-per-prax-i-a
hy-per-pres-by-o-pi-a
hy-per-pro-te-in-e-mi-a
hy-per-py-rex-i-a
hy-per-re-flex-i-a
hy-per-res-o-nance
hy-per-se-cre-tion
hy-per-sen-si-tiv-i-ty
hy-per-som-ni-a
hy-per-sple-nism
hy-per-sthe-ni-a
hy-per-sus-cep-ti-bil-i-ty
hy-per-syn-chro-ny
hy-per-tel-or-ism
hy-per-ten-sin
hy-per-ten-sin-ase
hy-per-ten-sin-o-gen
hy-per-ten-sion
hy-per-ten-sive car-di-o-vas-cu-lar dis-ease
hy-per-the-li-a
hy-per-ther-my
hy-per-thy-mi-a

hy-per-thy-roid-ism
hy-per-to-ni-a
hy-per-ton-ic
hy-per-tri-cho-sis
hy-per-tro-phy
hy-per-tro-pi-a
hy-per-u-ri-ce-mi-a
hy-per-vas-cu-lar
hy-per-veg-e-ta-tive
hy-per-ven-ti-la-tion
hy-per-vi-ta-min-o-sis
hy-per-vo-le-mi-a
hyp-es-the-si-a
hy-pha
hy-phe-ma
hy-phe-mi-a
hyp-hi-dro-sis
hyp-i-no-sis
hyp-na-gog-ic
hyp-na-gogue
hyp-nal-gi-a
hyp-nic
hyp-no-a-nal-y-sis
hyp-no-gen-ic
hyp-noid
hyp-no-lep-sy
hyp-nol-o-gy
hyp-no-nar-co-sis
hyp-no-pho-bi-a
hyp-no-phre-no-sis
hyp-no-pom-pic
hyp-no-si-gen-e-sis
hyp-no-sis
hyp-no-ther-a-py
hyp-not-ic
hyp-no-tism
hyp-no-tize
hy-po
hy-po-a-cid-i-ty
hy-po-ac-tiv-i-ty
hy-po-ad-re-nal-ism
hy-po-ad-re-ni-a

hy-po-al-bu-min-e-mi-a
hy-po-al-i-men-ta-tion
hy-po-al-ler-gen-ic
hy-po-az-o-tu-ri-a
hy-po-bar-ic
hy-po-bar-ism
hy-po-bran-chi-al
hy-po-bro-mite
hy-po-bro-mous ac-id
hy-po-bu-li-a
hy-po-cal-ce-mi-a
hy-po-cal-ci-fi-ca-tion
hy-po-cap-ni-a
hy-po-ca-thex-is
hy-po-chlo-re-mi-a
hy-po-chlor-hy-dri-a
hy-po-chlo-rite
hy-po-chlo-ri-za-tion
hy-po-chlo-rous ac-id
hy-po-chlor-u-ri-a
hy-po-cho-les-ter-e-mi-a
hy-po-chon-dri-a
hy-po-chon-dri-ac
hy-po-chon-dri-a-sis
hy-po-chon-dri-um
hy-po-chor-dal
hy-po-chro-mat-ic
hy-po-chro-mic
hy-po-chy-li-a
hy-po-cone
hy-po-con-id
hy-po-con-ule
hy-po-con-u-lid
hy-po-cy-clo-sis
Hy-po-der-ma
hy-po-der-ma-toc-ly-sis
hy-po-der-mi-a-sis
hy-po-der-mic
hy-po-der-mis
hy-po-der-moc-ly-sis
hy-po-don-ti-a
hy-po-er-gy

hy-po-es-o-pho-ri-a
hy-po-es-trin-ism
hy-po-ex-o-pho-ri-a
hy-po-fi-brin-o-gen-e-
    mi-a
hy-po-func-tion
hy-po-gas-tric
hy-po-gas-tri-um
hy-po-gen-i-tal-ism
hy-po-geu-si-a
hy-po-glos-sal
hy-po-glos-sus
hy-po-glot-tis
hy-po-gly-ce-mi-a
hy-po-gly-co-ge-nol-y-sis
hy-po-gnath-ous
hy-po-gon-ad-ism
hy-po-gran-u-lo-cy-to-sis
hy-po-hi-dro-sis
hy-po-in-su-lin-ism
hy-po-kal-i-e-mi-a
hy-po-ki-ne-si-a
hy-po-lem-mal
hy-po-ley-dig-ism
hy-po-lo-gi-a
hy-po-ma-ni-a
hy-po-ma-nic
hy-po-mas-ti-a
hy-po-men-or-rhe-a
hy-po-me-tab-o-lism
hy-po-me-tro-pi-a
hy-po-mi-cro-gnath-us
hy-po-mi-cron
hy-pom-ne-si-a
hy-po-mo-til-i-ty
hy-po-nat-re-mi-a
hy-po-no-ic
hy-po-nych-i-um
hy-po-os-to-sis
hy-po-par-a-thy-roid-ism
hy-po-per-me-a-bil-i-ty
hy-po-pha-lan-gism

hy-po-phar-yn-gos-co-py
hy-po-phar-ynx
hy-po-pho-ri-a
hy-po-phos-pha-te-mi-a
hy-po-phos-phite
hy-po-phos-pho-rous
   ac-id
hy-po-phre-ni-a
hy-poph-y-sec-to-mized
hy-poph-y-sec-to-my
hy-poph-y-sis
hy-po-pi-tu-i-ta-rism
hy-po-pla-si-a
hy-pop-nea
hy-po-pot-as-se-mi-a
hy-po-prax-i-a
hy-po-pro-sex-i-a
hy-po-pro-te-i-ne-mi-a
hy-po-pro-throm-bi-ne-
   mi-a
hy-po-py-on
hy-po-sal-i-va-tion
hy-o-scle-ral
hy-po-se-cre-tion
hy-po-sen-si-tiv-i-ty
hy-po-sen-si-ti-za-tion
hy-pos-mi-a
hy-po-som-ni-a
hy-po-spa-di-as
hy-po-sper-ma-to-gen-e-
   sis
hy-po-spray
hy-pos-ta-sis
hy-po-stat-ic
hy-pos-the-ni-a
hy-pos-the-nu-ri-a
hy-po-sul-fite
hy-po-tax-is
hy-po-tel-or-ism
hy-po-ten-sion
hy-po-ten-sor
hy-po-thal-am-ic

hy-po-thal-a-mus
hy-po-the-nar
hy-po-ther-mi-a
hy-poth-e-sis
hy-po-thy-roid-ism
hy-po-to-ni-a
hy-po-ton-ic
hy-po-tri-cho-sis
hy-po-tro-pi-a
hy-po-tym-pan-ic
hy-po-vi-ta-min-o-sis
hy-po-vo-le-mi-a
hy-po-xan-thine
hy-po-xan-thyl-ic ac-id
hy-pox-i-a
hyp-so-chro-mic ef-fect
hyp-so-pho-bi-a
hys-sop
hys-ter-al-gi-a
hys-ter-ec-to-my
hys-ter-e-sis
hys-te-ri-a
hys-ter-ics
hys-ter-i-form
hys-ter-o-cele
hys-ter-o-dyn-i-a
hys-ter-o-fren-ic
hys-ter-og-ra-phy
hys-ter-oid
hys-ter-o-lap-a-rot-o-my
hys-ter-ol-y-sis
hys-ter-o-my-o-ma
hys-ter-o-my-o-mec-
   to-my
hys-ter-o-my-ot-o-my
hys-ter-o—o-o-pho-rec-
   to-my
hys-ter-o-pex-y
hys-ter-o-plas-ty
hys-ter-op-to-sis
hys-ter-or-rha-phy
hys-ter-or-rhex-is

hys-ter-o-sal-pin-gec-to-
   my
hys-ter-o-sal-pin-gog-ra-
   phy
hys-ter-o-sal-pin-go—o-
   o-pho-rec-to-my
hys-ter-o-sal-pin-gos-to-
   my
hys-ter-os-cop-y
hys-ter-ot-o-my
hys-ter-o-tra-che-lec-to-
   my
hys-ter-o-tra-che-lo-
   plas-ty
hys-ter-o-tra-che-lor-rha-
   phy
hys-ter-o-tra-che-lot-
   o-my
hy-ther

I

i-at-ro-gen-ic
ice-land spar
ich-no-gram
i-chor
ich-tham-mol
ich-thy-ism
ich-thy-oid
ich-thy-oph-a-gous
ich-thy-o-sis
ich-thy-o-tox-in
i-con
i-co-nog-ra-phy
ic-ter-ic
ic-ter-o-gen-ic
ic-ter-oid
ic-ter-us
ic-ter-us in-dex
ic-ter-us ne-o-na-to-rum

ic-tus
id
i-de-a
i-de-al-i-za-tion
i-de-a-tion
i-den-ti-fi-ca-tion
id-e-o-ge-net-ic
id-e-ol-o-gy
id-e-o-pec-tis-tic
id-e-o-vas-cu-lar
id-i-o-chro-mo-some
id-i-oc-ra-sy
id-i-o-cy
id-i-o-gen-e-sis
id-i-o-glos-si-a
id-i-o-glot-tic
id-i-ol-o-gism
id-i-o-path-ic
id-i-op-a-thy
id-i-o-psy-chol-o-gy
id-i-o-re-flex
id-i-o-ret-i-nal
id-i-o-some
id-i-o-spasm
id-i-o-syn-cra-sy
id-i-o-syn-crat-ic
id-i-ot
id-i-o-ven-tric-u-lar
ig-ni-tion
il-e-ec-to-my
il-e-i-tis
il-e-o-ce-cos-to-my
il-e-o-ce-cum
il-e-o-col-ic
il-e-o-co-li-tis
il-e-o-co-los-to-my
il-e-o-il-e-os-to-my
il-e-o-sig-moid-os-to-my
il-e-os-to-my
il-e-ot-o-my
il-e-um
il-e-us

il-i-a
il-i-ac
i-li-a-cus
il-i-o-coc-cyg-e-al
il-i-o-coc-cyg-e-us
il-i-o-fem-o-ral
il-i-o-hy-po-gas-tric
il-i-o-in-gui-nal
il-i-o-pec-tin-e-al
il-i-o-pso-as
il-i-o-sac-ral-is
il-i-um
il-le-git-i-mate
il-le-git-i-ma-cy
il-li-ni-tion
il-lin-i-um
ill-ness
il-lu-mi-nance
il-lu-mi-na-tion
il-lu-mi-nism
il-lu-sion
i-ma
im-age
im-ag-i-na-tion
i-ma-go
im-a-zine
im-bal-ance
im-be-cile
im-be-cil-i-ty
im-bibe
im-bi-bi-tion
im-bri-ca-tion
im-id-az-ole
im-id-az-ole-py-ru-vic
  ac-id
im-ide
i-min-a-zole
i-mi-no ac-id
i-mi-no-glu-tar-ic ac-id
im-i-ta-tion
im-ma-ture
im-me-di-ate

im-med-i-ca-ble
im-mer-sion
im-mer-sion foot
im-mer-sion lens
im-mer-sion oil
im-mis-ci-ble
im-mo-bi-li-za-tion
im-mor-tal-i-ty
im-mune
im-mu-ni-ty
im-mu-ni-za-tion
im-mu-no-chem-is-try
im-mu-no-gen-ic
im-mu-no—he-ma-tol-o-gy
im-mu-nol-o-gist
im-mu-nol-o-gy
im-mu-no-ther-a-py
im-pac-tion
im-pal-pa-ble
im-par-i-dig-i-tate
im-passé
im-pe-dance
im-pe-din
im-per-a-tive
im-per-cep-tion
im-per-fo-rate
im-pe-ri-al green
im-per-me-a-ble
im-per-vi-ous
im-pe-tig-i-ni-za-tion
im-pe-ti-go
im-pe-ti-go cir-cin-at-a
im-pe-ti-go con-ta-gi-o-sa
im-pe-ti-go fol-li-cu-lar-
  is
im-pe-ti-go ne-o-na-
  to-rum
im-pin-ger
im-plan-ta-tion
im-plants
im-pon-der-able
im-po-tence

im-preg-nate
im-preg-na-tion
im-pres-sion
im-pulse
im-pul-sion
im-pu-ta-bil-i-ty
in-a-cid-i-ty
in-ac-ti-vate
in-ad-e-qua-cy
in-an-i-mate
in-a-ni-tion
in-ar-tic-u-late
in ar-tic-u-lo mor-tis
in-as-sim-i-la-ble
in-born
in-breed-ing
in-ca-nous
in-car-cer-at-ed
in-car-cer-a-tion
in-car-nant
in-car-na-tion
in-cest
in-ci-dence
in-ci-dent
in-cin-er-a-tion
in-cip-i-ent
in-ci-sal
in-cised
in-ci-sion
in-ci-sive
in-ci-sor
in-ci-su-ra
in-ci-sure
in-cli-na-tion
in-cli-nom-e-ter
in-co-ag-u-la-ble
in-co-her-ence
in-co-her-ent
in-com-bus-ti-ble
in-com-pat-i-ble
in-com-pat-i-bil-i-ty
in-com-pe-tence

in-com-pe-tent
in-con-gru-ence
in-con-gru-i-ty
in-con-ti-nence
in-co-or-di-na-tion
in-cor-po-ra-tion
in-cre-ment
in-cre-tin
in-cre-tion
in-crus-ta-tion
in-cu-ba-tion
in-cu-ba-tor
in-cu-dec-to-my
in-cu-do-mal-le-al
in-cu-do-sta-pe-di-al
in-cur-a-ble
in-cus
in-cy-clo-pho-ri-a
in-cy-clo-tro-pi-a
in-da-mine
in-de-cent
in-de-ci-sion
in-den-ta-tion
in-de-pend-ent
in-dex
in-di-can
in-di-cant
in-di-ca-nu-ri-a
in-di-ca-tion
in-di-ca-tor
in-di-ces
in-dif-fer-ent
in-dig-e-nous
in-di-ges-tion
in-dig-i-ta-tion
in-di-go
in-di-go-u-ri-a
in-di-rect
in-di-um
in-dol-ac-e-tu-ri-a
in-dole
in-dole-a-ce-tic ac-id

in-do-lent
in-dole-pro-pi-on-ic
    ac-id
in-dole-py-ru-vic ac-id
in-do-lu-ri-a
in-do-phe-nol
in-do-phe-nol ox-i-dase
in-dox-yl
in-dox-yl-glu-cu-ron-ic
    ac-id
in-dox-yl-u-ri-a
in-duc-tion
in-du-lin
in-du-ra-tion
in-du-si-um
in-e-bri-ant
in-e-bri-a-tion
in-e-bri-e-ty
in-ef-fi-ca-cy
in-er-ti-a
in ex-tre-mis
in-fan-cy
in-fant
in-fan-ti-cide
in-fan-tile
in-fan-ti-lism
in-farct
in-farc-tion
in-fec-tion
in-fe-cun-di-ty
in-fe-ri-or
in-fe-ri-or-i-ty
in-fer-til-i-ty
in-fes-ta-tion
in-fil-trate
in-fil-tra-tion
in-fin-i-ty
in-firm
in-fir-ma-ry
in-fir-mi-ty
in-flam-ma-tion
in-fla-tion

in-flec-tion
in-flu-en-za
in-fold
in-fra-car-di-ac
in-fra-cla-vic-u-lar
in-fra-cla-vic-u-lar-is
in-fra-cos-tal
in-frac-tion
in-fra-di-a-phrag-mat-ic
in-fra-glenoid
in-fra-hy-oid
in-fra-oc-clu-sion
in-fra-or-bit-al
in-fra-pa-tel-lar
in-fra-red
in-fra-scap-u-lar
in-fra-spi-na-tus
in-fra-spi-nous
in-fra-ster-nal
in-fra-tem-po-ra-le
in-fra-ten-to-ri-al
in-fra-troch-le-ar
in-fric-tion
in-fun-dib-u-li-form
in-fun-dib-u-lo-ma
in-fun-dib-u-lum
in-fu-sion
in-fu-so-ri-a
in-ges-ta
in-ges-tion
in-gra-ves-cent
in-gre-di-ent
in-guen
in-gui-nal
in-gui-no-scro-tal
in-ha-lant
in-ha-la-tion
in-ha-la-tor
in-ha-ler
in-her-ent
in-her-it-ance
in-her-it-ed

in-hib-in
in-hi-bi-tion
in-hib-i-tor
in-i-on
in-i-tial
in-ject
in-jec-tion
in-ju-ry
in-ju-ry po-ten-tial
in-lay
in-let
in-nate
in-ner-va-tion
in-no-cent
in-noc-u-ous
in-nom-i-nate
in-nox-ious
in-nom-i-nate
in-nox-ious
in-o-chon-dri-tis
in-oc-u-la-tion
in-oc-u-la-tor
in-oc-u-lum
in-op-er-a-ble
in-or-gan-ic
in-os-cu-la-tion
in-o-sine
in-o-sin-ic ac-id
in-o-si-tol
in-o-trop-ic
in-quest
in-qui-si-tion
in-sa-lu-bri-ous
in-sa-lu-bri-ty
in-san-i-tar-y
in-san-i-ty
in-scrip-tion
in-scrip-ti-o-nes
    ten-din-e-ae
in-sect
in-sec-ti-cide
in-sec-ti-fuge

in-se-cu-ri-ty
in-sem-i-na-tion
in-sen-si-ble
in-ser-tion
in-sheathed
in-sid-i-ous
in-sight
in-sip-id
in si-tu
in-so-la-tion
in-sol-u-bil-i-ty
in-sol-u-ble
in-spec-tion
in-spi-ra-tion
in-spi-ra-tor
in-spi-ra-to-ry
in-spire
in-spi-rom-e-ter
in-spis-sant
in-spis-sate
in-spis-sat-ed
in-sta-bil-i-ty
in-stance
in-step
in-stil-la-tion
in-stinct
in-stinc-tive
in-stru-ment
in-stru-men-ta-tion
in-suf-fi-cien-cy
in-suf-fla-tion
in-suf-fla-tor
in-su-la
in-su-lin
in-su-lin-e-mi-a
in-sult
in-sus-cep-ti-bil-i-ty
in-te-gra-tion
in-teg-u-ment
in-tel-lect
in-tel-li-gence quo-
    tient

in-tem-per-ance
in-tense
in-ten-si-fi-ca-tion
in-ten-sim-e-ter
in-ten-si-ty
in-ten-tion
in-ter-ac-i-nous
in-ter-al-ve-o-lar
in-ter-a-tri-al
in-ter-ca-la-ted
in-ter-cap-il-lar-y
    glo-mer-u-lo-scle-ro-sis
in-ter-car-pal
in-ter-cav-ern-ous
in-ter-cel-lu-lar
in-ter-con-dy-lar
in-ter-cos-tal
in-ter-cos-to-bra-chi-al
in-ter-coup-ler
in-ter-course
in-ter-cris-tal
in-ter-cru-ral
in-ter-cur-rent
in-ter-cusp-ing
in-ter-den-tal
in-ter-den-ti-um
in-ter-dic-tion
in-ter-dig-i-ta-tion
in-ter-face
in-ter-fere
in-ter-fer-ence
in-ter-fer-om-e-ter
in-ter-fer-om-e-try
in-ter-fi-bril-lar
in-ter-fol-lic-u-lar
in-ter-glob-u-lar
in-ter-go-ni-al
in-te-ri-or
in-ter-la-bi-al
in-ter-la-mel-lar
in-ter-lam-i-nar

in-ter-lin-gua
in-ter-lo-bar
in-ter-lob-u-lar
in-ter-mar-riage
in-ter-max-il-lar-y
in-ter-me-di-o-lat-er-al
in-ter-mem-bra-nous
in-ter-me-nin-ge-al
in-ter-men-stru-al
in-ter-ment
in-ter-mi-cel-lar flu-id
in-ter-mi-tot-ic
in-ter-mit-tent
in-ter-mu-ral
in-ter-mus-cu-lar
in-tern
in-ter-nal
in-ter-neu-ron
in-ter-nist
in-ter-no-dal
in-ter-nun-ci-al
in-ter-nus
in-ter-o-cep-tor
in-ter-o-fec-tive
in-ter-ol-i-var-y
in-ter-os-se-ous
in-ter-os-se-us
in-ter-pal-pe-bral
in-ter-pa-ri-e-tal
in-ter-pe-dun-cu-lar
in-ter-pha-lan-ge-al
in-ter-phase
in-ter-prox-i-mal
in-ter-prox-i-mate
in-ter-pu-pil-la-ry
    dis-tance
in-ter-sex
in-ter-space
in-ter-spi-nal-es
in-ter-spi-nous
in-ter-sti-ces
in-ter-sti-tial

in-ter-tar-sal
in-ter-trans-ver-sa-ri-i
in-ter-trans-verse
in-ter-tri-go
in-ter-tri-gi-nous
in-ter-tro-chan-ter-ic
in-ter-tu-bu-lar
in-ter-val
in-ter-vas-cu-lar
in-ter-ven-tric-u-lar
in-ter-ver-te-bral
in-ter-vil-lous
in-ter-zo-nal
in-tes-tine
in-tes-ti-num
in-ti-ma
in-toe-ing
in-tol-er-ance
in-tort-er
in-tox-i-cant
in-tox-i-ca-tion
in-tox-im-e-ter
in-tra-ab-dom-i-nal
in-tra-ac-i-nar
in-tra-ar-tic-u-lar
in-tra-a-tri-al
in-tra-cap-su-lar
in-tra-car-ti-lag-i-nous
in-tra-cav-i-ta-ry
in-tra-cel-lu-lar
in-tra-cra-ni-al
in-tra-cu-ta-ne-ous
in-tra-cys-tic
in-tra-der-mal
in-tra-du-ral
in-tra-fu-sal
in-tra-gem-mal
in-tra-he-pat-ic
in-tra-lo-bar
in-tra-lob-u-lar
in-tra-lu-mi-nal
in-tra-med-ul-lar-y

in-tra-mem-bra-nous
in-tra-mu-ral
in-tra-mus-cu-lar
in-tra-na-sal
in-tra-nu-cle-ar
in-tra-oc-u-lar
in-tra-o-ral
in-tra-or-bit-al
in-tra-pa-ri-e-tal
in-tra-pel-vic
in-tra-per-i-to-ne-al
in-tra-pleu-ral
in-tra-scro-tal
in-tra-spi-nal
in-tra-stro-mal
in-tra-the-cal
in-tra-tra-che-al
in-tra-tu-bal
in-tra-u-re-thral
in-tra-u-ter-ine
in-tra-vas-cu-lar
in-tra-ve-nous
in-tra-ven-tric-u-lar
in-tra-ves-i-cal
in-tra-vi-tal
in-trin-sic
in-tro-ces-sion
in-tro-flex-ion
in-tro-i-tus
in-tro-jec-tion
in-tro-mis-sion
in-tro-mit-tent
in-tro-spec-tion
in-tro-sus-cep-tion
in-tro-ver-sion
in-tro-vert
in-tu-ba-tion
in-tu-ba-tor
in-tu-mes-cence
in-tus-sus-cep-tion
in-u-lase
in-u-lin

in-unc-tion
in u-te-ro
in vac-u-o
in-vag-i-na-tion
in-va-lid
in-va-sion
in-ver-sion
in-vert
in-ver-tase
in-ver-te-bral
in-ver-te-bra-ta
in-ver-te-brate
in-vert sug-ar
in-vest-ing
in-vest-ment
in-vet-er-ate
in-vi-ril-i-ty
in vit-ro
in vi-vo
in-vol-un-tar-y
in-vo-lute
in-vo-lu-tion
in-vo-lu-tion-al
in-ward
i-o-da-moe-ba butsch-li-i
i-od-ic ac-id
i-o-dide
i-o-dine
i-o-dism
i-o-dized
i-o-do-a-ce-tic ac-id
i-o-do-der-ma
i-o-do-form
i-o-do-phthal-ein
so-di-um
i-o-do-thy-rine
i-o-do-thy-ro-glob-u-lin
i-on
i-o-ni-um
i-on-i-za-tion
i-on-om-e-ter
i-on-to-pho-re-sis

ip-e-cac
"i"—per-so-na
i-pro-ni-a-zid
ip-si-lat-er-al
i-ral-gi-a
i-ras-ci-bil-i-ty
i-ri-dal
ir-i-dal-gi-a
ir-i-dec-tome
ir-i-dec-to-mize
ir-i-dec-to-my
ir-i-dec-tro-pi-um
ir-i-den-tro-pi-um
ir-i-des-cence
i-rid-i-um
ir-i-di-za-tion
ir-i-do-cap-su-li-tis
ir-i-do-cap-su-lot-o-my
ir-i-do-cho-roid-i-tis
ir-i-do-cy-clec-to-my
ir-i-do-cy-cli-tis
ir-i-do-cy-clo-cho-roid-i-tis
ir-i-do-cys-tec-to-my
ir-i-do-di-al-y-sis
ir-i-do-pa-ral-y-sis
ir-i-do-ple-gi-a
ir-i-do-scle-rot-o-my
ir-i-do-tome
ir-i-dot-o-my
i-ris
i-rish moss
i-ri-tis
ir-i-to-ec-to-my
i-rit-o-my
i-ron
i-ron lung
i-rot-o-my
ir-ra-di-ate
ir-ra-di-a-ting
ir-ra-di-a-tion
ir-ra-tion-al

ir-re-du-ci-ble
ir-reg-u-lar-i-ty
ir-re-ver-si-ble
ir-ri-ga-tion
ir-ri-ga-tor
ir-ri-ta-bil-i-ty
ir-ri-ta-ble
ir-ri-tant
ir-ri-ta-tion
is-che-mi-a
is-chi-al-gi-a
is-chi-o-cap-su-lar
is-chi-o-cav-er-no-sus
is-chi-o-coc-cyg-e-us
is-chi-o-my-e-li-tis
is-chi-o-pu-bic
is-chi-o-rec-tal
is-chi-um
is-cho-ga-lac-tic
is-cho-me-ni-a
is-chu-ri-a
Ishihara col-or test
i-sin-glass
is-land
is-let
i-so-ag-glu-ti-nin
i-so-am-yl al-co-hol
i-so-an-ti-bod-ies
i-so-an-ti-gen
i-so-bar
i-so-bes-tic point
i-so-bu-tyl al-co-hol
i-so-cel-lu-lar
i-so-chor-ic
i-so-chro-mat-ic
i-so-chro-mat-o-phil
i-soch-ro-nal
i-so-chro-ni-a
i-so-cit-ric ac-id
i-so-co-ri-a
i-so-cor-tex
i-so-cy-a-nide

i-so-dac-ty-lism
i-so-dont
i-so-do-ses
i-so-dy-nam-ic
i-so-e-lec-tric
i-so-gam-ete
i-sog-a-mous
i-so-gen-e-sis
i-so-graft
i-so-he-mol-y-sin
i-so-he-mol-y-sis
i-so-hy-dric shift
i-so-i-co-ni-a
i-so-im-mu-ni-za-tion
i-so-i-on-ic point
i-so-la-tion
i-so-lec-i-thal
i-so-leu-cine
i-so-log
i-so-ly-ser-gic ac-id
i-so-mer
i-so-mer-ase
i-so-mer-ic
i-som-er-ism
i-so-met-ric
i-so-me-tro-pi-a
i-so-morph
i-so-mor-phic
i-so-ni-a-zid
i-so-os-mot-ic
i-so-phen-ic
i-so-pho-ri-a
i-so-pi-a
i-so-plas-tic
i-so-pre-cip-i-tin
i-so-prene
i-so-pro-pa-nol
i-so-pro-pyl al-co-hol
i-so-pro-pyl-ar-ter-e-nol
i-sop-ters
i-so-scope
i-so-ser-ine

i-sos-po-ra hom-i-nis
i-so-therm
i-so-ther-mal
i-so-ton-ic
i-so-tope
is-sue
isth-mus
itch
itch-ing
itch mite
i-ter
i-vo-ry
ix-o-des
ix-od-i-dae

J

jack bean
jack-et
jack-screw
Jacksonian ep-i-lep-sy
jac-ti-ta-tion
jac-u-lif-er-ous
Jaeger's test types
Jaffé's test
jal-ap
Janeway's nodes
Ja-nus green B
Ja-pan wax
ja-ra-ra-ca
Jarcho's press-o-me-ter
jar-gon
jar-gon-ize
Jarisch—Herxheimer re-
    ac-tion
Jarvis' snare
jaun-dice
jej-u-nec-to-my
jej-u-ni-tis
jej-u-no-ce-cos-to-my

156

jej-u-no-co-los-to-my
jej-u-no-gas-tric
jej-u-no-il-e-i-tis
jej-u-no-il-e-os-to-my
jej-u-no-il-e-um
jej-u-no-jej-u-nos-to-my
jej-u-nor-rha-phy
jej-u-nos-to-my
jej-u-not-o-my
je-ju-num
jel-ly
jel-ly boot
jerk
Jes-u-its' bal-sam
Jim-son weed
jock-ey strap
joh-nin
joint
joint fu-sion
joint mouse
Jolly bod-ies
Jones splint
joule
judg-ment
ju-do
ju-gal
jug-u-lar
juice
ju-jit-su
ju-jube
ju-men-tous
junc-tion
junc-tu-ra
jung-le rot
ju-ni-per oil
ju-ris-pru-dence
ju-ry
jury mast
jus-to-ma-jor
jus-to mi-nor
jute
ju-ve-nile

jux-ta—ar-tic-u-lar
jux-ta-glo-mer-u-lar
jux-ta-po-si-tion
jux-ta-py-lor-ic

K

Kahn test
kai-no-pho-bi-a
kak-or-rhaph-i-o-pho-bi-a
ka-la-a-zar
ka-le-mi-a
kal-li-kre-in
Kammerer—Battle in-ci-
    sion
Kan-da-har sore
kan-ga-roo ten-don
ka-o-lin
ka-o-li-no-sis
Kaposi's sar-co-ma
ka-ra-ya gum
Karell di-et
ka-ry-en-chy-ma
ka-ry-o-blast
ka-ry-o-chrome
ka-ry-o-cyte
ka-ry-og-am-ic
ka-ry-o-ki-ne-sis
ka-ry-o-lo-bic
ka-ry-o-lymph
ka-ry-ol-y-sis
ka-ry-o-mere
ka-ry-o-mi-to-sis
ka-ry-o-phage
ka-ry-o-some
ka-ry-os-ta-sis
kar-y-o-type
kat-a-did-y-mus
kat-a-ther-mom-e-ter
Kat-a-ya-ma

ka-va
ka-wine
keep-er
kef-ir
Kelly's for-ceps
ke-loid
kelp
Kelso test
kel-vin
Kel-vin scale
ke-nes-the-si-a
Kenny treat-ment
ken-o-pho-bi-a
Kent, bun-dle of
ker-a-sin
ker-a-tal-gi-a
ker-a-tec-ta-si-a
ker-a-tec-to-my
ker-a-tin
ker-a-tin-i-za-tion
ke-rat-i-nous
ker-a-ti-tis bul-lo-sa
ker-a-ti-tis dis-ci-form-is
ker-a-ti-tis hy-po-py-on
ker-a-ti-tis neu-ro-par-
    a-lyt-i-ca
ker-a-ti-tis punc-ta-ta
ker-a-ti-tis ro-sa-ce-a
ker-a-to-ac-an-tho-ma
ker-a-to-cele
ker-a-to-cen-te-sis
ker-a-to-chro-ma-to-sis
ker-a-to-con-junc-ti-vi-
    tis
ker-a-to-co-nus
ker-a-to-der-ma
ker-a-to-gen-e-sis
ker-a-to-glo-bus
ker-a-to-hel-co-sis
ker-a-to-hy-a-lin
ker-a-toid
ker-a-to-i-ri-tis

157

ker-a-to-leu-ko-ma
ker-a-tol-y-sis
ker-a-to-lyt-ic
ker-a-to-ma
ker-a-to-ma-la-ci-a
ker-a-tome
ker-a-tom-e-ter
ker-a-to-my-co-sis
ker-a-to-nyx-is
ker-a-to-plas-ty
ker-a-tor-rhex-is
ker-a-to-scle-ri-tis
ker-a-to-scope
ker-a-tos-co-py
ker-a-tose
ker-a-to-sis
ker-a-to-sis fol-li-cu-
    lar-is
ker-a-to-sis punc-ta-ta
ker-a-to-sis seb-or-rhei-
    ca
ker-a-to-sis se-ni-lis
ker-a-tot-o-my
ke-rau-no-pho-bi-a
ke-ri-on cel-si
ker-nic-ter-us
Kernig's sign
ker-o-sene
ke-tene
ke-to ac-id
ke-to-a-dip-ic ac-id
ke-to-gen-e-sis
ke-to-glu-tar-ic ac-id
ke-to-hep-tose
ke-to-hex-ose
ke-tol
ke-tol-y-sis
ke-to-lyt-ic
ke-tone
ke-to-ne-mi-a
ke-to-nu-ri-a
ke-to-re-duc-tase

ke-tose
ke-to-side
ke-to-sis
ke-to-ster-oid
kid-ney
Kielland's for-ceps
Kienbock's dis-ease
Kiesselbach's tri-an-gle
Kiliani's re-ac-tion
kil-o-cal-o-rie
kil-o-gram
kil-o-gram—me-ter
kil-o-joule
kil-o-li-ter
kil-o-me-ter
kil-o-nem
kil-o-volt
kil-o-watt
Kimmelstiel—Wilson
    syn-drome
ki-nase
kin-e-ma-di-ag-ra-phy
kin-e-mat-ics
kin-e-mat-o-graph
kin-e-ra-di-o-ther-a-py
kin-e-scope
ki-ne-si-at-rics
ki-ne-si-es-the-si-om-
    e-ter
kin-e-sim-e-ter
ki-ne-si-ol-o-gy
ki-ne-si-om-e-ter
ki-ne-sis
ki-ne-sis par-a-dox-a
ki-ne-si-ther-a-py
kin-es-the-si-a
kin-es-the-si-om-e-ter
kin-es-thet-ic
ki-net-ic
ki-net-ics
ki-ne-to-chore
ki-ne-to-plast

king's yel-low
ki-no-cen-trum
ki-o-tome
ki-ot-o-my
Kirschner's wires
Kjeldahl meth-od
Klebs—Loeffler ba-cil-
    lus
Kleb-si-el-la pneu-mo-
    ni-ae
klep-to-ma-ni-a
Kline test
Klippel—Feil syn-drome
knead-ing
knee
knee-cap
knee—jerk
knee—sprung
knife
knit-ting
knob
knock—knee
knot
knuck-le
Koch's pos-tu-late
Kohler's dis-ease
koi-lo-nych-i-a
Kojewnikoff's ep-i-lep-sy
ko-la
Kolmer's test
ko-ni-me-ter
ko-ni-o-cor-tex
Koplik's spots
Korsakov's psy-cho-sis
kra-tom-e-ter
krau-ro-sis
Krebs cy-cle
kre-o-tox-ism
Krukenberg tu-mor
kryp-ton
Kupffer cells
Kurlov bod-ies

158

Kussmaul's res-pir-a-tion
kwash-i-or-kor
ky-mo-gram
ky-mo-graph
ky-mog-ra-phy
ky-pho-ra-chi-tis
ky-pho-sco-li-o-ra-chi-
   tis
ky-pho-sco-li-o-sis
ky-pho-sis

L

la-bi-a
la-bile
la-bil-i-ty
la-bi-o-al-ve-o-lar
la-bi-o-cer-vi-cal
la-bi-o-den-tal
la-bi-o-gin-gi-val
la-bi-o-glos-so-la-ryn-
   ge-al
la-bi-o-gres-sion
la-bi-o-men-tal
la-bi-o-pal-a-tine
la-bi-o-plas-ty
la-bi-um
la-bor
lab-o-ra-to-ry
la-brum
lab-y-rinth
lab-y-rin-thec-to-my
lab-y-rin-thi-tis
lab-y-rin-thot-o-my
lac-er-at-ed
lac-er-a-tion
la-cer-tus
Lach-e-sis mu-tus
lach-ry-mal
la-cin-i-ate

lac-ri-mal
lac-ri-ma-tion
lac-ri-ma-tor
lac-ri-mo-tome
lac-ri-mot-o-my
lac-ta-gogue
lac-tal-bu-min
lac-tam
lac-tam-ide
lac-tase
lac-tate
lac-ta-tion
lac-te-al
lac-tes-cence
lac-tic
lac-tide
lac-tif-er-ous
lac-ti-fuge
lac-tig-e-nous
lac-tim
lac-tiv-o-rous
Lac-to-ba-cil-lus
   a-cid-o-phil-us
lac-to-crit
lac-to-gen
lac-to-gen-ic
lac-to-glob-u-lin
lac-tom-e-ter
lac-tone
lac-to-per-ox-i-dase
lac-to-phos-phate
lac-to-pro-te-in
lac-tor-rhe-a
lac-to-sa-zone
lac-tose
lac-to-su-ri-a
lac-tyl
la-cu-na
la-cu-nu-la
Laennec's cir-rho-sis
lag
la-ge-na

la-ge-ni-form
lag-oph-thal-mos
la grippe
la-i-ty
lake
la-ky
lal-la-tion
lal-og-no-sis
la-lop-a-thy
lal-o-pho-mi-a-trist
lal-or-rhe-a
lamb-da
lamb-doid
lam-bert
lam-bli-a-sis
la-mel-la
la-mel-lar
lame-ness
lam-i-na
lam-i-na-gram
lam-i-nat-ed
lam-i-na-tion
lam-i-nec-to-my
lam-i-nog-ra-phy
lam-i-not-o-my
lamp
lamp-black
la-na
lan-a-to-side
lance
lan-cet
lan-ci-na-ting
land-marks
Landolt ring
Landouzy—Dejerine at-
   ro-phy
Landry's pa-ral-y-sis
Landsteiner clas-si-fi-
   ca-tion
Langerhans, is-lets of
lan-guor
lan-o-ce-ric ac-id

lan-o-lin
lan-os-ter-ol
lan-tha-nide
lan-tha-num
lan-thi-o-nine
la-nu-go
lan-u-lous
la-pac-tic
lap-a-rot-o-my
lap-a-ro-tra-che-lot-o-my
la-pis
lap-sus
lard
lar-da-ceous
lark-spur
lar-va
lar-va mi-grans
lar-val
lar-vate
lar-vi-cide
lar-yn-gal-gi-a
la-ryn-ge-al cri-sis
lar-yn-gec-to-my
lar-yn-gis-mus
lar-yn-gi-tis
la-ryn-go-cele
lar-yn-gol-o-gist
lar-yn-gol-o-gy
la-ryn-go-pa-ral-y-sis
lar-yn-gop-a-thy
la-ryn-go-pha-ryn-ge-al
la-ryn-go-phar-yn-gec-to-my
la-ryn-go-pha-ryn-ge-us
la-ryn-go-phar-yn-gi-tis
la-ryn-go-phar-ynx
la-ryn-go-plas-ty
la-ryn-go-ple-gi-a
la-ryn-go-rhi-nol-o-gy
la-ryn-go-scope
lar-yn-gos-co-pist

lar-yn-gos-co-py
la-ryn-go-spasm
la-ryn-go-ste-no-sis
lar-yn-gos-to-my
la-ryn-go-stro-bo-scope
la-ryn-go-syr-inx
lar-yn-got-o-my
la-ryn-go-tra-che-al
la-ryn-go-tra-che-i-tis
la-ryn-go-tra-che-o-bron-chi-tis
la-ryn-go-tra-che-os-co-py
la-ryn-go-tra-che-ot-o-my
la-ryn-go-xe-ro-sis
lar-ynx
las-civ-i-ous
Lasegue's sign
lash
Lassar's paste
las-si-tude
la-tent
lat-er-ad
lat-er-al
lat-er-i-tious
lat-er-o-ab-dom-i-nal
lat-er-o-duc-tion
lat-er-o-flex-ion
lat-er-o-mar-gin-al
lat-er-o-pul-sion
lat-er-o-tor-sion
lat-er-o-ver-sion
la-tex
la-tis-si-mus dor-si
la-trine
Lat-ro-dec-tus mac-tans
la-tus
laud-a-ble
lau-da-num
laugh
Laughlen test

laugh-ter
Launois—Cléret syn-drome
Laurence—Moon—Biedl syn-drome
lau-ric ac-id
la-vage
la-va-tion
lav-en-der
lax-a-tive
lax-i-ty
lay-er
lay-ette
lay-man
la-zar
laz-a-ret-to
leach-ing
lead
lead-er
lead poi-son-ing
leaf
lec-i-thal
lec-ith-al-bu-min
lec-i-thin
lec-i-thi-nase
lec-i-tho-blast
lec-i-tho-pro-te-in
lec-i-tho-vi-tel-lin
lec-tin
Lederer's a-ne-mi-a
Leduc's cur-rent
Lee—White meth-od
leech
left—hand-ed
Legg—Calvé—Perthes dis-ease
le-git-i-ma-cy
le-gu-me-lin
le-gu-min
Leiner's dis-ease
lei-o-der-mi-a
lei-o-my-o-fi-bro-ma

lei-o-my-o-ma
lei-o-my-o-sar-co-ma
lei-ot-ri-chous
lei-po-me-ri-a
Leishman—Donovan bod-ies
Leish-ma-ni-a
leish-man-i-a-sis
le-ma
Lembert's su-ture
lem-mo-cyte
lem-nis-cus
lem-no-blast
lem-on
le-mo-pa-ral-y-sis
le-mo-ste-no-sis
Lempert's op-er-a-tion
len-i-ceps
len-i-tive
lens-om-e-ter
len-ti-co-nus
len-tic-u-lar
len-tic-u-late
len-tic-u-lo-stri-ate
len-tic-u-lo-tha-lam-ic
len-ti-form
len-tig-i-nous
len-ti-go
le-on-ti-a-sis
lep-er
Lep-i-dop-ter-a
lep-o-thrix
lep-rid
lep-rol-o-gist
lep-rol-o-gy
lep-ro-ma
lep-ro-pho-bi-a
lep-ro-sar-i-um
lep-ro-sy
lep-ro-tene
lep-rous
lep-to-ce-pha-li-a

lep-to-ceph-a-lus
lep-to-chro-mat-ic
lep-to-cyte
lep-to-cy-tic
lep-to-cy-to-sis
lep-to-dac-ty-lous
lep-to-don-tous
lep-to-me-nin-ges
lep-to-me-nin-gi-o-ma
lep-to-men-in-gi-tis
lep-to-men-in-gop-a-thy
lep-to-me-ninx
lep-to-mi-cro-gnath-i-a
Lep-to-mi-cru-rus
Lep-to-mo-nas
lep-ton
lep-to-pel-lic
lep-to-pho-ni-a
lep-to-pro-so-pi-a
lep-tor-rhine
lep-to-scope
Lep-to-spi-ra au-tumn-al-is
Lep-to-spi-ra ic-ter-o-haem-or-rha-gi-ae
lep-to-spi-ro-sis
lep-to-tene
Lep-to-thrix buc-cal-is
lep-to-tri-cho-sis
Les-bi-an-ism
le-sion
le-thal
leth-ar-gy
Letterer—Siwe dis-ease
leu-cine
leu-ci-no-sis
leu-ci-nu-ri-a
leu-co-fla-vin
leu-co-ma-ine
Leu-co-nos-toc
leu-co-ri-bo-fla-vin
leu-co-sin

leu-co-tax-in
leu-ka-ne-mi-a
leu-ke-mi-a
leu-kem-id
leu-ke-moid
leu-ko-blast
leu-ko-blas-to-sis
leu-ko-ci-din
leu-ko-cyte
leu-ko-cy-the-mi-a
leu-ko-cy-to-blast
leu-ko-cy-to-gen-e-sis
leu-ko-cy-to-ly-sin
leu-ko-cy-tol-y-sis
leu-ko-cy-to-ma
leu-ko-cy-tom-e-ter
leu-ko-cy-to-pe-ni-a
leu-ko-cy-to-poi-e-sis
leu-ko-cy-to-sis
leu-ko-der-ma
leu-ko-ma
leu-ko-nych-i-a
leu-kop-a-thy
leu-ko-pe-de-sis
leu-ko-pe-ni-a
leu-ko-pla-ki-a
leu-ko-pro-te-ase
leu-kop-sin
leu-kor-rha-gi-a
leu-kor-rhe-a
leu-ko-sar-co-ma
leu-ko-sar-co-ma-to-sis
leu-ko-tome
leu-kot-o-my
leu-ko-tox-ic
leu-ko-trich-i-a
lev-an
le-va-tor
le-va-tor a-ni
le-va-tor pal-pe-brae su-pe-ri-or-is
le-va-tor scap-u-lae

le-va-tor ve-li pal-a-
    tin-i
lev-i-ga-tion
Levin tube
lev-i-ta-tion
le-vo-duc-tion
le-vo-ro-ta-tion
le-vo-ro-ta-to-ry
le-vo-tar-tar-ic ac-id
lev-u-lin
lev-u-lo-san
lev-u-lose
lev-u-lo-su-ri-a
Lévy—Roussy syn-drome
lew-is-ite
Leyden's a-tax-i-a
Layden jar
Leydig cells
lib-er-a-tion
li-bi-do
li-bra
lice
li-cense
li-cen-ti-ate
li-chen
li-chen chron-ic-us
    sim-plex
li-chen pla-nus
li-chen spin-u-lo-sus
li-chen-if-i-ca-tion
li-chen-i-za-tion
lic-o-rice
lid lag
li-en
li-e-ni-tis
li-e-no-cele
li-en-og-ra-phy
li-e-no-re-nal
li-en-un-cu-lus
life ex-pec-tan-cy
lig-a-ment
lig-a-men-tous

lig-a-men-to-pex-y
lig-a-men-tum
lig-a-men-tum ar-te-ri-
    o-sum
lig-a-men-tum fla-vum
lig-a-men-tum te-res
    u-ter-i
lig-a-men-tum tes-tis
lig-a-men-tum ve-no-sum
li-gate
li-ga-tion
lig-a-ture
light
light-en-ing
light-ning pains
lig-ne-ous
lig-nin
lig-num
lig-ro-in
Lilienthal's op-er-a-tion
limb
lim-ber-neck
lim-bus
lime milk
lime wa-ter
li-men
li-mes death
li-mes ze-ro
lim-i-na
lim-i-nal
lim-i-troph-ic
Lim-na-tis ni-lo-ti-ca
lim-nol-o-gy
lim-o-nene
li-mo-nite
li-moph-thi-sis
limp
lin-al-o-ol
lin-a-ma-rin
lin-dane
Lindau's tu-mor
Lindberg flask

line of de-mar-ca-tion
line of fix-a-tion
line of oc-clu-sion
line of sight
lin-e-a
lin-e-a al-ba
line-a lin-e-ae al-bi-
    can-tes
lin-e-a lin-e-ae grav-
    i-dar-um
lin-e-a ni-gra
lin-e-ar-cor-re-la-tion
lin-gua
lin-gua ni-gra
lin-gua pli-ca-ta
lin-gual
lin-gu-la
lin-guo-dis-tal
lin-guo-gin-gi-val
lin-i-ment
li-nin
li-ni-tis plas-ti-ca
link-age
lin-o-le-ic ac-id
lin-o-le-nic ac-id
li-no-lic ac-id
lin-seed oil
lint
lin-tin
li-pa
lip-a-ro-trich-i-a
lip-a-rous
li-pase
lip-a-su-ri-a
lip-ec-to-my
li-pe-mi-a
li-pem-ic
lip-fan-o-gen
lip-id
lip-i-do-sis
li-pin
lip-o-blast

162

lip-o-blas-to-ma
lip-o-blas-to-sis
lip-o-ca-ic
lip-o-cal-ci-no-gran-u-lo-
  ma-to-sis
lip-o-chon-dro-dys-
  tro-phy
lip-o-chon-dro-ma
lip-o-chrome
lip-o-cyte
lip-o-dys-tro-phy
lip-o-fi-bro-ma
lip-o-fi-bro-myx-o-ma
lip-o-fi-bro-sar-co-ma
lip-o-fus-cin
lip-o-gen-e-sis
li-pog-e-nous
lip-o-gran-u-lo-ma
lip-o-gran-u-lo-ma-to-sis
lip-o-he-mar-thro-sis
lip-o-ic ac-id
lip-oid
lip-oi-do-sis
li-pol-y-sis
li-po-ma
li-po-ma-to-sis
lip-o-me-tab-o-lism
lip-o-my-o-ma
lip-o-my-o-sar-co-ma
lip-o-myx-o-ma
Lip-o-nys-sus bac-o-ti
lip-o-pe-ni-a
lip-o-pep-tide
lip-o-pha-gic
lip-o-phil
lip-o-phil-i-a
lip-o-phre-ni-a
lip-o-pro-te-in
lip-o-rho-din
lip-o-sar-co-ma
li-po-sis
lip-o-sol-u-ble

lip-o-thi-am-ide py-ro-
  phos-phate
lip-o-tro-pic
lip-o-vac-cine
lip-o-vi-tel-lin
lip-o-xan-thin
li-pox-e-nous
li-pox-i-dase
lip-ping
lip-pi-tu-do
lip read-ing
li-pu-ri-a
liq-ue-fac-tion
liq-uid
liq-uo-gel
liq-uor
liq-uor am-ni-i
liq-uor fol-li-cu-li
Lisfranc's am-pu-ta-tion
lisp
Lissauer's tract
lis-sen-ceph-a-lous
Lis-te-ri-a mon-o-cy-to-
  genes
li-ter
lith-arge
lith-ec-to-my
li-the-mi-a
lith-i-a
li-thi-a-sis
lith-ic ac-id
lith-i-co-sis
lith-i-um
lith-o-chol-ic ac-id
lith-o-di-al-y-sis
lith-o-gen-e-sis
lith-oid
lith-o-kel-y-pho-pe-di-on
lith-o-ne-phri-tis
lith-o-ne-phrot-o-my
lith-o-pe-di-on
li-thot-o-my

lith-o-trip-sy
lith-o-trite
li-thox-y-du-ri-a
lith-u-re-sis
li-thu-ri-a
lit-mus
lit-ter
Little's dis-ease
Littre's glands
li-ve-do-re-tic-u-lar-is
liv-er
liv-er ex-tract
liv-er fluke
liv-er in-jec-tion
liv-er spot
liv-er-wort
liv-e-tin
liv-id
li-vid-i-ty
Livierato's sign
li-vor mor-tis
Lo-a lo-a
lo-a-i-a-sis
lo-bar
lo-bate
lobe
lo-bec-to-my
lo-be-line
lo-bot-o-my
lob-ster—claw
lob-ule
lob-u-lus
lo-bus
lo-cal
lo-cal-i-za-tion
lo-cal-ized
lo-cal-i-zer
lo-chi-a
lo-chi-a al-ba
lo-chi-a ru-bra
lo-chi-o-me-tra
lo-chi-o-me-tri-tis

lo-chi-or-rhe-a
lo-cho-me-tri-tis
lo-ci
Locke—Ringer's so-lu-
    tion
lock-jaw
lo-co dis-ease
lo-co-mo-tion
lo-co weed
loc-u-lat-ed
loc-u-la-tion
loc-u-lus
lo-cum-te-nens
lo-cus
Loeffler's syn-drome
Loef-fler-el-la mal-le-i
Loewenberg's for-ceps
log-a-do-blen-nor-rhe-a
log-ag-no-sis
log-a-graph-i-a
log-am-ne-si-a
log-a-pha-si-a
log-o-ko-pho-sis
log-o-ma-ni-a
log-op-a-thy
log-o-pe-dics
log-o-pha-si-a
log-o-ple-gi-a
log-or-rhe-a
lo-i-a-sis
loin
lon-gev-i-ty
long-ing
lon-gis-si-mus
lon-gi-tu-di-nal
lon-gus
loop
loop of Henle
loose
loose-ness
lo-pho-dont
lo-phoph-o-rine

lo-quac-i-ty
Lorain dwarf-ism
lor-do-sis
lo-ri-ca
lo-ti-o
lo-tion
Lo-tus
lo-tus-in
loupe
loup-ing ill
louse
lous-y
Lowenstein's me-di-um
lox-ot-ic
loz-enge
lu-can-thone
lu-cid
lu-cid-i-ty
lu-ci-dum
lu-cif-er-ase
lu-cif-er-in
lu-cite
Ludwig's an-gi-na
lu-es
lu-et-ic
lu-e-tin
Lugol's so-lu-tion
luke-warm
lum-ba-go
lum-bar
lum-bar-i-za-tion
lum-bo-co-los-to-my
lum-bo-co-lot-o-my
lum-bo-cos-tal
lum-bo-dor-sal
lum-bo-in-gui-nal
lum-bo-is-chi-al
lum-bo-sa-cral
lum-bri-cal
Lum-bri-cus
lu-men
lu-mi-chrome

lu-mi-fla-vin
lu-mi-nance
lu-mi-nes-cence
lu-mi-nif-er-ous
lu-mi-nos-i-ty
lump
lump-y jaw
lu-na-cy
lu-nar
lu-nar caus-tic
lu-nate
lu-na-tic
lung
lung-wort
lu-nu-la
lu-pine
lu-po-ma
lu-pus
lu-pus er-y-the-ma-to-
    sus
lu-pus per-ni-o
lu-pus vul-gar-is
Luschka's for-a-men
Lusk's con-trac-tion
    ring
lu-sus na-tu-rae
lute
lu-te-al
lu-te-in
Lutembacher's com-plex
lu-te-o-blas-to-ma
lu-te-o-lin
lu-te-o-ma
lu-te-ti-um
lu-ti-din
lux-a-tion
lux-u-ri-ant
lux-us
ly-can-thro-py
ly-cine
ly-co-pene
ly-co-po-di-um

164

ly-co-rex-i-a
lye
ly-go-phil-i-a
ly-ing—in
lymph
lymph fol-li-cle
lymph nodes
lym-phad-e-nec-to-my
lym-phad-e-ni-tis
lym-phad-e-no-ma
lym-phad-e-no-ma-to-sis
lym-phad-e-nop-a-thy
lym-pha-gogue
lym-phan-gi-ec-ta-sis
lym-phan-gi-ec-to-my
lym-phan-gi-o-en-do-the-
  li-o-ma
lym-phan-gi-o-ma
lym-phan-gi-o-sar-co-ma
lym-phan-gi-ot-o-my
lym-phan-gi-tis
lym-phat-ic
lym-pho-blast
lym-pho-blas-to-ma
lym-pho-cyte
lym-pho-cy-the-mi-a
lym-pho-cy-to-ma
lym-pho-cy-to-pe-ni-a
lym-pho-cy-to-poi-e-sis
lym-pho-cy-to-sis
lym-pho-der-mi-a
lym-pho-ep-i-the-li-o-ma
lym-phog-en-ous
lym-pho-go-ni-a
lym-pho-gran-u-lo-ma
lym-pho-gran-u-lo-ma
  in-gui-nale
lym-pho-gran-u-lo-ma
  ve-ne-re-um
lym-pho-gran-u-lo-ma-
  to-sis
lym-pho-ken-tric ac-id

lym-pho-ma
lym-pho-ma-to-sis
lym-pho-path-i-a ve-ne-
  re-um
lym-pho-pe-ni-a
lym-pho-poi-e-sis
lym-pho-pro-te-ase
lym-pho-re-tic-u-lo-ma
lym-pho-re-tic-u-lo-sis
lym-phor-rhage
lym-phor-rhe-a
lym-pho-sar-co-ma
lym-pho-sar-co-ma-to-sis
lym-phu-ri-a
ly-o-gel
ly-o-gly-co-gen
ly-o-phile
ly-o-phil-ic
ly-o-phil-i-za-tion
ly-o-phil-i-zed
ly-o-phobe
ly-o-pho-bic
ly-o-sol
ly-o-sorp-tion
ly-o-trop-ic
lyse
ly-ser-gic ac-id
ly-sim-e-ter
ly-sin
ly-sine
ly-sis
ly-tic
ly-so-ceph-a-lin
ly-so-gen-ic
ly-so-lec-i-thin
ly-so-zyme
ly-so-zy-mu-ri-a
lys-sic
lys-soid
Lyt-ta ves-i-ca-to-ri-a
ly-xo-fla-vin
lyx-ose

M

McBurney's in-ci-sion
McClintock's sign
mace
mac-er-ate
mac-er-a-tion
mac-er-a-ter
Macewen's sign
Mache u-nit
mac-ra-cu-si-a
mac-ren-ce-phal-ic
mac-ren-ceph-a-ly
mac-ro-bac-ter-ri-um
mac-ro-ble-phar-i-a
mac-ro-bra-chi-a
mac-ro-ceph-a-lous
mac-ro-chei-li-a
mac-ro-chei-ri-a
mac-ro-cyte
mac-ro-cyt-ic
mac-ro-cy-to-sis
mac-ro-dac-ty-ly
mac-ro-don-ti-a
mac-ro-gam-ete
mac-ro-ga-me-to-cyte
mac-ro-glob-u-lin-e-mi-a
mac-ro-glos-si-a
mac-ro-gnath-ic
mac-ro-gy-ri-a
mac-ro-lymph-o-cyte
mac-ro-mas-ti-a
mac-ro-me-li-a
mac-ro-mer-o-zo-ite
mac-ro-mo-lec-u-lar
mac-ro-mon-o-cyte
mac-ro-my-e-lo-blast
mac-ro-nor-mo-blast
mac-ro-nu-cle-us
mac-ro-phage
mac-ro-po-di-a

mac-ro-pol-y-cytes
ma-crop-si-a
mac-ro-scop-ic
mac-ro-so-mi-a
mac-ro-spore
mac-ro-sto-mi-a
ma-cro-ti-a
mac-u-la
mac-ule
mac-u-lo-pap-u-lar
mad-a-ro-sis
Maddox rod
Madelung's de-form-i-ty
mad-ness
ma-du-ra foot
Mad-u-rel-la
mad-u-ro-my-co-sis
ma-gen-bla-se
mag-en-stras-se
ma-gen-ta
mag-got
mag-ma
mag-na-li-um
Magnan's sign
mag-ne-sia
mag-ne-si-um
mag-ne-si-um car-bo-
   nate
mag-ne-si-um hy-
   drox-ide
mag-ne-si-um ox-ide
mag-ne-si-um sul-fate
mag-ne-si-um tri-sil-
   i-cate
mag-net
mag-net-ism
mag-net-ite
mag-ne-tron
mag-ni-fi-ca-tion
mag-num
maid-en-head
maim

maize
mal
mal-a-chite green
ma-la-ci-a
mal-a-co-pla-ki-a
mal-ad-just-ment
mal-a-dy
ma-laise
mal-an-ders
ma-lar
ma-lar-i-a
ma-lar-i-ol-o-gist
ma-lar-i-o-ther-a-py
Mal-as-se-zi-a fur-fur
mal-as-sim-i-la-tion
mal-ate
ma-le-ate
male fern
ma-le-ic ac-id
mal-for-ma-tion
mal-ic ac-id
ma-lig-nan-cy
ma-lig-nant
ma-lin-ger-er
ma-lin-ger-ing
mal-in-ter-dig-i-ta-tion
mal-le-a-ble
mal-le-o-lus
Mal-le-o-my-ces mal-lei
Mal-le-o-my-ces pseu-do-
   mal-lei
mal-le-ot-o-my
mal-let fin-ger
mal-le-us
mal-nu-tri-tion
mal-oc-clu-sion
ma-lo-nic ac-id
Malpighian cor-pus-cles
Malpighian lay-er
mal-po-si-tion
mal-pos-ture
mal-prac-tice

mal-pres-en-ta-tion
mal-re-duc-tion
malt
Mal-ta fe-ver
malt-ase
Malthusian doc-trine
mal-to-dex-trin
malt-ose
mal-to-su-ri-a
mal-un-ion
mam-ba
mam-e-lon
mam-ma
mam-mal
mam-mal-gi-a
Mam-ma-li-a
mam-ma-li-an
mam-ma-plas-ty
mam-ma-ry
mam-mec-to-my
mam-mi-form
mam-mil-la
mam-mil-lar-y
mam-mil-la-tion
mam-mil-li-form
mam-mil-li-plas-ty
mam-mil-li-tis
mam-mil-lo-tha-lam-ic
mam-mog-ra-phy
mam-mose
mam-mot-o-my
man-del-ic ac-id
man-di-ble
man-drake
ma-neu-ver
man-ga-nese
man-gan-ic
man-ga-nous
mange
man-go
ma-ni-a

man-ic—depres-sive
re-ac-tion
man-i-kin
man-i-oc
ma-nip-u-la-tion
Mann's sign
manna
man-ni-no-tri-ose
man-ni-tol
man-nose
man-no-tri-ose
ma-nom-e-ter
man-om-e-try
man-o-scope
Man-so-nel-la
Man-so-ni-a
man-tle
Mantoux test
ma-nu-bri-um
ma-nus
man-y-plies
ma-ras-mic
ma-ras-muc
mar-ble-i-za-tion
marche—à—pet-it—pas
Marfan's syn-drome
mar-ga-rin
mar-gin
mar-gi-na-tion
mar-gi-no-plas-ty
Marie—Strumpell ar-
thri-tis
ma-ri-hua-na
Marjolin's ul-cer
mar-jo-ram
mar-row
mar-ru-bi-um
marsh gas
marsh-mal-low
mar-su-pi-al-i-za-tion
Mar-ti-us yel-low
mas-cu-line

mas-cu-lin-i-za-tion
mas-cu-lin-o-ma
mas-cu-lin-o-vo-blas-
to-ma
mask
mask of preg-nan-cy
mask-ing
mas-o-chism
Mason's in-ci-sion
masque bil-i-are
mass
mas-sage
mas-se-ter
mas-seur
mas-seuse
mast-ad-e-ni-tis
mast-ad-e-no-ma
mas-tal-gi-a
mast-a-tro-phi-a
mas-taux-y
mas-tec-chy-mo-sis
mas-tec-to-my
mas-tic
mas-ti-ca-tion
mas-ti-ca-tor
mas-ti-ca-to-ry
Mas-ti-goph-o-ra
mas-ti-tis
mas-to-car-ci-no-ma
mas-to-dyn-i-a
mas-toid
mas-toid-i-tis
mas-toid-ot-o-my
mas-ton-cus
mas-top-a-thy
mas-to-pex-y
mas-to-pla-si-a
mas-to-plas-ty
mas-to-scir-rhus
mas-to-sis
mas-tos-to-my
mas-tot-o-my

mas-tous
mas-tur-ba-tion
ma-te-ri-a al-ba
ma-te-ri-a med-i-ca
ma-ter-nal
ma-ter-ni-ty
ma-ting
mat-la-za-hua-ti
ma-trix
mat-ter
mat-u-rate
mat-u-ra-tion
ma-ture
ma-tu-ri-ty
ma-tu-ti-nal
Mau-rer's dots
max-il-la
max-il-lo-fa-cial
max-il-lo—fron-ta-le
max-il-lo-tur-bi-nal
max-i-mal
Maximow's meth-od
max-i-mum
Maxwell's law
may-hem
Mayo Clin-ic
maze
Mazzini test
mean cor-pus-cu-lar
he-mo-glo-bin
mean cor-pus-cu-lar
he-mo-glo-bin con-
cen-tra-tion
mean cor-pus-cu-lar vol-
ume
mea-sles
meas-ly
meas-ure
me-a-ti-tis
me-a-tot-o-my
me-a-tus
mech-a-nism

mech-a-no-ther-a-py
Meckel's di-ver-tic-
    u-lum
me-co-nal-gi-a
mec-o-neu-ro-path-i-a
me-con-i-dine
mec-o-nin
me-co-ni-um
me-cys-ta-sis
me-di-a
me-di-ad
me-di-al
me-di-an
me-di-as-ti-ni-tis
me-di-as-ti-no-per-i-car-
    di-tis
me-di-as-ti-not-o-my
me-di-as-ti-num
me-di-ate
med-i-ca-ble
med-i-cal
med-i-cal cen-ter
me-dic-a-ment
med-i-ca-men-to-sus
med-i-ca-ted
med-i-ca-tion
me-dic-i-nal
med-i-cine
med-i-co-le-gal
Me-di-na worm
me-di-o-car-pal
me-di-o-dor-sal
me-di-o-fron-tal
me-di-o-ne-cro-sis
me-di-o-tar-sal
Med-i-ter-ra-ne-an
    fe-ver
me-di-um
me-di-us
me-dul-la
me-dul-la ob-lon-
    ga-ta

med-ul-lar-y
med-ul-la-ted
med-ul-la-tion
med-ul-li-za-tion
med-ul-lo-blast
med-ul-lo-blas-to-ma
meg-a-car-di-a
meg-a-ce-cum
meg-a-co-lon
meg-a-dont
meg-a-du-o-de-num
meg-a-e-soph-a-gus
meg-a-kar-y-o-blast
meg-a-kar-y-o-cy-te
meg-a-lec-i-thal
meg-a-lo-blast
meg-a-lo-car-di-a
meg-a-lo-ce-phal-ic
meg-a-lo-ceph-a-ly
meg-a-lo-cy-te
meg-a-lo-cy-to-sis
meg-a-lo-dac-ty-ly
meg-a-lo-glos-si-a
meg-a-lo-kar-y-o-cy-te
meg-a-lo-ma-ni-a
meg-a-lo-ma-ni-ac
meg-a-lo-ny-cho-sis
meg-a-lo-pe-nis
meg-a-loph-thal-mus
meg-a-lo-po-di-a
meg-a-lo-spore
meg-a-lo-u-re-ter
meg-a-phone
meg-a-sig-moid
meg-a-volt
meg-ohm
Meibomian cyst
Meigs's syn-drome
mei-o-sis
Meissner's cor-pus-cle
me-lal-gi-a
mel-an-cho-li-a

mel-an-chol-y
Me-la-ni-a
mel-a-nif-er-ous
mel-a-nin
mel-a-nism
mel-a-no-blast
mel-a-no-blas-to-ma
mel-a-no-car-ci-no-ma
mel-a-no-cyte
mel-a-no-der-ma
mel-a-no-der-ma-ti-tis
    tox-i-ca
mel-a-no-der-ma-to-sis
mel-a-no-ep-i-the-li-o-
    ma
me-lan-o-gen
mel-a-no-gen-e-sis
mel-a-no-glos-si-a
mel-a-noid
mel-a-no-ma
mel-a-no-ma-to-sis
mel-a-no-nych-i-a
mel-a-no-phage
mel-a-no-phore
mel-a-no-pla-ki-a
mel-a-no-sar-co-ma
mel-a-no-sis
mel-a-no-trich-i-a
    lin-guae
mel-a-not-ri-chous
mel-a-nu-ri-a
me-las-ma
me-le-na
mel-i-bi-ose
me-li-tis
mel-i-tu-ri-a
mel-i-tum
mel-o-ma-ni-a
Me-loph-a-gus
melt-ing point
mem-ber
mem-brane

mem-brane po-ten-tial
mem-o-ry
me-nac-me
men-ad-i-one
me-nar-che
Mendel's laws
Mendeléev's law
Men-del-ism
Meniéré's syn-drome
me-nin-ge-al
me-nin-ges
me-nin-gi-o-blas-to-ma
me-nin-gi-o-ma
men-in-gis-mus
men-in-git-i-des
men-in-gi-tis
me-nin-go-ar-te-ri-tis
me-nin-go-cele
me-nin-go-ceph-a-li-tis
me-nin-go-cer-e-bri-tis
me-nin-go-coc-ce-mi-a
me-nin-go-coc-cal
me-nin-go-coc-cus
me-nin-go-cor-ti-cal
me-nin-go-cyte
me-nin-go—en-ceph-a-
    li-tis
me-nin-go—en-ceph-a-
    lo-cele
me-nin-go—en-ceph-a-lo-
    my-e-li-tis
me-nin-go—en-ceph-a-
    lop-a-thy
me-nin-go-my-e-li-tis
me-nin-go-my-e-lo-cele
men-in-gop-a-thy
me-nin-go-vas-cu-lar
me-ninx
men-is-cec-to-my
men-is-ci-tis
me-nis-co-cyte
me-nis-cus

men-o-lip-sis
men-o-pause
men-or-rha-gi-a
men-or-rhal-gi-a
men-or-rhe-a
men-o-stax-is
men-ses
men-stru-ate
men-stru-a-tion
men-stru-um
men-su-al
men-su-ra-tion
men-tal
men-ta-lis
men-tal-i-ty
men-ta-tion
men-thol
men-tum
mep-a-crine
me-per-i-dine
me-phen-e-sin
me-phit-ic
me-pro-bam-ate
me-ra-lo-pi-a
mer-cap-tal
mer-cap-tan
mer-cap-tide
mer-cap-tol
mer-cap-to-pu-rine
Mercier's bar
mer-cu-ma-til-in
mer-cu-ri-al
mer-cu-ri-al-ism
mer-cu-ric
mer-cu-rous
mer-cu-ry
mer-er-ga-si-a
me-rid-i-an
mer-i-spore
me-ris-tic
Merkel's cor-pus-cles
mer-o-blas-tic

mer-o-crine
me-ro-pi-a
mer-o-ra-chis-chi-sis
me-ros-mi-a
mer-o-some
me-rot-o-my
mer-o-zo-ite
mer-sa-lyl
mer-y-cism
mes-a-me-boid
mes-a-or-ti-tis
mes-ar-te-ri-tis
mes-a-ti-pel-vic
mes-cal
mes-ca-line
mes-ec-to-derm
mes-em-brin
mes-en-ceph-al-ic
mes-en-ceph-al-i-tis
mes-en-ceph-a-lon
mes-en-chy-mal
mes-en-chyme
mes-en-chy-mo-ma
mes-en-ter-ec-to-my
mes-en-ter-i-or-rha-phy
mes-en-ter-i-pli-ca-tion
mes-en-te-ri-um
mes-en-ter-on
mes-en-ter-y
me-sen-to-derm
mes-en-tor-rha-phy
me-si-al
me-si-o-buc-cal
me-si-o-buc-co-oc-clu-sal
me-si-o-clu-sion
me-si-o-dis-tal
me-si-o-gres-sion
me-si-o-in-ci-sal
me-si-o-la-bi-al
me-si-o-lin-gual
me-si-o-lin-guo-oc-clu-sal
me-si-o-oc-clu-sal

me-si-o-oc-clu-sion
Mesmerism
mes-o-ap-pen-dix
mes-o-bil-i-ru-bin
mes-o-bil-i-ru-bin-o-gen
mes-o-blast
mes-o-blas-te-ma
mes-o-car-di-um
mes-o-carp
mes-o-ce-cum
mes-o-ce-phal-ic
mes-o-co-lon
mes-o-derm
mes-o-du-o-de-num
mes-o-e-soph-a-gus
mes-o-gas-ter
me-sog-li-a
mes-o-gna-thi-on
mes-o-lec-i-thal
mes-o-mere
mes-o-me-tri-um
mes-o-morph
mes-on
mes-o-ne-phro-ma
mes-o-neph-ros
mes-o-pic
me-so-por-phyr-in
mes-or-chi-um
mes-o-rec-tum
mes-o-rop-ter
mes-o-sal-pinx
mes-o-sig-moid
mes-o-ten-don
mes-o-the-li-o-ma
mes-o-the-li-um
mes-o-tho-ri-um
me-sot-o-my
mes-o-tron
mes-o-var-i-um
mes-quite
met-a-bi-o-sis
met-a-bol-ic

met-a-bo-lim-e-ter
me-tab-o-lism
me-tab-o-lite
me-tab-o-lize
met-a-car-pal
met-a-car-po-pha-lan-
ge-al
met-a-car-pus
met-a-chro-mat-ic
met-a-chro-sis
met-a-cone
met-a-con-id
met-a-con-ule
met-a-cre-sol
met-a-cy-e-sis
met-a-fil-tra-tion
met-a-gen-e-sis
met-a-gran-u-lo-cyte
met-a-kar-y-o-cyte
met-al
met-al-de-hyde
me-tal-lic
met-al-loid
met-a-mere
me-tam-er-ism
met-a-mor-phic
met-a-mor-phop-si-a
met-a-mor-pho-sis
met-a-mor-phous
met-a-my-e-lo-cyte
met-a-neph-ros
met-a-phase
met-a-phos-phor-ic ac-id
me-taph-y-sis
met-a-phys-i-tis
met-a-pla-si-a
met-a-plasm
met-a-pro-te-in
met-a-sta-ble
me-tas-ta-sis
me-tas-tat-ic
me-tas-ta-size

Met-a-stron-gy-lus
met-a-tar-sal
met-a-tar-sal-gi-a
met-a-tar-sec-to-my
met-a-tar-so-pha-lan-ge-al
met-a-tar-sus
met-a-thal-a-mus
Met-a-zo-a
met-en-ceph-a-lon
me-te-or-ic
me-te-or-ism
me-te-or-ol-o-gy
me-ter
me-tes-trus
meth-a-don
meth-am-phet-a-mine
   hy-dro-chlo-ride
meth-ane
meth-a-nol
meth-an-thel-ine bro-
   mide
meth-ar-bi-tal
met-he-mal-bu-mi-ne-
   mi-a
met-he-mo-glo-bin
met-he-mo-glo-bi-ne-
   mi-a
met-he-mo-glo-bi-nu-ri-a
me-the-na-mine
me-thim-a-zole
meth-i-o-dal so-di-um
meth-i-o-nine
meth-od
meth-o-in
me-tho-ni-um
meth-ox-a-mine hy-dro-
   chlo-ride
meth-ox-y-chlor
meth-yl
meth-yl al-co-hol
meth-yl al-de-hyde
meth-yl-am-ine

170

meth-yl-ated
meth-yl-a-tion
meth-yl blue
meth-yl bro-mide
meth-yl-cel-lu-lose
meth-yl chlo-ride
meth-yl-cho-lan-threne
meth-yl-ene blue
meth-yl-ene chlo-ride
meth-yl-ene vi-o-let
meth-yl e-ther
meth-yl for-mate
meth-yl-gly-ox-al
meth-yl green
meth-yl i-o-dide
meth-yl meth-ac-ryl-ate
meth-yl or-ange
meth-yl-phe-nol
meth-yl-pu-rine
meth-yl red
meth-yl sal-i-cyl-ate
meth-yl-tes-tos-ter-one
meth-yl-thi-o-u-ra-cil
meth-yl vi-o-let
met-my-o-glo-bin
me-top-ic
met-o-pon
met-o-pryl
met-ra-pec-tic
me-tri-a
met-ric sys-tem
me-tri-tis
me-tro-cele
me-tro-col-po-cele
me-tro-dyn-i-a
met-rog-ra-phy
me-tro-ma-la-ci-a
met-ro-nome
me-tro-pa-ral-y-sis
me-trop-a-thy
me-tro-per-i-to-ni-tis
me-tro-phle-bi-tis

me-trop-to-sis
me-tror-rha-gi-a
me-tror-rhex-is
me-tro-sal-pin-gi-tis
me-tro-sal-pin-gog-ra-phy
me-tro-stax-is
Meulengracht di-et
Meynet's no-dos-i-ties
mi-ca
mi-ca-ce-ous
mi-celle
Michel clip
mi-cra-cous-tic
mi-cren-ceph-a-ly
mi-cro-ab-scess
mi-cro-a-nal-y-sis
mi-cro-a-nat-o-mist
Mi-cro-bac-te-ri-um
mi-crobe
mi-cro-bi-al
mi-cro-bi-cide
mi-cro-bi-ol-o-gist
mi-cro-bi-ol-o-gy
mi-cro-bi-ot-ic
mi-cro-blast
mi-cro-bleph-a-ron
mi-cro-bra-chi-a
mi-cro-bu-ret
mi-cro-car-di-a
mi-cro-cen-trum
mi-cro-ceph-al-ic
mi-cro-ceph-a-lus
mi-cro-ceph-a-ly
mi-cro-chem-is-try
Mi-cro-coc-ca-ce-ae
Mi-cro-coc-cus
mi-cro-co-lon
mi-cro-co-nid-i-um
mi-cro-cor-ne-a
mi-cro-cou-lomb
mi-cro-crys-tal-line
mi-cro-cu-rie

mi-cro-cyte
mi-cro-cyt-ic
mi-cro-cy-to-sis
mi-cro-dac-ty-ly
mi-cro-de-ter-mi-na-tion
mi-cro-dis-sec-tion
mi-cro-don-ti-a
mi-cro-drep-a-no-cyt-ic dis-ease
mi-cro-e-lec-tro-pho-ret-ic cells
mi-cro-far-ad
mi-cro-fi-lar-i-a
mi-cro-flu-o-ro-met-ric scan-ner
mi-cro-gam-ete
mi-cro-ga-me-to-cyte
mi-cro-gas-tri-a
mi-crog-li-a
mi-cro-glos-si-a
mi-cro-gna-thi-a
mi-cro-go-ni-o-scope
mi-cro-graph
mi-crohm
mi-cro-in-jec-tion
mi-cro-li-ter
mi-cro-ma-nip-u-la-tive tech-nique
mi-cro-ma-nip-u-la-tor
mi-cro-mas-ti-a
mi-crom-e-ter
mi-crom-e-ter disk
mi-cro-meth-od
mi-cro-mi-cron
mi-cron
mi-cro-nee-dles
mi-cro-nu-cle-us
mi-cro-nu-tri-ents
mi-cro-or-gan-ism
mi-cro-par-a-site
mi-cro-phage

mi-cro-phone
mi-cro-pho-ni-a
mi-cro-pho-to-graph
mi-cro-pho-tom-e-ter
mi-cro-phys-ics
mi-cro-pi-pet
mi-cro-pla-nar
mi-cro-pro-jec-tion
mi-crop-si-a
mi-cro-pyle
mi-cro-ra-di-og-ra-phy
mi-cro-res-pi-ra-tor
mi-cro-ruth-er-ford
mi-cro-scope
mi-cro-scop-ic
mi-cros-co-pist
mi-cros-co-py
mi-cro-some
mi-cro-spec-trog-ra-phy
mi-cro-spec-tro-pho-
    tom-e-try
mi-cro-spec-tro-scope
mi-cro-spher-o-cyte
Mi-cro-spo-rid-i-a
mi-cro-spo-rin
Mi-cro-spo-rum
mi-cro-steth-o-scope
mi-cro-sto-mi-a
mi-cro-sur-ger-y
mi-cro-the-li-a
mi-cro-therm
mi-cro-tome
mi-crot-o-my
mi-cro-volt
mi-cro-wave
mi-cro-zo-on
mi-crur-gy
Mi-cru-roi-des
Mi-cru-rus
mic-tu-rate
mic-tu-ri-tion
mid-ax-il-lar-y

mid-bod-y
mid-brain
mid-fron-tal
midge
midg-et
mid-gut
mid-pain
mid-riff
mid-wife
mid-wife-ry
mi-graine
mi-grate
mi-gra-tion
Mikulicz op-er-a-tion
Mikulicz's dis-ease
mil-dew
Miles's op-er-a-tion
mil-i-a-ri-a
mil-i-ar-y tu-ber-cu-
    lo-sis
mi-lieu ex-té-rieur
mi-lieu in-té-rieur
mil-i-um
milk a-gent
milk fe-ver
milk-ing
Millard—Gubler
    syn-drome
Miller—Abbott tube
mil-let seed
mil-li-am-me-ter
mil-li-am-pere
mil-li-bar
mil-li-cu-rie
mil-li-cu-rie—hour
mil-li-e-quiv-a-lent
mil-li-gram
mil-li-gram—hour
mil-li-grams per cent
mil-li-li-ter
mil-li-me-ter
mil-li-mi-cron

mil-li-mol
mil-li-mol-ar
mil-li-nor-mal
mil-li-os-mol
mil-li-pedes
mil-li-ruth-er-ford
mil-li-volt
Milroy's dis-ease
mi-met-ic
mind
min-er-al
min-im
min-i-mal
min-i-mum
mi-nom-e-ter
mi-nor
mint
mi-o-sis
mi-ot-ic
mi-ra-cid-i-um
mire
mir-ror
mis-an-thro-py
mis-car-riage
mis-car-ry
mis-ce-ge-na-tion
mis-ci-ble
mis-sog-a-my
mi-sog-y-nist
mis-tle-toe
mite
mi-ti-ci-dal
mit-i-gate
mi-tis
mit-o-chon-dri-a
mi-to-sis
mit-o-some
mi-tral
mit-tel-schmerz
mix-ture
mne-mon-ics
moan

mo-bile
mo-bil-i-ty
mo-bi-li-za-tion
mo-dal-i-ty
mode
mod-el
mod-er-a-tor
mo-di-o-lus
mod-u-la-tor
mod-u-lus
mo-dus op-er-an-di
mog-i-la-li-a
moi-e-ty
mo-lar
mo-las-ses
mold
mold-ing
mole
mo-lec-u-lar
mol-e-cule
mol-lus-cum con-ta-gi-o-sum
molt
mo-lyb-date
mo-lyb-de-num
mo-lyb-dic
mo-lyb-dic ac-id
mo-lyb-dous
mo-ment
mo-men-tum
mon-ad
Monaldi drain-age
mon-am-ide
mon-am-ine
mon-ar-thri-tis
mon-ar-tic-u-lar
mon-as-ter
mon-a-tom-ic
Monckeberg's dis-ease
mo-nes-trus
mon-go-lism

mon-go-loid
mo-nil-e-thrix
Mo-nil-i-a
mo-ni-li-a-sis
mon-i-lid
mo-nil-i-form
mo-nil-i-id
mon-i-tor-ing
monks-hood
mon-o-bas-ic
mon-o-blast
mon-o-blep-si-a
mon-o-bra-chi-us
mon-o-cel-lu-lar
mon-o-chlo-ro-ac-e-tone
mon-o-chlor-o-meth-ane
mon-o-chro-ma-sy
mon-o-chro-mat-ic
mon-o-chro-ma-tism
mon-o-chro-mat-o-phil
mon-o-chro-ma-tor
mon-o-chro-mic
mon-o-clin-ic
mon-o-coc-cus
mon-o-crot-ic
mon-oc-u-lar
mon-oc-u-lus
mon-o-cy-e-sis
mon-o-cys-tic
mon-o-cyte
mon-o-cy-to-ma
mon-o-cy-to-pe-ni-a
mon-o-cy-to-sis
mon-o-dro-mi-a
mo-nog-a-my
mon-o-gas-tric
mo-nog-o-nous
mon-o-hy-brid
mon-o-hy-drate
mon-o-hy-dric
mon-o—i-de-ism
mon-o-loc-u-lar

mon-o-ma-ni-a
mon-o-mer
mon-o-mer-ic
mon-o-mor-phic
mon-o-mor-phous
mon-o-nu-cle-ar
mon-o-nu-cle-o-sis
mon-o-nu-cle-o-tide
mon-o-pha-gi-a
mon-o-pha-si-a
mon-o-pha-sic
mon-o-pho-bi-a
mon-o-phos-phate
mon-o-phy-let-ic
mon-o-phy-o-dont
mon-o-ple-gi-a
mon-o-po-di-a
mon-o-pty-chi-al
mon-o-ra-dic-u-lar
mon-or-chid-ism
mon-o-sac-cha-ride
mon-o-so-di-um glu-ta-mate
mon-o-some
mon-o-symp-to-mat-ic
mo-not-o-cous
mo-not-ri-chous
mon-ox-ide
mon-o-zy-got-ic
Monro's bur-sa
mons pu-bis
mons ve-ner-is
mon-ster
mon-stros-i-ty
mon-tan wax
Monteggia's dis-lo-ca-tion
Montgomery's glands
mon-tic-u-lus
mood
Morax—Axenfeld ba-cil-lus

173

mor-bid
mor-bid-i-ty
mor-bil-li-form
mor-da-cious
mor-dant
Morgagni's valves
morgue
mor-i-bund
morn-ing sick-ness
Moro re-flex
mo-ron
mor-phi-a
mor-phine
mor-phin-ism
mor-pho-gen-e-sis
mor-pho-log-i-cal
mor-phol-og-y
mors su-bi-ta
mor-sal
mor-sus
mor-tal
mor-tal-i-ty
mor-tar
mor-ti-fi-ca-tion
Morton's syn-drome
mor-tu-ar-y
mor-u-la
Morvan's dis-ease
mo-sa-ic
mos-qui-to
moss
Mossman fe-ver
mos-sy foot
Moszkowicz's test
moth-er
mo-tile
mo-til-i-ty
mo-tion
mo-tor
mot-tled en-am-el
mot-tling
mou-lage

mound
moun-tain sick-ness
mouse-pox
mouth
move-ment
Moynihan's clamp
mu-cic ac-id
mu-cif-er-ous
mu-ci-gen
mu-ci-lage
mu-cin
mu-cin-oid
mu-cip-a-rous
mu-co-cele
mu-co-co-li-tis
mu-co-cu-ta-ne-ous
mu-co-en-ter-i-tis
mu-coid
mu-con-ic ac-id
mu-co-pol-y-sac-cha-
   ride
mu-co-pro-te-in
mu-co-pu-ru-lent
Mu-cor
mu-co-rif-er-ous
mu-cor-in
mu-cor-my-co-sis
mu-co-sa
mu-co-sal
mu-co-san-guin-e-ous
mu-co-se-rous
mu-co-sin
mu-co-si-tis
mu-cos-i-ty
mu-cous
mu-co-vis-ci-do-sis
mu-cus
mul-ber-ry cal-cu-lus
mul-ber-ry mark
Mullerian ducts
Muller's fix-ing flu-id
mul-tan-gu-lum

mul-ti-cap-su-lar
mul-ti-cel-lu-lar
Mul-ti-ceps mul-ti-ceps
Mul-ti-ceps se-ri-al-is
mul-ti-cus-pid
mul-ti-den-tate
mul-ti-dig-i-tate
mul-ti-fa-mil-i-al
mul-tif-i-dus
mul-ti-flag-el-late
mul-ti-form
mul-ti-gan-gli-on-ate
mul-ti-glan-du-lar
mul-ti-grav-i-da
mul-ti-lo-bar
mul-ti-lob-u-lar
mul-ti-loc-u-lar
mul-ti-nod-u-lar
mul-ti-nu-cle-ar
mul-tip-a-ra
mul-tip-a-rous
mul-ti-ple
mul-ti-po-lar
mul-ti-va-lent
mum-mi-fi-ca-tion
mum-mi-fied
mumps
mun-dif-i-cant
Munson—Walker val-ues
mu-on
mu-ral
mu-ri-at-ic ac-id
mur-mur
Murphy's sign
Mus mus-cu-lus
Mus-ca do-mes-ti-ca
mus-cae vol-i-tan-tes
mus-ca-rine
mus-ca-rin-ism
Mus-ci-dae
mus-cle
mus-cle splint-ing

mus-cu-lar-is mu-co-sae
mus-cu-lar-i-ty
mus-cu-la-ture
mus-cu-lo-ap-o-neu-rot-
ic
mus-cu-lo-cu-ta-ne-ous
mus-cu-lo-fas-ci-al
mus-cu-lo-fi-brous
mus-cu-lo-phren-ic
mus-cu-lo-spi-ral
mus-cu-lo-ten-di-nous
mush-room
mu-si-co-ther-a-py
musk
mus-si-ta-tion
mus-tard
mus-tine hy-dro-chlo-
ride
mu-ta-gen
mu-tant
mu-ta-ro-ta-tion
mu-tase
mu-ta-tion
mute
mu-ti-la-tion
mu-tism
muz-zle
my-al-gi-a
my-as-the-ni-a grav-is
my-as-then-ic
my-a-to-ni-a con-gen-i-
ta
my-ce-li-al
my-ce-li-um
my-ce-tes
my-ce-toid
my-ce-to-ma
My-co-bac-ter-i-a-ce-ae
My-co-bac-te-ri-um lep-
rae
My-co-bac-te-ri-um tu-
ber-cu-lo-sis

my-coid
my-col-o-gy
my-coph-thal-mi-a
my-co-sis
my-co-sis fun-goid-es
my-cot-ic
myc-ter-o-pho-ni-a
my-de-sis
my-dri-a-sis
my-dri-at-ic
my-ec-to-my
my-e-len-ceph-a-lon
my-e-lin
my-e-li-nat-ed
my-e-li-na-tion
my-e-li-ni-za-tion
my-e-lin-o-cla-sis
my-e-li-no-gen-e-sis
my-e-li-nop-a-thy
my-e-li-no-sis
my-e-li-tis
my-e-lo-blast
my-e-lo-blas-tic
my-e-lo-blas-to-ma
my-e-lo-blas-to-sis
my-e-lo-cele
my-e-lo-cys-to-cele
my-e-lo-cyte
my-e-lo-cy-to-sis
my-e-lo-dys-pla-si-a
my-e-lo-en-ceph-a-li-tis
my-e-lo-fi-bro-sis
my-el-o-gen-e-sis
my-e-lo-gen-ic
my-e-lo-gram
my-e-lo-gra-phy
my-e-loid
my-e-lo-ken-tric ac-id
my-e-lo-ma
my-e-lo-ma-la-ci-a
my-e-lo-ma-to-sis
my-e-lo-men-in-gi-tis

my-e-lo-me-nin-go-cele
my-e-lo-mere
my-e-lo-mon-o-cyte
my-e-lo-neu-ri-tis
my-e-lop-a-thy
my-e-lo-ple-gi-a
my-e-lo-pro-lif-er-a-tive
dis-or-ders
my-e-lo-ra-dic-u-li-tis
my-e-lo-ra-dic-u-lop-a-thy
my-e-lo-rrha-gi-a
my-e-lo-sar-co-ma
my-e-los-chi-sis
my-e-lo-scin-to-gram
my-e-lo-scin-tog-ra-phy
my-e-lo-scle-ro-sis
my-e-lo-sis
my-en-ter-ic
my-en-ter-on
my-es-the-si-a
my-ia-sis
my-io-de-op-si-a
my-ler-an
my-lo-glos-sus
my-lo-hy-oid
my-lo-phar-yn-ge-al
my-o-arch-i-tec-ton-ic
my-o-blas-tic
my-o-blas-to-ma
my-o-car-di-al in-suf-fi-
cien-cy
my-o-car-di-tis
my-o-car-di-um
my-o-car-do-sis
my-o-clo-ni-a
my-o-clon-ic
my-o-clo-nus
my-o-dys-to-ni-a
my-o-dys-tro-phy
my-o-e-las-tic
my-o-ep-i-the-li-o-ma
my-o-fas-ci-al

175

my-o-fas-ci-tis
my-o-fi-bril
my-o-fi-bro-ma
my-o-fi-bro-sar-co-ma
my-o-ge-lo-sis
my-o-gen
my-o-gen-ic
my-o-glo-bin
my-o-glo-bin-u-ri-a
my-o-gram
my-o-graph
my-o-he-ma-tin
my-o-he-mo-glo-bin
my-o-he-mo-glo-bin-
   u-ri-a
my-o-ki-nase
my-o-kin-es-i-og-ra-
   phy
my-o-li-po-ma
my-ol-o-gy
my-o-ma
my-o-ma-la-ci-a cor-
   dis
my-om-a-tous
my-o-mec-to-my
my-o-me-tri-tis
my-o-me-tri-um
my-o-neu-ral
my-o-pa-re-sis
my-o-path-i-a ra-chit-
   i-ca
my-op-a-thy
my-ope
my-o-per-i-car-di-tis
my-o-pi-a
my-op-ic
my-o-plasm
my-o-plas-ty
my-o-psy-cho-sis
my-o-sar-co-ma
my-o-scle-ro-sis
my-o-sin

my-o-si-tis
my-o-stat-ic
my-o-syn-o-vi-tis
my-o-ten-o-si-tis
my-o-te-not-o-my
my-o-tome
my-ot-o-my
my-o-to-ni-a con-gen-
   i-ta
my-o-to-ni-a dys-tro-
   phi-ca
my-rin-ga
myr-in-gec-to-my
myr-in-gi-tis
my-rin-go-dec-to-my
my-rin-go-my-co-sis
my-rin-go-plas-ty
my-rin-go-tome
myr-in-got-o-my
my-rinx
my-ris-tic ac-id
my-ris-tin
myrrh
myr-til-lin
myr-tle
my-so-pho-bi-a
myth-o-ma-ni-a
myth-o-pho-bi-a
myt-i-lo-tox-ism
myx-ad-e-ni-tis
myx-ad-e-no-ma
myx-e-de-ma
myx-e-dem-a-tous
myx-o-ad-e-no-ma
myx-o-chon-dro-fi-bro-
   sar-co-ma
myx-o-chon-dro-ma
myx-o-chon-dro-sar-
   co-ma
myx-o-fi-bro-ma
myx-o-fi-bro-sar-co-ma
myx-o-gli-o-ma

myx-oid
myx-o-li-po-ma
myx-o-li-po-sar-co-ma
myx-o-ma
myx-o-ma-to-sis
Myx-o-my-ce-tes
myx-o-neu-ro-ma
myx-o-sar-co-ma
myx-o-spore

N

Nabothian glands
Naffziger's syn-drome
nail
Na-ja na-ja
na-ked
nal-or-phine hy-dro-
   chlo-ride
na-nism
na-no-ceph-a-lus
na-noid
nan-oph-thal-mos
na-no-som-i-a pi-tu-i-
   ta-ri-a
na-nus
na-palm
nape
na-pex
naph-tha
naph-tha-lene
naph-thene
naph-thol
naph-thol-ate
naph-tho-qui-none
na-pi-form
nar-cis-sism
nar-cis-sis-tic
nar-co-an-al-y-sis
nar-co-hyp-no-sis

nar-co-lep-sy
nar-com-a-tous
nar-co-ma-ni-a
nar-co-sis
nar-co-syn-the-sis
nar-co-ther-a-py
nar-cot-ic
nar-co-tism
nar-co-tize
na-ris
na-sal
na-sa-lis
nas-cent
na-si-o-al-ve-o-lar
na-si-on
na-so-cil-i-ar-y
na-so-fron-tal
na-so-gen-i-tal
na-so-la-bi-al
na-so-la-bi-a-lis
na-so-lac-ri-mal
na-so-max-il-lar-y
na-so-pal-a-tine
na-so-phar-yn-gi-tis
na-so-pha-ryn-go-scope
na-so-phar-ynx
na-so-pha-ryn-ge-al
na-sus
na-tal
na-tal-i-ty
na-tant
Na-tion-al In-sti-tutes
    of Health
na-tive
nat-re-mi-a
na-tri-um
na-tri-u-ret-ic
nat-u-ral
na-tur-o-path
nau-se-a
nau-seous
nau-se-ant

na-vel
na-vic-u-lar
near point
near—sight-ed
ne-ar-thro-sis
neb-u-la
neb-u-li-za-tion
neb-u-lize
neb-u-li-zer
Ne-ca-tor a-mer-i-can-us
nec-a-to-ri-a-sis
neck
Nec-ro-ba-cil-lus
nec-ro-bi-o-sis lip-oid-
    i-ca
nec-ro-cy-to-sis
nec-ro-gen-ic
nec-ro-ma-ni-a
nec-ro-mi-me-sis
nec-ro-phil-i-a
ne-croph-i-lous
nec-ro-pho-bi-a
nec-rop-sy
ne-crose
ne-cro-sis
ne-crot-ic
nec-ro-sper-mi-a
nee-dle
nee-dle hold-er
nee-dling
Neelsen stain
neg-a-tive
neg-a-tiv-ism
neg-a-tron
neg-li-gence
Negri bod-ies
Neis-se-ri-a ca-tarrh-
    al-is
Neis-se-ri-a gon-or-rhoe-
    ae
Neis-se-ri-a in-tra-cel-
    lu-lar-is

Neis-se-ri-a men-in-gi-
    ti-dis
Nélaton's line
Nem-a-thel-min-thes
Nem-a-to-da
nem-a-tode
ne-o-ars-phen-a-mine
ne-o-ar-thro-sis
ne-o-blas-tic
ne-o-cal-a-mine
ne-o-cer-e-bel-lum
ne-o-cor-tex
ne-o-dym-i-um
ne-o-gen-e-sis
ne-o-mor-phism
ne-o-my-cin
ne-on
ne-o-na-tal
ne-o-nate
ne-o-pal-li-um
ne-o-pho-bi-a
ne-o-phren-i-a
ne-o-pla-si-a
ne-o-plasm
ne-o-plast-ic
ne-o-prene
ne-o-sal-var-san
ne-o-stig-mine
ne-ot-e-ny
neph-a-lism
neph-e-lom-e-ter
ne-phral-gi-a
ne-phrec-to-mize
ne-phrec-to-my
neph-ric
ne-phrid-i-um
ne-phri-tis
neph-ro-cal-ci-no-sis
neph-ro-cap-sec-to-my
neph-ro-col-o-pex-y
neph-ro-cys-ti-tis
neph-ro-gen-ic

ne-phrog-e-nous
neph-roid
neph-ro-lith
neph-ro-li-thi-a-sis
neph-ro-li-thot-o-my
ne-phrol-y-sis
neph-ro-ma
neph-ron
neph-ro-path-ic
neph-ro-pex-y
neph-rop-to-sis
neph-ro-py-e-li-tis
neph-ror-rha-phy
neph-ros
neph-ro-scle-ro-sis
ne-phro-sis
ne-phrot-o-my
neph-ro-tox-ic
neph-ro-tu-ber-cu-lo-sis
neph-ro-u-re-ter-ec-to-my
nep-tu-ni-um
nerve
ner-vos-i-ty
nerv-ous ex-haus-tion
nerv-ous-ness
nerv-ous sys-tem
ner-vus
Nessler's re-a-gent
nest
net-tle rash
net-work
Neubauer's cham-ber
neu-ral
neu-ral-gi-a
neu-ral-gic
neu-ra-poph-y-sis
neu-ra-prax-i-a
neu-ras-the-ni-a
neu-rec-to-my
neu-ri-lem-ma
neu-ri-lem-mi-tis
neu-ri-lem-mo-ma

neu-ri-no-ma
neu-ri-no-ma-to-sis
neu-ri-tis
neu-ro-a-nas-to-mo-sis
neu-ro-a-nat-o-my
neu-ro-as-the-ni-a
neu-ro-as-tro-cy-to-ma
neu-ro-bi-ol-o-gy
neu-ro-blast
neu-ro-blas-to-ma
neu-ro-blas-to-ma-to-sis
neu-ro-ca-nal
neu-ro-chem-is-try
neu-ro-cho-ri-o-ret-i-
ni-tis
neu-ro-cho-roid-i-tis
neu-ro-cir-cu-la-to-ry
neu-ro-cu-ta-ne-ous
neu-ro-cy-to-ma
neu-ro-den-drite
neu-ro-den-dron
neu-ro-der-ma-ti-tis
neu-ro-der-ma-ti-tis
cir-cum-scrip-ta
neu-ro-der-ma-ti-tis
dis-sem-i-na-ta
neu-ro-der-ma-to-my-o-
si-tis
neu-ro-der-ma-to-sis
neu-ro-dyn-i-a
neu-ro-en-do-crine
neu-ro-ep-i-der-mal
neu-ro-ep-i-the-li-o-ma
neu-ro-ep-i-the-li-um
neu-ro-fi-bril
neu-ro-fi-bro-ma
neu-ro-fi-bro-ma-to-sis
neu-ro-fi-bro-sar-co-ma
neu-ro-fi-bro-si-tis
neu-ro-gas-tric
neu-ro-gen-ic
neu-rog-e-nous

neu-rog-li-a
neu-rog-li-o-ma
neu-rog-li-o-sis
neu-ro-his-tol-o-gy
neu-ro-hu-mor-al
neu-ro-hy-poph-y-sis
neu-roid
neu-ro-in-duc-tion
neu-ro-lem-ma
neu-rol-o-gist
neu-ro-log-ic
neu-rol-o-gy
neu-rol-y-sin
neu-rol-y-sis
neu-ro-ma
neu-ro-ma-to-sis
neu-ro-mech-a-nism
neu-ro-mere
neu-ro-mi-met-ic
neu-ro-mus-cu-lar
neu-ro-my-e-li-tis
neu-ro-my-o-si-tis
neu-ron
neu-ro-ni-tis
neu-ro-path-ic
neu-ro-path-o-gen-e-sis
neu-ro-pa-thol-o-gy
neu-rop-a-thy
neu-ro-phys-i-ol-o-gy
neu-ro-plasm
neu-ro-plas-ty
neu-ro-pore
neu-ro-psy-chi-a-try
neu-ro-psy-cho-path-ic
neu-ro-ret-i-ni-tis
neu-ror-rha-phy
neu-ro-sar-co-ma
neu-ro-scle-ro-sis
neu-ro-sis
neu-ro-skel-e-tal
neu-ro-spasm
Neu-ros-po-ra

neu-ro-sur-geon
neu-ro-sur-ger-y
neu-ro-syph-i-lis
neu-ro-the-ci-tis
neu-ro-ther-a-py
neu-rot-ic
neu-rot-i-ca
neu-rot-i-cism
neu-ro-tome
neu-rot-o-my
neu-ro-ton-ic
neu-ro-tox-in
neu-ro-trau-ma
neu-ro-trip-sy
neu-ro-troph-ic
neu-ro-trop-ic
neu-ro-vas-cu-lar
neu-ru-la
neu-tral
neu-tra-li-za-tion
neu-tral-ize
neu-tri-no
neut-ro-clu-sion
neu-tro-cyte
neu-tron
neu-tro-pe-ni-a
neu-tro-phil
ne-vose
ne-vus
new-born
Newcastle dis-ease
Newton's law
nex-us
nib-ble
nic-co-lum
niche
nick-el
nick-ing
nic-o-tin-am-ide
nic-o-tine
nic-o-tin-ic ac-id
nic-ta-tion

nic-ti-ta-ting
nic-ti-ta-ti-o
nic-ti-ta-tion
ni-da-tion
ni-dus
Niemann—Pick dis-ease
night blind-ness
night-mare
night pal-sy
night-shade
night sweat
night vi-sion
nig-ri-cans
ni-gri-ti-es
ni-gro-sine
ni-hil-ism
ni-keth-a-mide
ni-o-bi-um
niph-a-blep-si-a
nip-pers
nip-ple
Nissl bod-ies
ni-sus
nit
ni-ter
ni-ton
ni-trate
ni-tra-tion
ni-tric ac-id
ni-tri-fi-ca-tion
ni-tri-fi-er
ni-trile
ni-trite
ni-tro-ben-zene
ni-tro-ben-zol
ni-tro-cel-lu-lose
ni-tro-er-y-throl
ni-tro-gen
ni-trog-e-nous
ni-tro-glyc-er-in
ni-tro-mer-sol
ni-trom-e-ter

ni-tron
ni-tro-prus-side
ni-tro-so-ni-tric ac-id
ni-trous
ni-trous ac-id
Nobel lau-re-ate
Nobel prize
no-ble gas-es
No-car-di-a
no-car-di-o-sis
no-ci-cep-tive
no-ci-per-cep-tion
no-ci-per-cep-tor
noc-tal-bu-mi-nu-ri-a
noc-tam-bu-la-tion
noc-ti-pho-bi-a
noc-tu-ri-a
noc-tur-nal
noc-u-ous
node
no-dose
no-dos-i-ty
nod-ule
nod-u-lus
no-dus
no-ma
no-mad-ic
no-men-cla-ture
nom-o-graph
non-ac-cess
non-ad-he-rent
non-al-ler-gic
non-a-que-ous
non com-pos men-tis
non-con-duc-tor
non-dis-junc-tion
non-ma-lig-nant
non-med-ul-la-ted
non-mo-tile
non-nu-cle-a-ted
non-pro-te-in ni-tro-gen
non-py-o-gen-ic

non-re-frac-tive
non-sex-u-al
non-spe-cif-ic
non-sup-pu-ra-tive
non-sur-gi-cal
non-vi-a-ble
nor-a-dren-a-lin
nor-bi-o-tin
nor-e-phed-rine
nor-ep-i-neph-rine
nor-leu-cine
norm
nor-mal
nor-mo-blast
nor-mo-chro-mat-ic
nor-mo-chro-mic
nor-mo-cyte
nor-mo-cy-to-sis
nor-mo-gly-ce-mi-a
nor-mo-ten-sive
nor-mo-ther-mi-a
nor-mo-ton-ic
nor-mo-vo-le-mi-a
nor-val-ine
nose
nose-bleed
nose drops
nose-piece
nos-och-tho-nog-ra-phy
no-sog-e-ny
no-sol-o-gy
nos-o-ma-ni-a
nos-o-pho-bi-a
No-sop-syl-lus
nos-tal-gi-a
nos-tal-gic
nos-to-pho-bi-a
nos-tril
nos-trum
no-tan-en-ce-pha-li-a
no-ta-tion
notch

note
No-te-chis
no-ten-ceph-a-lo-cele
no-ti-fi-a-ble
no-to-chord
No-to-ed-res
nox-ious
nu-bile
nu-cha
nu-chal
nu-cle-ar dis-in-te-gra-tion
nu-cle-ar fis-sion
nu-cle-ar re-ac-tor
nu-cle-ase
nu-cle-a-ted
nu-cle-a-tion
nu-cle-i
nu-cle-ic ac-id
nu-cle-ide
nu-cle-in-ase
nu-cle-o-cy-to-plas-mic
nu-cle-o-his-tone
nu-cle-oid
nu-cle-o-lin
nu-cle-o-lus
nu-cle-on
nu-cle-on-ics
nu-cle-o-pro-te-in
nu-cle-o-si-dase
nu-cle-o-side
nu-cle-o-spin-dle
nu-cle-o-ti-dase
nu-cle-o-tide
nu-cle-o-tox-in
nu-cle-us
nu-clide
nud-ism
nui-sance
nul-lip-a-ra
nul-lip-a-rous

numb
num-ber
numb-ness
num-mi-form
num-mu-lar
nurse
nurs-ing
nurs-ling
nu-ta-tion
nut-meg liv-er
nu-tri-ent
nu-tri-ment
nu-tri-tion
nu-tri-tion-al
nu-tri-tious
nu-tri-tive
nux vom-i-ca
nyc-tal-gi-a
nyc-ter-ine
nyc-to-phil-i-a
nyc-to-pho-bi-a
nymph
nym-pha
nym-phi-tis
nym-pho-ma-ni-a
nym-pho-ma-ni-ac
nys-tag-mic
nys-tag-mi-form
nys-tag-moid
nys-tag-mus

O

oa-kum
o-a-sis
o-bese
o-be-si-ty
ob-fus-ca-tion
ob-jec-tive
ob-li-gate

ob-lique
ob-liq-ui-ty
ob-li-quus
ob-lit-er-a-tion
ob-ses-sion
ob-ses-sive com-pul-
  sive re-ac-tion
ob-so-les-cence
ob-ste-tri-cian
ob-stet-rics
ob-sti-pa-tion
ob-struc-tion
ob-stru-ent
ob-tund
ob-tu-ra-tion
ob-tu-ra-tor
ob-tuse
ob-tu-sion
oc-cip-i-tal
oc-cip-i-ta-lis
oc-cip-i-tal-ize
oc-cip-i-to-an-te-ri-
  or
oc-cip-i-to-fron-tal
oc-cip-i-to-pos-te-
  ri-or
oc-ci-put
oc-clude
oc-clu-sion
oc-clu-sive
oc-cult
oc-cu-pa-tion-al
  dis-ease
oc-cu-pa-tion-al
  ther-a-py
oc-cu-pied
o-cel-lus
och-lo-pho-bi-a
o-chro-no-sis
oc-ta-meth-yl py-ro-
  phos-phor-am-ide
oc-tane

oc-ta-ri-us
oc-tyl ni-trite
oc-u-lar
oc-u-len-tum
oc-u-list
oc-u-lo-gy-ra-tion
oc-u-lo-gy-ric cri-sis
oc-u-lo-mo-tor
oc-u-lo-my-co-sis
oc-u-lus
o-dax-es-mus
o-don-tal-gi-a
o-don-tec-to-my
o-don-tex-e-sis
o-don-tic
o-don-to-blas-to-ma
o-don-to-cele
o-don-to-gen-e-sis
o-don-to-glyph
o-don-tog-ra-phy
o-don-toid
o-don-tol-o-gist
o-don-tol-o-gy
o-don-to-lox-i-a
o-don-to-ma
o-don-to-ne-cro-sis
o-don-to-par-al-lax-is
o-don-to-pri-sis
o-don-to-ra-di-o-graph
o-don-tos-chi-sis
o-dor
o-dor-if-er-ous
o-dyn-a-cou-sis
oed-i-pal
Oed-i-pus com-plex
Oes-trus o-vis
of-fal
of-fi-cial
ohm
ohm-me-ter
O-id-i-um
oi-ko-site

oi-no-ma-ni-a
oint-ment
o-le-ag-i-nous
o-le-an-der
o-le-ate
o-le-cra-nar-thri-tis
o-lec-ra-non
o-le-fine
o-le-ic ac-id
o-le-in
o-le-o-mar-ga-rine
o-le-om-e-ter
o-le-o-res-in
o-le-o-vi-ta-min
o-le-um
o-le-yl al-co-hol
ol-fac-tion
ol-fac-tor-y
o-lib-a-num
ol-i-ge-mi-a
ol-ig-hid-ri-a
ol-i-go-am-ni-os
ol-i-go-cho-li-a
ol-i-go-cy-the-mi-a
ol-i-go-dac-ry-a
ol-i-go-dac-tyl-i-a
ol-i-go-den-dro-blas-
  to-ma
ol-i-go-den-drog-li-a
ol-i-go-den-dro-gli-o-
  ma
ol-i-go-den-dro-gli-o-
  ma-to-sis
ol-i-go-den-dro-ma
ol-i-go-don-ti-a
ol-i-go-gen-ic
ol-i-go-hy-dram-ni-os
ol-i-go-lec-i-thal
ol-i-go-men-or-rhe-a
ol-i-go-nu-cle-o-tide
ol-i-go-phos-pha-tu-ri-a
ol-i-go-phre-ni-a

ol-i-gop-noe-a
ol-i-go-sper-mi-a
ol-i-go-trich-i-a
ol-i-gu-ri-a
o-lis-ther-o-chro-ma-tin
o-lis-ther-o-zone
ol-ive
ol-i-vo-pon-to-cer-e-bel-lar
o-lym-pi-an fore-head
o-mar-thri-tis
o-ma-sum
o-men-tec-to-my
o-men-to-pex-y
o-men-tor-rha-phy
o-men-tum
om-ma-tid-i-um
om-niv-o-rous
o-mo-hy-oid
om-pha-lec-to-my
om-phal-ic
om-pha-li-tis
om-phal-o-cele
om-pha-lo-mes-en-ter-ic
om-pha-lo-prop-to-sis
om-pha-los
o-nan-ism
On-cho-cer-ca vol-vu-lus
on-cho-cer-ci-a-sis
on-cho-cer-co-ma
on-cho-der-ma-ti-tis
on-co-cyte
on-co-cy-to-ma
on-co-gen-e-sis
on-col-o-gy
on-com-e-ter
on-co-met-ric
on-co-sis
one—min-ute de-na-tur-a-tion val-ue
o-ni-o-ma-ni-a

on-ion
on-o-mat-o-ma-ni-a
on-o-mat-o-poi-e-sis
on-tog-e-ny
on-y-chec-to-my
o-nych-i-a
on-y-cho-gry-po-sis
on-y-chol-y-sis
on-y-cho-ma
on-y-cho-ma-la-ci-a
on-y-cho-my-co-sis
on-y-chop-a-thy
on-y-cho-pha-gi-a
on-y-chot-o-my
o-nyx-i-tis
o-o-cyst
o-o-cyte
o-o-gen-e-sis
o-o-ge-net-ic
o-o-go-ni-um
o-o-ki-nete
o-o-pho-rec-to-my
o-o-pho-ri-tis
o-oph-o-ro-cys-tec-to-my
o-oph-o-ro-hys-ter-ec-to-my
o-oph-o-ron
o-oph-o-ro-sal-pin-gec-to-my
o-oph-o-ro-sal-pin-gi-tis
o-o-pho-ros-to-my
o-o-tid
o-pac-i-fi-ca-tion
o-pac-i-ty
o-pal-es-cent
o-paque
o-pen
o-pen-ing
op-er-a-bil-i-ty
op-er-a-ble
op-e-ra-tion
op-er-a-tor

o-per-cu-lum
o-phi-a-sis
o-phid-i-o-pho-bi-a
oph-ry-i-tis
oph-ryt-ic
oph-thal-ma-cro-sis
oph-thal-mal-gi-a
oph-thal-mec-chy-mo-sis
oph-thal-mec-to-my
oph-thal-mi-a
oph-thal-mic
oph-thal-mi-tis
oph-thal-mo-blen-nor-rhe-a
oph-thal-mo-cen-te-sis
oph-thal-mo-do-ne-sis
oph-thal-mo-dy-na-mom-e-ter
oph-thal-mo-dyn-i-a
oph-thal-mo-fun-do-scope
oph-thal-mog-ra-phy
oph-thal-mo-gy-ric
oph-thal-mo-lith
oph-thal-mo-log-ic
oph-thal-mol-o-gist
oph-thal-mol-o-gy
oph-thal-mo-ma-cro-sis
oph-thal-mo-ma-la-ci-a
oph-thal-mo-mel-a-no-ma
oph-thal-mom-e-ter
oph-thal-mom-e-try
oph-thal-mo-my-co-sis
oph-thal-mo-my-i-tis
oph-thal-mop-a-thy
oph-thal-mo-phy-ma
oph-thal-mo-plas-ty
oph-thal-mo-ple-gi-a
oph-thal-mor-rhex-is
oph-thal-mos
oph-thal-mo-scope
oph-thal-mo-scop-ic

oph-thal-mos-co-py
oph-thal-mo-spasm
oph-thal-mos-ta-sis
oph-thal-mo-stat
oph-thal-mot-o-my
oph-thal-mo-to-nom-
e-ter
oph-thal-mo-tro-pom-
e-try
oph-thal-mus
o-pi-ate
o-pi-o-ma-ni-a
o-pis-the-nar
o-pis-thi-on
op-is-thog-na-thism
o-pis-tho-po-rei-a
Op-is-thor-chis
op-is-thot-o-nos
o-pi-um
op-po-nens
op-por-tu-nist
op-sin-o-gen
op-si-nog-e-nous
op-so-nin
op-son-i-za-tion
op-so-no-cy-to-pha-gic
op-tic
op-ti-cal
op-ti-cian
op-ti-co-cil-i-ar-y
op-ti-co-pu-pil-lar-y
op-tics
op-ti-mum
op-tom-e-ter
op-tom-e-trist
op-tom-e-try
op-to-my-om-e-ter
o-ral
or-ange
or-bic-u-lar
or-bic-u-lar-is
or-bit

or-bi-tal
or-bi-to-na-sal
or-chi-dot-o-my
or-chi-ec-to-my
or-chi-ep-i-did-y-mi-tis
or-chi-o-cele
or-chi-o-pa-thy
or-chi-o-pex-y
or-chi-o-plas-ty
or-chi-tis
or-chot-o-my
or-cin
or-der
or-der-ly
or-di-nate
o-rex-is
orf
or-gan
or-gan-elle
or-gan-ic
or-gan-ism
or-gan-i-za-tion
or-gan-i-zer
or-gan-o-gel
or-ga-no-gen-e-sis
or-ga-no-me-tal-lic
or-gan-o-sol
or-ga-no-trop-ic
or-gasm
or-gas-tic
o-ri-en-tal sore
o-ri-en-ta-tion
or-i-fice
or-i-gin
or-ni-thine
Or-ni-thod-o-rus
or-ni-tho-sis
o-ro-phar-ynx
O-ro-ya val-ley fe-ver
or-ris
or-tho-caine
or-tho-chlo-ro-phe-nol

or-tho-chro-mat-ic
or-tho-cre-sol
or-tho-di-a-graph
or-tho-don-tics
or-tho-dont-ist
or-tho-gen-e-sis
or-tho-grade
or-tho-ki-net-ic
or-thom-e-ter
or-tho-pe-dic
or-tho-pe-dist
or-tho-phe-nan-thro-
line
or-tho-pho-ri-a
or-thop-ne-a
or-tho-psy-chi-a-try
or-thop-tic
or-thop-tics
or-thop-to-scope
or-tho-scop-ic
or-tho-stat-ic
or-thot-ic
or-thot-o-nus
or-thot-ro-pism
os cal-cis
os pu-bis
o-sa-zone
os-cil-la-tion
os-cil-la-tor
os-cil-lo-graph
os-cil-lom-e-ter
os-cil-lo-scope
Os-cin-i-dae
Os-ci-nis
os-ci-ta-tion
os-cu-la-tion
Osgood—Schlatter dis-
ease
os-mat-ic
os-mic ac-id
os-mi-um
os-mol

183

os-mo-lar-i-ty
os-mol-o-gy
os-mom-e-ter
os-mo-sis
os-mot-ic
os-sa
os-se-o-car-ti-lag-i-nous
os-se-o-fi-brous
os-se-ous
os-si-cle
os-sif-er-ous
os-sif-ic
os-si-fi-ca-tion
os-si-form
os-si-fy
os-tal-gi-a
os-tal-gi-tis
os-te-al
os-tec-to-my
os-te-i-tis
os-te-o-ar-threc-to-my
os-te-o-ar-thri-tis
os-te-o-ar-throp-a-thy
os-te-o-ar-throt-o-my
os-te-o-blast
os-te-o-blas-to-ma
os-te-o-car-ci-no-ma
os-te-o-car-ti-lag-i-nous
os-te-o-chon-dral
os-te-o-chon-dri-tis
os-te-o-chon-dro-dys-pla-si-a
os-te-o-chon-dro-dys-tro-phi-a
os-te-o-chon-dro-ma
os-te-o-chon-dro-ma-to-sis
os-te-o-chon-dro-myx-o-ma

os-te-o-chon-dro-myx-o-sar-co-ma
os-te-o-chon-dro-sar-co-ma
os-te-o-chon-dro-sis
os-te-oc-la-sis
os-te-o-clast
os-te-o-cys-to-ma
os-te-o-cyte
os-te-o-dyn-i-a
os-te-o-dys-tro-phy
os-te-o-fi-bro-chon-dro-ma
os-te-o-fi-bro-ma
os-te-o-fi-bro-sar-co-ma
os-te-o-fi-bro-sis
os-te-o-gen-e-sis im-per-fec-ta
os-te-o-gen-ic
os-te-o-hy-per-troph-ic
os-te-oid
os-te-o-lip-o-chon-dro-ma
os-te-ol-o-gy
os-te-ol-y-sis
os-te-o-ma
os-te-o-ma-la-ci-a
os-te-o-met-ric
os-te-o-my-e-li-tis
os-te-o-myx-o-chon-dro-ma
os-te-o-ne-cro-sis
os-te-o-neph-rop-a-thy
os-te-o-neu-ral-gia
os-te-o-path
os-te-op-a-thy
os-te-o-per-i-os-ti-tis
os-te-o-pe-tro-sis
os-te-o-phage
os-te-o-plas-ty
os-te-o-po-ro-sis
os-te-o-sar-co-ma

os-te-o-scle-ro-sis
os-te-o-spon-gi-o-ma
os-te-o-syn-o-vi-tis
os-te-o-syn-the-sis
os-te-o-tome
os-te-ot-o-my
os-te-o-tribe
os-ti-tis
os-ti-um
os-to-sis
o-tal-gi-a
o-the-ma-to-ma
o-tic
o-ti-tis
o-to-dyn-i-a
o-to-gen-ic
o-to-lar-yn-gol-o-gist
o-to-lar-yn-gol-o-gy
o-to-lith
o-tol-o-gist
o-tol-o-gy
o-to-my-co-sis
o-to-pha-ryn-ge-al
o-to-plas-ty
o-to-rhi-nol-o-gy
o-tor-rha-gi-a
o-tor-rhe-a
o-to-scle-ro-sis
o-to-scope
o-to-scop-ic
o-tot-o-my
ot-ri-vin
oua-ba-in
ounce
out-flow
out-let
out-pa-tient
o-va
o-val
o-val-bu-min
o-val-o-cyte
o-va-ri-an

o-va-ri-ec-to-my
o-va-ri-o-gen-ic
o-va-ri-o-hys-ter-ec-
    to-my
o-va-ri-o-sal pin-gec-
    to-my
o-va-ri-tis
o-va-ri-um
o-va-ry
o-ver-bite
o-ver-cor-rec-tion
o-ver-de-pen-den-cy
o-ver-de-ter-mi-na-tion
o-ver-ex-ten-sion
o-ver-flow
o-ver-growth
o-ver-ly-ing
o-ver-rid-ing
o-ver-tone
o-ver-weight
o-vi-duct
o-vif-er-ous
o-vi-form
o-vine
o-vip-a-rous
o-vi-pos-i-tor
o-vi vi-tel-lus
o-vo-cen-ter
o-void
o-vo-tes-tis
o-vo-vi-vip-a-rous
ov-u-lar
ov-u-la-tion
ov-ule
o-vum
ox-a-late
ox-al-ic
ox-al-o-a-ce-tic ac-id
ox-al-o-suc-cin-ic
    ac-id
ox-a-lu-ri-a
ox bile

ox-i-dant
ox-i-dase
ox-i-da-tion
ox-ide
ox-i-dize
ox-i-do—re-duc-tase
ox-im-e-ter
ox-o-i-som-er-ase
ox-y-ac-id
ox-y-ceph-a-ly
ox-y-chro-ma-tin
ox-y-gen
ox-y-gen-ase
ox-y-ge-na-ted
ox-y-ge-na-tion
ox-y-hem-a-tin
ox-y-he-mo-glo-bin
ox-y-op-ter
ox-y-phe-non-i-um
    bro-mide
ox-y-phil
ox-y-ster-oid
ox-y-tet-ra-cy-cline
ox-y-thi-a-mine
ox-y-to-cic
ox-y-to-cin
Ox-y-u-ris ver-mic-u-
    la-ris
o-ze-na
o-zone

P

pab-u-lum
pace-mak-er
pach-y-bleph-a-ro-sis
pach-y-ceph-a-ly
pach-y-der-ma-tous
pach-y-lep-to-men-in-
    gi-tis

pach-y-lo-sis
pach-y-men-in-gi-tis
pach-y-me-ninx
pa-chyn-tic
pach-y-o-nych-i-a
pach-y-pel-vi-per-i-
    to-ni-tis
pach-y-per-i-to-ni-tis
pa-chyt-ic
pac-i-fi-er
Pacinian cor-pus-cle
pack
pack-er
Padgett's der-ma-tome
Paget's dis-ease
pain
pair pro-duc-tion
pal-a-ta
pal-ate
pal-ate—hook
pal-a-tine
pal-a-ti-tis
pal-a-to-glos-sal
pal-a-to-glos-sus
pal-a-to-max-il-lar-y
pal-a-to-na-sal
pal-a-to-pha-ryn-ge-us
pal-a-to-plas-ty
pal-a-to-ple-gi-a
pal-a-tor-rha-phy
pal-a-tum
pa-le-o-cer-e-bel-lum
pa-le-on-tol-o-gy
pa-le-o-pa-thol-o-gy
pa-le-o-thal-a-mus
pal-i-ki-ne-si-a
pal-in-gen-e-sis
pal-i-op-si-a
pal-la-di-um
pal-les-the-si-a
pal-li-a-tion
pal-li-a-tive

185

pal-lor
pal-mar
pal-ma-ris
pal-ma-ture
Palmer meth-od
pal-mi-ped
pal-mi-tate
pal-mit-ic ac-id
pal-mi-tin
pal-mo-plan-tar
pal-mus
pal-pa-ble
pal-pate
pal-pa-tion
pal-pe-bra
pal-pe-bral
pal-pi-tate
pal-pi-ta-tion
pal-sy
pam-a-quine
pam-pin-i-form
pan-a-ce-a
pan-ag-glu-ti-nin
pan-ar-te-ri-tis
pan-ar-thri-tis
pan-at-ro-phy
pan-car-di-tis
Pancoast syn-drome
pan-co-lec-to-my
pan-cre-as
pan-cre-a-ta
pan-cre-at-i-co-du-o-de-
nal
pan-cre-at-i-co-en-ter-
os-to-my
pan-cre-at-i-co-je-ju-
nos-to-my
pan-cre-at-i-co-li-thot-
o-my
pan-cre-at-i-co-splen-ic
pan-cre-a-tin
pan-cre-a-ti-tis

pan-cre-a-to-du-o-de-nec-
to-my
pan-cre-a-to-en-ter-os-to-
my
pan-cre-a-to-li-thot-o-my
pan-cre-a-tot-o-my
pan-cre-ec-to-my
pan-cre-o-lith
pan-cre-o-zy-min
pan-cy-to-pe-ni-a
pan-de-mi-a
pan-dem-ic
Pandy's test
pan-en-do-scope
pang
pan-hy-po-pi-tu-i-ta-
rism
pan-hys-ter-ec-to-my
pan-hys-ter-o-col-pec-
to-my
pan-hys-ter-o-sal-pin-
gec-to-my
pan-hys-ter-o-sal-pin-
go—o-o-pho-rec-
to-my
pan-ic
pan-me-tri-tis
pan-nic-u-li-tis
pan-nic-u-lus
pan-nus
pan-oph-thal-mi-tis
pan-o-ti-tis
pan-si-nus-i-tis
Pan-stron-gy-lus meg-is-
tus
pan-ta-pho-bi-a
pan-to-pho-bi-a
pan-to-then-ic ac-id
pan-trop-ic
pa-nus
pan-zo-ot-ic
pa-pa-in

Papanicolau stain
pa-pav-er-ine
pa-paw
pa-pa-ya
pa-per
pa-pes-cent
pa-pil-la
pap-il-lar-y
pap-il-late
pa-pil-le-de-ma
pap-il-lif-er-ous
pa-pil-li-form
pap-il-li-tis
pap-il-lo-ma
pap-il-lo-ma-to-sis
pa-pil-lo-ret-i-ni-tis
pap-pose
pap-pus
pa-pri-ka
Pap's smear
pap-u-la-tion
pap-ule
pap-u-lif-er-ous
pap-u-lo-er-y-them-a-
tous
pap-u-lo-pus-tu-lar
pap-u-lo-squa-mous
pap-u-lo-ve-sic-u-lar
pap-y-ra-ce-ous
par-a—a-mi-no-ben-zo-ic
ac-id
par-a—a-mi-no-hip-pu-ric
ac-id
par-a—a-mi-no-sal-i-cyl-
ic ac-id
par-a—an-es-the-si-a
par-a—ap-pen-di-ci-tis
par-a-bi-o-sis
par-ac-an-tho-sis
par-a-ca-se-in
par-a-cen-te-sis
par-a-cen-tral

par-a-chol-er-a
par-a-chor-dal
par-a-chro-ma-tism
par-a-chro-ma-top-si-a
par-a-chro-mo-phor-ic
par-a-coc-cid-i-oi-do-my-co-sis
par-a-co-li-tis
par-a-co-lon
par-a-col-pi-tis
par-a-con-dy-lar
par-a-cu-si-a
par-a-cy-e-sis
par-a-cys-tic
par-a-cys-ti-tis
par-a—di-chlo-ro-ben-zene
par-a-dox-i-a-sex-u-al-is
par-a-du-o-de-nal
par-a-dys-en-ter-y
par-a-ep-i-lep-sy
par-af-fin
par-af-fi-no-ma
par-a-form-al-de-hyde
par-a-gan-gli-o-ma
par-a-gan-gli-ons
par-a-geu-si-a
par-ag-glu-ti-na-tion
Par-a-gon-i-mus wes-ter-man-i
par-a-gran-u-lo-ma
par-a-graph-i-a
par-a-he-mo-phil-i-a
par-a-he-pat-ic
par-a-hy-drox-y-ben-zo-ic ac-id
par-a-in-flu-en-za
par-a-ker-a-to-sis
par-al-de-hyde
par-a-lex-i-a
par-al-ge-si-a
par-al-lax

par-al-lel-ism
par-al-lel-om-e-ter
pa-ral-o-gism
pa-ral-y-sis
par-a-lyt-ic
par-a-ly-zant
par-a-ly-zer
par-a-mag-net-ic
par-a-mas-ti-tis
par-a-mas-toid-i-tis
Par-a-me-ci-um
par-a-me-di-an
pa-ram-e-ter
par-a-meth-a-di-one
par-a-me-tri-tis
par-a-me-tri-um
par-am-ne-si-a
par-a-mo-lar
par-a-mu-cin
par-a-my-e-lo-blast
par-a-my-oc-lo-nus mul-ti-plex
par-a-my-o-to-ni-a con-gen-i-ta
par-a-na-sal
par-a-ne-phri-tis
par-a-neu-ral
par-a—ni-tro-sul-fa-thi-a-zole
par-a-noi-a
par-a-noid state
par-a-nu-cle-us
par-a-per-tus-sis
par-a-pha-si-a
par-a-phen-yl-ene-di-am-ine
par-a-phi-mo-sis
par-a-pho-bi-a
par-a-pho-ni-a
par-a-phra-si-a
par-a-plas-tic
par-a-pneu-mo-ni-a

par-a-pso-ri-a-sis
par-a-psy-chol-o-gy
par-a-rec-tal
par-a-sa-cral
par-a-sag-it-tal
par-a-site
par-a-sit-ic cap-ture
par-a-sit-i-cide
par-a-sit-ism
par-a-si-tize
par-a-si-to-gen-ic
par-a-si-tol-o-gist
par-a-si-tol-o-gy
par-a-si-to-sis
par-a-some
par-a-spasm
par-a—sprue
par-a-ster-nal
par-a-sym-pa-thet-ic
par-a-sym-pa-tho-lyt-ic
par-a-sym-pa-tho-mi-met-ic
par-a-syn-ap-sis
par-a-thor-mone
par-a-thy-rin
par-a-thy-roid
par-a-thy-roid-ec-to-my
par-a-thy-ro-tro-pic hor-mone
par-a-ton-sil-lar
par-a-tri-cho-sis
par-a-troph-ic
par-a-ty-phoid
par-a-u-re-thral
par-a-vag-i-nal
par-a-ver-te-bral
par-ax-i-al
parch-ment skin
Pardee's sign
par-e-gor-ic
pa-ren-chy-ma
pa-ren-chym-a-tous

par-e-nol
par-ent
par-en-ter-al
pa-re-sis
par-es-the-si-a
pa-reu-ni-a
par-fo-cal
par-hi-dro-sis
pa-ri-e-tal
pa-ri-e-to-fron-tal
pa-ri-e-to-mas-toid
pa-ri-e-to—oc-cip-i-tal
Par-is green
par-i-ty
Parker's flu-id
Parkinson's dis-ease
par-kin-son-ism
par-o-don-ti-tis
par-o-don-ti-um
par-o-nych-i-a
par-o-nych-o-my-co-sis
pa-ro-pi-on
par-op-tic
par-o-rex-i-a
par-os-mi-a
par-os-ti-tis
par-os-to-sis
pa-rot-id
pa-rot-id-ec-to-my
par-o-ti-tis
par-ous
par-o-va-ri-an
par-o-va-ri-um
par-ox-ysm
par-rot fe-ver
pars an-te-ri-or
pars in-ter-me-di-a
pars ner-vo-sa
pars pos-te-ri-or
pars-ley
par-the-no-gen-e-sis
par-tial

par-tic-i-pa-tion
par-ti-cle
par-tic-u-late
par-ti-tion
par-tu-ri-ent
par-tu-ri-tion
pa-ru-lis
par-um-bil-i-cal
par-vule
Pascal's law
pas-sage
pas-sion
pas-sive
pas-siv-ism
pas-ta
paste boot
pas-tern
Pasteur treat-ment
Pas-teur-el-la pes-tis
Pas-teur-el-la tu-la-ren-sis
pas-teur-i-za-tion
pas-til
past point-ing
patch test
pate
pa-tel-la
pa-ten-cy
pa-tent
pa-thet-ic
path-o-don-ti-a
path-o-gen
path-o-gen-e-sis
path-o-gen-ic
path-o-ge-nic-i-ty
pa-thog-no-mon-ic
path-o-log-ic
pa-thol-o-gist
pa-thol-o-gy
pa-tho-met-ric
path-o-mim-ic-ry
path-o-phor-ic

path-o-psy-chol-o-gy
pa-tient
pat-ri-lin-e-al
pat-ten
pat-tern
pat-u-lous
Paul—Bunnell test
paunch
pause
Pavlovian re-sponse
pa-vor
paw-paw
Payr's clamp
pearl
peat
pec-tase
pec-tin
pec-tin-ase
pec-ti-nate
pec-tin-e-al
pec-tin-e-us
pec-to-ral
pec-to-ra-lis
pec-to-ril-o-quy
pec-tose
pec-tus ca-ri-na-tum
pec-tus ex-ca-va-tum
pe-di-at-rics
pe-di-a-tri-cian
ped-i-cle
pe-dic-te-rus
pe-dic-u-lar
pe-dic-u-li-cide
pe-dic-u-lo-sis cap-i-tis
pe-dic-u-lo-sis cor-po-ris
pe-dic-u-lo-sis pu-bis
Pe-dic-u-lus
ped-i-cure
pe-do-don-tics
pe-do-don-tist
pe-dol-o-gy
pe-dom-e-ter

pe-dun-cle
pe-dun-cu-la-ted
peel-ing
peg
Pel—Ebstein's dis-ease
pel-age
pel-lag-ra
Pellegrini—Stieda
    dis-ease
pel-let
pel-li-cle
pel-lic-u-la
pel-lo-tine
pel-lu-cid
pe-loid
pel-vim-e-ter
pel-vim-e-try
pel-vi-o-ra-di-og-ra-phy
pel-vis
pem-mi-can
pem-phi-goid
pem-phi-gus
pen-du-lous
pen-e-tra-ting
pen-e-tra-tion
pen-i-cil-late
pen-i-cil-li-form
pen-i-cil-lin
pen-i-cil-lin-ase
Pen-i-cil-li-um
pe-nis
pen-nate
pen-ni-form
pen-ny-weight
pe-nol-o-gist
pe-nol-o-gy
Penrose drain
pen-ta-chlo-ro-phe-nol
pen-ta-dac-tyl
pen-ta-e-ry-th-ri-tyl
    tet-ra-ni-trate
pen-ta-me-tho-ni-um

pen-tam-i-dine
pen-tane
pen-ta-quine
pen-tas-tomes
pen-ta-va-lent
pen-te-no-lac-tone
pen-to-bar-bi-tal
pen-to-lin-i-um bi-tar-
    trate
pen-to-sa-zone
pen-tose
pen-to-side
pep-per
pep-per-mint
pep-si-gogue
pep-sin
pep-sin-o-gen
pep-tic
pep-ti-dase
pep-tide
pep-ti-za-tion
pep-to-gen-ic
pep-tone
pep-to-nize
pep-to-nol-y-sis
pep-to-nu-ri-a
per-a-cute
per a-num
per-ben-zo-ic ac-id
per-bo-rate
per cent
per-cen-tile
per-cep-tion
per-cep-tiv-i-ty
per-chlo-rate
per-chlo-ric ac-id
per-chlo-ro-eth-yl-ene
per-co-la-tion
per-co-la-tor
per-cus-sion
per-cu-ta-ne-ous
per-for-ans

per-for-ate
per-fo-ra-ted
per-fo-ra-tion
per-fo-ra-tor
per-fu-sion
per-i-a-nal
per-i-an-gi-i-tis
per-i-an-gi-o-cho-li-tis
per-i-ap-i-cal
per-i-ap-pen-di-ci-tis
per-i-ar-te-ri-al
per-i-ar-te-ri-tis
per-i-ar-thri-tis
per-i-ar-tic-u-lar
per-i-a-tri-al
per-i-bron-chi-al
per-i-bron-chi-tis
per-i-car-di-o-cen-te-
    sis
per-i-car-di-tis
per-i-car-di-um
per-i-carp
per-i-cel-lu-lar
per-i-chol-an-gi-tis
per-i-chol-e-cys-ti-tis
per-i-chon-dri-tis
per-i-cho-roid
per-i-co-li-tis
per-i-cor-ne-al
per-i-cor-o-ni-tis
per-i-cys-tic
per-i-cyte
per-i-den-tal
per-i-du-o-de-ni-tis
per-i-du-ral
per-i-en-ter-i-tis
per-i-e-so-phag-e-al
per-i-fol-lic-u-li-tis
per-i-glot-tic
per-i-he-pat-ic
per-i-hi-lar
per-i-kar-y-on

per-i-lymph
per-im-e-ter
per-i-me-tri-tis
per-im-e-try
per-i-ne-al
per-i-ne-o-plas-ty
per-i-ne-or-rha-phy
per-i-ne-ot-o-my
per-i-neph-ric
per-i-ne-phrit-ic
per-i-ne-um
per-i-neu-ri-tis
per-i-nu-cle-ar
per-i-oc-u-lar
pe-ri-od
pe-ri-od-ic
pe-ri-o-dic-i-ty
pe-ri-od-ic ta-ble
per-i-o-don-tal
per-i-o-don-tics
per-i-o-don-tist
per-i-o-don-ti-tis
per-i-o-don-ti-um
per-i-o-don-tol-o-gy
per-i-om-phal-ic
per-i-o-nych-i-a
per-i-o-nych-i-um
per-i-or-al
per-i-or-bi-tal
per-i-os-te-al
per-i-os-te-um
per-i-os-ti-tis
per-i-os-to-sis
per-i-o-tic
per-i-phak-us
pe-riph-er-al
pe-riph-er-y
per-i-phle-bi-tis
Per-i-pla-ne-ta
per-i-por-tal
per-i-proc-ti-tis
per-i-pros-ta-ti-tis

per-i-rec-tal
per-i-re-nal
per-i-sal-pin-gi-tis
per-i-splen-ic
per-i-spon-dy-li-tis
per-i-stal-sis
per-i-stal-tic
per-i-syn-o-vi-al
per-i-ten-di-ni-tis
per-i-thy-roid-i-tis
per-i-to-ne-al
per-i-to-ne-o-cen-te-sis
per-i-to-ne-os-cop-y
per-i-to-ne-um
per-i-to-ni-tis
per-i-ton-sil-lar
per-i-tra-che-al
pe-rit-ri-chous
per-i-typh-lic
per-i-um-bil-i-cal
per-i-un-gual
per-i-u-re-thral
per-i-u-ter-ine
per-i-vag-i-nal
per-i-vas-cu-lar
per-i-ve-nous
per-i-ves-i-cal
per-i-vi-tel-line
perle
per-lèché
per-ma-nent
per-man-ga-nate
per-me-a-bil-i-ty
per-me-a-ble
per-me-a-tion
per-ni-cious
pe-rom-e-ly
per-o-ne-al
per-o-ne-us bre-vis
per-o-ne-us lon-gus
per-o-ral
per os

per-ox-i-dase
per-ox-ide
per-pen-dic-u-lar
per pri-mam
per rec-tum
per-sev-er-a-tion
per-sim-mon
per-son-al
per-son-al-i-ty
per-spi-ra-tion
per-spire
Perthes dis-ease
per-tur-ba-tion
per-tus-sis
per-ver-sion
per-vert
pes ca-vus
pes pla-nus
pes-sa-ry
pes-ti-cide
pes-tis
pes-tle
pe-te-chi-a
pe-te-chi-al
peth-i-dine
pe-tit-mal
Petragnani's me-di-um
Petri dish
pet-ri-fac-tion
pet-ro-chem-i-cal
pet-ro-la-tum
pe-tro-le-um
pe-tro-sal
pet-ro-si-tis
pet-rous
Peyer's patches
Peyronie's dis-ease
Pfannenstiel's in-ci-
    sion
pha-ci-tis
phac-o-cys-tec-to-my
phac-o-er-i-sis

190

pha-col-y-sis
phac-o-met-a-cho-re-sis
phac-o-scle-ro-sis
phac-os-cop-y
phage
phag-o-cyte
phag-o-cy-tol-y-sis
phag-o-cy-to-sis
phag-o-ma-ni-a
pha-lan-ge-al
pha-lan-ges
pha-lanx
phal-lic
phal-lus
phan-tasm
phan-ta-sy
phan-tom
phar-ma-ceu-ti-cal
phar-ma-cist
phar-ma-cog-no-sist
phar-ma-cog-no-sy
phar-ma-col-o-gist
phar-ma-col-o-gy
phar-ma-co-pe-ia
phar-ma-cy
phar-yn-gal-gi-a
phar-yn-ge-al
phar-yn-gec-to-my
phar-yn-gi-tis
pha-ryn-go-cele
pha-ryn-go-ep-i-glot-
tic
pha-ryn-go-e-so-phag-
e-al
pha-ryn-go-la-ryn-ge-
al
pha-ryn-go-lar-yn-gi-
tis
phar-yn-gol-o-gy
pha-ryn-go-na-sal
pha-ryn-go-pal-a-tine
pha-ryn-go-rhi-ni-tis

pha-ryn-go-scope
pha-ryn-go-spasm
phar-yn-got-o-my
pha-ryn-go-ton-sil-li-
tis
phar-ynx
phase
phe-nac-e-tin
phe-nan-threne
phen-in-di-one
phe-no-bar-bi-tal
phe-nol
phe-nol-phthal-ein
phe-nol-sul-fon-phthal-
ein
phe-no-lu-ri-a
phe-nom-e-non
phe-no-thi-a-zine
phe-no-type
phen-tol-a-mine
phen-yl-a-ce-tic ac-id
phen-yl-al-a-nine
phen-yl-bu-ta-zone
phen-yl-ene-di-a-mine
phen-yl-eph-rine
hy-dro-chlo-ride
phen-yl-hy-dra-zine
phen-yl-ke-to-nu-ri-a
phen-yl-mer-cu-ric
ac-e-tate
phen-yl-pro-pa-nol-a-
mine
phen-yl-py-ru-vic
ac-id
phen-yl-py-ru-vic ol-i-
go-phre-ni-a
phe-o-chro-mo-blas-to-
ma
phe-o-chro-mo-cy-to-ma
phil-ter
phil-trum
phi-mo-sis

phle-bec-to-my
phle-bi-tis
phleb-o-gram
phleb-o-lith
phleb-o-li-thi-a-sis
phleb-or-rhex-is
phleb-o-scle-ro-sis
phleb-o-throm-bo-sis
Phle-bot-o-mus
phle-bot-o-my
phlegm
phleg-ma-si-a
phleg-mat-ic
phleg-mon
phlyc-ten-u-lar
pho-bi-a
pho-bic
pho-nal
pho-na-tion
phon-au-to-graph
pho-net-ic
phon-ic
phon-ics
pho-no-car-di-o-gram
pho-no-car-di-o-graph
pho-no-car-di-og-ra-phy
pho-no-gram
pho-no-graph
pho-nom-e-ter
pho-rom-e-ter
phor-op-ter
phor-o-scope
phose
phos-gene
phos-pha-tase
phos-phate
phos-pha-te-mi-a
phos-phene
phos-phide
phos-pho-cre-a-tine
phos-pho-e-nol-py-ru-
vic ac-id

phos-pho-fruc-to-mu-tase
phos-pho-ga-lac-to-i-so-mer-ase
phos-pho-glu-co-mu-tase
phos-pho-glu-con-ic ac-id
phos-pho-glyc-er-al-de-hyde
phos-pho-hex-o-i-som-er-ase
phos-pho-hex-o-ki-nase
phos-pho-lip-id
phos-pho-mo-lyb-dic ac-id
phos-pho-nu-cle-ase
phos-pho-pro-te-in
phos-pho-pyr-i-dine nu-cle-o-tides
phos-pho-py-ru-vic ac-id
phos-phor
phos-phor-es-cence
phos-phor-ic ac-id
phos-pho-rism
phos-pho-rous ac-id
phos-pho-rus
phos-phor-yl-ase
phos-pho-ryl-a-tion
phos-pho-ser-ine
phos-sy jaw
pho-tal-gi-a
pho-tic
pho-to-chem-i-cal
pho-to-chem-is-try
pho-to-col-or-im-e-ter
pho-to-con-junc-ti-vi-tis
pho-to-der-ma-to-sis
pho-to-dy-nam-ic
pho-to-e-lec-tric col-or-im-e-ter

pho-to-e-lec-tron
pho-to-flu-or-os-co-py
pho-to-gen-ic
pho-tol-y-sis
pho-to-mes-on
pho-tom-e-ter
pho-tom-e-try
pho-to-mi-cro-graph
pho-ton
pho-to-neu-tron
pho-to-nu-cle-ar re-ac-tion
pho-to-per-cep-tive
pho-to-pho-bi-a
pho-toph-thal-mi-a
pho-to-po-lym-er-i-za-tion
pho-to-pro-ton
pho-top-si-a
pho-top-tom-e-ter
pho-to-re-cep-tive
pho-to-sen-si-tiv-i-ty
pho-to-sen-si-ti-za-tion
pho-to-syn-the-sis
pho-to-tax-is
pho-to-ti-mer
pho-to-troph-ic
pho-tot-ro-pism
phren-as-the-ni-a
phre-net-ic
phren-ic
phren-i-cec-to-my
phren-i-co-splen-ic
phren-i-cot-o-my
phren-i-co-trip-sy
phren-o-car-di-a
phre-nol-o-gy
phren-o-ple-gi-a
phren-o-splen-ic
phryn-o-der-ma
phthal-ic ac-id

phthal-ic an-hy-dride
Phthir-i-us pu-bis
phthi-sis
Phy-co-my-ce-tes
phyg-o-ga-lac-tic
phy-let-ic
phy-log-e-ny
phy-lum
phy-ma
phys-i-at-rics
phys-i-at-rist
phys-ic
phys-i-cal
phy-si-cian
phys-i-cist
phys-i-co-chem-i-cal
phys-ics
phys-i-og-no-my
phys-i-o-log-ic
phys-i-ol-o-gist
phys-i-ol-o-gy
phys-i-o-ther-a-py
phy-sique
phy-so-stig-mine
phy-to-be-zoar
phy-to-chem-is-try
phy-to-gen-e-sis
phy-tog-e-nous
phy-to-par-a-site
phy-to-path-o-gen-ic
phy-to-pa-thol-o-gy
phy-toph-a-gous
phy-to-pneu-mo-no-co-ni-o-sis
phy-to-sis
phy-to-tox-ic
pi-a
pi-a-rach-noid
pi-ca
Pick's dis-ease
pic-rate
pic-ric ac-id

pic-ro-car-mine
pic-ro-tox-in
pi-e-zo-e-lec-tric
    ef-fect
pi-e-zom-e-ter
pi-geon—toed
pig-ment
pig-men-tar-y
pig-men-ta-tion
pig-men-tum
pi-lar
pi-las-tered
pile
pi-le-ous
piles
pil-i-a-tion
pil-i-form
pill
pil-lar
pi-lo-car-pine
pi-lo-e-rec-tion
pi-lo-mo-tor
pi-lo-ni-dal
pi-lose
pi-lo-se-ba-ceous
pi-lo-sis
pi-lus
pim-e-lo-pte-ryg-i-um
pim-e-lor-thop-ne-a
pim-ple
pin-a-coid
Pinard's ma-neu-ver
pin-cers
pine oil
pin-e-al
pin-e-a-lo-ma
pine tar
pin-guec-u-la
pi-ni-form
pink-eye
pin-na
Pins's sign

pin-ta
pin-worm
Pi-oph-i-la
pi-per-a-zine
pi-per-i-dine
pip-er-ine
pi-per-i-tone
pip-er-o-caine hy-dro-
    chlo-ride
pip-er-o-nal
pip-er-ox-an hy-dro-
    chlo-ride
pi-pet
pir-i-form
pir-i-for-mis
pi-ro-plas-mo-sis
pis-iform
pitch-blende
pi-the-coid
pith-i-at-ric
pit-ted
pit-ting
pi-tu-i-tar-y
pit-y-ri-a-sis cap-i-tis
pit-y-ri-a-sis ro-se-a
pit-y-ri-a-sis ver-si-
    col-or
Pit-y-ro-spor-um o-vale
piv-ot-ing
pla-ce-bo
pla-cen-ta
pla-cen-ta ac-cre-ta
pla-cen-ta in-cre-ta
pla-cen-ta per-cre-ta
pla-cen-ta pre-vi-a
pla-cen-ta pre-vi-a
    cen-tral-is
pla-cen-ta pre-vi-a mar-
    gi-nal-is
pla-cen-ta pre-vi-a
    par-ti-al-is

pla-cen-ta suc-cen-tu-
    ri-ata
plac-en-ta-tion
plac-en-ti-tis
plac-ode
plad-a-ro-ma
pla-gi-o-ce-phal-ic
plague
pla-na
Planck's con-stant
pla-ni-ceps
pla-nig-ra-phy
plan-ing
plank-ton
pla-no-con-cave
pla-no-con-ic
pla-no-con-vex
pla-no-gram
Pla-nor-bis
plan-ta
Plan-ta-go psyl-li-um
plan-tar
plan-tar-is
plan-tar wart
plan-ta-tion
plan-ti-grade
pla-num
plaque
plasm
plas-ma-blast
plas-ma-cy-te
plas-ma-cy-to-ma
plas-ma-cy-to-sis
plas-ma-gel
plas-ma-lem-ma
plas-ma-some
plas-min
plas-min-o-gen
plas-mo-cy-to-ma
Plas-mo-di-um fal-ci-
    par-um

Plas-mo-di-um ma-lar-i-ae
Plas-mo-di-um o-vale
Plas-mo-di-um vi-vax
plas-mo-gen
plas-mol-y-sis
plas-mo-lyze
plas-mop-ty-sis
plas-mor-rhex-is
plas-mo-sin
plas-mo-some
plas-ter
plas-ter of Paris
plas-tic
plas-tic-i-ty
plas-ti-ciz-er
plas-tin
plas-to-some
pla-teau
plate cul-ture
plate-let
pla-ting
pla-tin-ic
plat-i-nous
plat-i-num
plat-ode
plat-y-ba-si-a
plat-y-ce-phal-ic
Plat-y-hel-min-thes
plat-y-mor-phi-a
plat-y-o-pic
plat-y-pel-lic
plat-yr-rhine
pla-tys-ma
pledg-et
plei-ot-rop-ic
ple-och-ro-mat-ic
ple-o-cy-to-sis
ple-o-mor-phic
ple-on-os-te-o-sis
pleth-o-ra
ple-thys-mo-graph

pleth-ys-mog-ra-phy
pleu-ra
pleu-ral-gi-a
pleu-rec-to-my
pleu-ri-sy
pleu-rit-ic
pleu-ri-tis
pleu-ro-cen-te-sis
pleu-ro-cu-ta-ne-ous
pleu-ro-dy-ni-a
pleu-ro-gen-ic
pleu-rol-y-sis
pleu-ro-per-i-car-di-al
pleu-ro-per-i-car-di-tis
pleu-ro-pneu-mo-ni-a
pleu-ro-pneu-mo-ni-tis
pleu-ro-pul-mo-nar-y
pleu-ros-co-py
pleu-rot-o-my
plex-i-form
plex-or
plex-us
pli-ca
pli-cate
pli-cot-o-my
plom-bage
plug-ger
plug-ging
plum-ba-go
plum-bic
plum-bism
plum-bum
Plummer—Vinson syn-drome
plu-to-ni-um
pne-o-dy-nam-ics
pne-om-e-ter
pneu-mar-thro-sis
pneu-mat-ic
pneu-ma-ti-za-tion
pneu-ma-to-car-di-a

pneu-ma-to-cele
pneu-ma-to-gram
pneu-ma-tol-o-gy
pneu-ma-tom-e-try
pneu-ma-tu-ri-a
pneu-mo-an-gi-og-ra-phy
pneu-mo—ar-throg-ra-phy
pneu-mo-cen-te-sis
pneu-mo-coc-cal
pneu-mo-coc-cus
pneu-mo-co-ni-o-sis
pneu-mo-cyst-o-gram
pneu-mo-en-ceph-a-lo-gram
pneu-mo-en-ceph-a-log-ra-phy
pneu-mo-graph
pneu-mog-ra-phy
pneu-mo-he-mo-per-i-car-di-um
pneu-mo-he-mo-tho-rax
pneu-mo-lith
pneu-mo-li-thi-a-sis
pneu-mo-me-di-as-ti-num
pneu-mom-e-try
pneu-mo-nec-to-my
pneu-mo-ni-a
pneu-mon-ic
pneu-mo-ni-tis
pneu-mo-nol-y-sis
pneu-mo-no-my-co-sis
pneu-mo-nor-rha-phy
pneu-mo-not-o-my
pneu-mop-a-thy
pneu-mo-per-i-car-di-um
pneu-mo-per-i-to-ne-um
pneu-mo-per-i-to-ni-tis
pneu-mo-ra-di-og-ra-phy
pneu-mo-roent-gen-og-ra-phy

pneu-mo-scle-ro-sis
pneu-mo-tax-ic
pneu-mo-tho-rax
pneu-mo-tox-in
pneu-mo-ven-tric-u-log-ra-phy
pock
pocked
pock-et
pock—marked
po-dal-gi-a
po-dal-ic
po-di-a-trist
po-di-a-try
po-dom-e-ter
pod-o-phyl-lin
pod-o-phyl-lum res-in
po-go-ni-on
poi-ki-lo-blast
poi-ki-lo-cyte
poi-ki-lo-cy-the-mi-a
poi-ki-lo-cy-to-sis
poi-ki-lo-der-ma
poi-ki-lo-der-ma-to-my-o-si-tis
poi-ki-lo-ther-mic
poi-ki-lo-zo-o-sper-mi-a
point-ing
poise
poi-son
poi-son-ing
poi-son i-vy
poi-son oak
poi-son-ous
poi-son su-mac
poke-ber-ry
po-ker back
po-lar
po-lar-im-e-ter
po-lar-i-scope
po-lar-i-ty
po-lar-i-za-tion

po-lar-ize
po-lar-o-gram
po-lar-og-ra-phy
po-li-o
po-li-o-en-ceph-a-li-tis
po-li-o-en-ceph-a-lo-me-nin-go-my-e-li-tis
po-li-o-en-ceph-a-lo-my-e-li-tis
po-li-o-my-e-len-ceph-a-li-tis
po-li-o-my-e-li-tis
Politzer bag
poll
pol-len
pol-le-no-sis
pol-lex
pol-lu-tion
po-lo-ni-um
Pólya's meth-od
pol-y-ac-id
pol-y-an-dry
pol-y-ar-te-ri-tis no-do-sa
pol-y-ar-thri-tis
pol-y-ar-tic-u-lar
pol-y-ba-sic
pol-y-cel-lu-lar
pol-y-cen-tric
pol-y-chro-ma-si-a
pol-y-chro-mat-ic
pol-y-chro-ma-to-phil
pol-y-chro-ma-to-phil-ic
pol-y-chro-mi-a
pol-y-clin-ic
pol-y-cy-clic
pol-y-cy-e-sis
pol-y-cys-tic
pol-y-cy-the-mi-a
pol-y-dac-tyl-ism

pol-y-dac-ty-ly
pol-y-dip-si-a
pol-y-e-lec-tro-lyte
pol-y-ene
pol-y-eth-yl-ene
pol-y-ga-lac-ti-a
po-lyg-a-mous
pol-y-gas-tric
pol-y-glan-du-lar
po-lyg-o-nal
pol-y-graph
pol-y-he-dral
pol-y-hy-dram-ni-os
pol-y-hy-dru-ri-a
pol-y-lec-i-thal
pol-y-lep-tic
pol-y-mas-ti-a
pol-y-mer
pol-y-mer-ic
po-lym-er-ide
po-lym-er-ism
pol-y-mer-i-za-tion
pol-y-mer-ize
pol-y-morph
pol-y-mor-phic
pol-y-mor-pho-cel-lu-lar
pol-y-mor-pho-nu-cle-ar
pol-y-my-o-si-tis
pol-y-myx-in
pol-y-ne-sic
pol-y-neu-ral-gi-a
pol-y-neu-ri-tis
pol-y-neu-rop-a-thy
pol-y-nu-cle-ar
pol-y-nu-cle-ot-i-dase
pol-y-nu-cle-o-tide
pol-y-o-don-ti-a
pol-y-o-pi-a
pol-y-or-chid-ism
pol-y-o-rex-i-a
pol-yp
pol-y-pa-re-sis

pol-y-pep-ti-dase
pol-y-pep-tide
pol-y-pha-gi-a
pol-y-pho-bi-a
pol-y-phy-o-dont
pol-y-ploid
pol-yp-ne-a
pol-yp-oid
pol-y-po-sis
pol-y-pus
pol-y-ra-dic-u-li-tis
pol-y-sac-cha-ride
pol-y-si-nus-i-tis
pol-y-so-mus
pol-y-sper-mi-a
pol-y-stom-a-tous
pol-y-sty-rene
pol-y-symp-to-mat-ic
pol-y-the-li-a
pol-y-trop-ic
pol-y-u-ri-a
pol-y-va-lent
pol-y-vi-nyl al-co-hol
pol-y-vi-nyl-pyr-rol-i-done
po-made
pome-gran-ate
pom-pho-lyx
pon-der-a-ble
pons
pon-tic
pon-tile
pon-tine
pop-li-te-al
pop-li-te-us
pop-py
pore
por-nog-ra-phy
Por-o-ceph-a-lus
por-o-ker-a-to-sis
por-o-plas-tic
po-ros-i-ty

po-rous
por-phin
por-pho-bi-lin-o-gen
por-phy-ri-a
por-phy-rin
por-phy-ri-nu-ri-a
por-phyr-u-ri-a
Porro's op-er-a-tion
por-ta
por-ta-ca-val
por-tal
por-ti-o
port—wine mark
Posadas' dis-ease
po-si-tion
pos-i-tive
pos-i-tron
pos-i-tro-ni-um
post-an-es-thet-ic
post-au-di-to-ry
post-ca-val
post-cen-tral
post-en-ceph-a-lit-ic
post-ep-i-lep-tic
pos-te-ri-or
pos-ter-o-an-te-ri-or
pos-ter-o-lat-er-al
pos-ter-o-me-di-al
pos-ter-o-su-pe-ri-or
post-e-rup-tive
post-fe-brile
post-gan-gli-on-ic
post-hem-or-rhag-ic
pos-thi-tis
post-hu-mous
post-hyp-not-ic
post-ic-ter-ic
post-mor-tem
post-na-tal
post—par-tum
post-pran-di-al
post-ro-ta-to-ry

post-trau-mat-ic
pos-tu-late
pos-tur-al
pos-ture
post-vac-ci-nal
po-ta-ble
pot-ash
pot-as-se-mi-a
po-tas-si-um
po-ten-cy
po-ten-tial
po-ten-ti-a-tion
po-tion
Pott's dis-ease
Pott's frac-ture
pouch
pou-drage
poul-tice
Poupart's lig-a-ment
pow-der
pow-er
pox
prac-tice
pran-di-al
pre-an-es-thet-ic
pre-au-ric-u-lar
pre-can-cer-ous
pre-cen-tral
pre-cip-i-tate
pre-cip-i-ta-tion
pre-cip-i-ta-tor
pre-cip-i-tin
pre-clin-i-cal
pre-co-cious
pre-coc-i-ty
pre-cog-ni-tion
pre-cor-di-um
pre-di-gest-ed
pre-dis-po-sing
pre-dis-po-si-tion
pre-ec-lamp-si-a
pre-e-rup-tive

pre-fron-tal
pre-gan-gli-on-ic
preg-nan-cy
preg-nane-di-ol
preg-nane-di-one
preg-nant
preg-nen-in-o-lone
preg-nen-o-lone
pre-hen-sile
pre-ma-lig-nant
pre-ma-ture
pre-max-il-lar-y
pre-med-i-ca-tion
pre-men-stru-al
pre-mo-lar
pre-mo-ni-tion
pre-mon-i-to-ry
pre-my-e-lo-blast
pre-nar-co-sis
pre-na-tal
pre-oc-cip-i-tal
prep-a-ra-tion
pre-pa-tel-lar
pre-pon-der-ance
pre-psy-chot-ic
pre-pu-ber-al
pre-puce
pre-py-lor-ic
pre-ret-i-nal
pre-sa-cral
pres-by-cu-sis
pres-by-o-phren-ic
pres-by-o-pi-a
pre-schiz-o-phren-ic
pre-scribe
pre-scrip-tion
pre-sent
pres-en-ta-tion
pre-sent-ing com-plaints
pres-sor
pres-so-re-cep-tor
pres-so-sen-si-tive

pres-sure
pre-sup-pu-ra-tive
pre-sys-to-le
pre-sys-tol-ic
prev-a-lence
pre-ven-tive med-i-cine
pre-ves-i-cal
pre-vi-a
pri-a-pism
prick-ly heat
pri-ma-quine phos-phate
pri-ma-ry
Pri-mates
pri-mi-grav-i-da
pri-mip-a-ra
prim-i-tive
pri-mor-di-al
pri-mor-di-um
prin-ceps
prin-ci-ple
prism
pris-mat-ic
pris-moid
pris-mop-tom-e-ter
priv-i-leged
pro-ac-cel-er-in
pro-ag-glu-ti-noid
prob-a-ble
probe
pro-ben-e-cid
pro-bit
pro-bos-cis
pro-caine
pro-caine am-ide hy-dro-
chlo-ride
proc-ess
pro-ces-sus
pro-chei-lon
pro-chon-dral
pro-chro-ma-tin
proc-i-den-ti-a
pro-con-ver-tin

pro-cre-ate
pro-cre-a-tion
proc-tal-gi-a
proc-ta-tre-si-a
proc-tec-ta-si-a
proc-tec-to-my
proc-ti-tis
proc-toc-ly-sis
proc-to-co-li-tis
proc-to-dyn-i-a
proc-tol-o-gist
proc-tol-o-gy
proc-to-scope
proc-tos-co-py
proc-to-sig-moid-ec-to-
my
proc-to-sig-moid-i-tis
proc-to-sig-moid-os-co-
py
pro-cum-bent
pro-cur-sive
prod-ro-mal
pro-drome
prod-uct
pro-duc-tive
pro-en-zyme
pro-e-ryth-ro-cyte
prc-es-trus
pro-fes-sion-al
pro-fla-vine
pro-flu-vi-um
pro-fun-da
pro-fun-dus
pro-gen-e-sis
pro-gen-i-tor
prog-e-ny
pro-ge-ri-a
pro-ges-ter-one
pro-glot-tid
pro-glot-tis
pro-gnath-ic
prog-na-thism

prog-nose
prog-no-sis
prog-nos-ti-cate
pro-gran-u-lo-cyte
pro-grav-id
pro-gres-sion
pro-gres-sive
pro-jec-tion
pro-ki-nase
pro-lac-tin
pro-lapse
pro-lap-sus
pro-lep-sis
pro-lif-er-ate
pro-lif-er-a-tion
pro-lif-ic
pro-line
pro-lym-pho-cyte
pro-meg-a-kar-y-o-cyte
pro-meth-a-zine hy-dro-
    chlo-ride
pro-me-thi-um
prom-i-nence
pro-mon-o-cyte
prom-on-to-ry
pro-my-e-lo-cyte
pro-nate
pro-na-tion
pro-na-tor
prone
pro-neph-ros
prong
pro-no-grade
pron-to-sil
pro-nu-cle-us
proof spir-it
prop-a-gate
pro-pam-i-dine
pro-pane
pro-pe-nyl eth-yl e-ther
pro-per-din
pro-per-i-to-ne-al

pro-phase
pro-phy-lac-tic
pro-phy-lax-is
pro-pi-o-nate
pro-pi-on-ic ac-id
pro-plas-ma-cyte
pro-pri-e-tar-y
pro-pri-o-cep-tion
pro-pri-o-cep-tive
pro-pri-o-cep-tor
pro-pri-us
prop-to-sis
pro-pul-sion
pro-pyl al-co-hol
pro-pyl-ene gly-col
pro-pyl-hex-e-drine
pro-pyl-thi-o-u-ra-cil
pro re na-ta
pro-ren-nin
pro-se-cre-tin
pro-sect
pro-sec-tor
pros-en-ceph-a-lon
pros-o-dem-ic
pros-o-pal-gi-a
pros-op-ic
pros-o-po-ple-gi-a
pros-o-pos-chi-sis
pros-tate
pros-ta-tec-to-my
pros-ta-tism
pros-ta-ti-tis
pros-ta-to-ve-sic-u-li-
    tis
pros-the-sis
pros-thet-ic
pros-the-tist
pros-tho-don-ti-a
pros-tho-don-tist
pros-ti-tu-tion
pros-trate
pros-trat-ed

pro-tac-tin-i-um
pro-ta-mine in-su-lin
pro-te-an
pro-te-ase
pro-tec-tive
pro-te-in
pro-te-in-ase
pro-te-in-e-mi-a
pro-te-in-u-ri-a
pro-te-o-lyt-ic
pro-te-ose
Pro-teus
pro-throm-bin
pro-throm-bi-ne-mi-a
pro-throm-bo-ki-nase
Pro-tis-ta
pro-ti-um
pro-to-col
pro-to-fi-bril
pro-tol-y-sis
pro-ton
pro-to-plasm
pro-to-plas-mic
pro-to-por-phy-rin
pro-to-ver-a-trine
pro-to-ver-ine
Pro-to-zo-a
pro-to-zo-an
pro-to-zo-ol-o-gy
pro-tract
pro-trac-tor
pro-trude
pro-tru-sion
pro-tu-ber-ance
proud flesh
pro-vi-ta-min
pro-voc-a-tive
prox-i-mal
prox-i-mate
prox-i-mo-buc-cal
prox-i-mo-la-bi-al
prox-i-mo-lin-gual

pru-rig-i-nous
pru-ri-go
pru-rit-ic
pru-ri-tus
pru-ri-tus a-ni
pru-ri-tus vul-vae
Prus-sian blue
prus-sic ac-id
psal-te-ri-um
psam-mo-ma
psel-lis-mus
pseu-dar-thro-sis
pseu-des-the-si-a
pseu-do-ag-glu-ti-na-tion
pseu-do-an-gi-na
pseu-do-cir-rho-sis
pseu-do-cy-e-sis
pseu-do-cyst
pseu-do-e-phed-rine
pseu-do-ep-i-lep-sy
pseu-do-glob-u-lin
pseu-do-he-mo-phil-i-a
pseu-do-her-maph-ro-dite
pseu-do-hy-per-tro-phy
pseu-do-hy-po-par-a-thy-roid-ism
pseu-do-ma-ni-a
pseu-do-mem-brane
pseu-do-men-stru-a-tion
Pseu-do-mo-nas ae-ru-gi-no-sa
Pseu-do-mo-nas cy-a-no-genes
pseu-do-mu-ci-nous
pseu-do-neu-ro-ma
pseu-do-pa-ral-y-sis
pseu-do-pod
pseu-do-pol-y-po-sis
pseu-do-scle-ro-sis
pseu-do-strat-i-fied

pseu-do-trun-cus ar-ter-i-o-sus
pseu-do-tu-ber-cu-lo-sis
pseu-do-xan-tho-ma e-las-ti-cum
psi phe-nom-e-na
psit-ta-co-sis
pso-as
pso-mo-pha-gi-a
pso-ri-a-sis
pso-ri-at-ic
psy-che
psy-chi-at-ric
psy-chi-a-trist
psy-chi-a-try
psy-chic
psy-cho-a-nal-y-sis
psy-cho-an-a-lyst
psy-cho-bi-ol-o-gy
psy-cho-cor-ti-cal
psy-cho-di-ag-nos-tics
psy-cho-dra-ma
psy-cho-dy-nam-ics
psy-cho-gen-ic o-ver-lay
psy-cho-gen-e-sis
psy-cho-gen-et-ic
psy-cho-lep-sy
psy-chol-o-gist
psy-chol-o-gy
psy-chom-e-try
psy-cho-mo-tor
psy-cho-neu-ro-sis
psy-cho-neu-rot-ic
psy-cho-path
psy-cho-path-i-a
psy-cho-pa-thol-o-gist
psy-cho-pa-thol-o-gy
psy-chop-a-thy
psy-cho-phys-i-o-log-ic
psy-cho-phys-i-ol-o-gy

psy-cho-ple-gic
psy-cho-sen-so-ry
psy-cho-sex-u-al
psy-cho-sis
psy-cho-so-mat-ic
psy-cho-sur-ger-y
psy-cho-ther-a-py
psy-chot-ic dis-or-der
psy-chrom-e-ter
psy-chro-phil-ic
psyl-li-um seed
ptar-mus
pter-i-on
pter-o-yl-glut-tam-ic ac-id
pte-ryg-i-um
pter-y-goid
pter-y-go-pal-a-tine
pter-y-go-pha-ryn-ge-us
pti-lo-sis
pto-maine
pto-sis
pty-a-lin
pty-a-lism
pty-a-lo-gen-ic
pty-al-o-gogue
pty-a-log-ra-phy
pu-ber-tas
pu-ber-ty
pu-bes
pu-bes-cence
pu-bic
pu-bis
pu-bo-coc-cyg-e-al
pu-den-dal
pu-den-dum
pu-er-ile
pu-er-per-al
pu-er-per-ant
pu-er-pe-ri-um
Pu-lex ir-ri-tans
pu-li-cide

pul-lu-la-tion
pul-mo-nar-y
pul-mon-ic
pul-mo-tor
pulp
pul-pa-tion
pul-pec-to-my
pulp-i-fac-tion
pulp-i-fy
pulp-i-tis
pulp-ot-o-my
pulp-y
pul-sate
pul-sa-tile
pul-sa-tion
pul-sa-tor
pulse
pulse def-i-cit
pulse-less
pulse pres-sure
pul-sion di-ver-tic-u-
    lum
pul-sus ir-reg-u-lar-is
pul-sus par-a-dox-us
pul-ver-ize
pul-vis
pum-ice
pump-kin seed
punc-tate
punc-ti-form
punc-tum
punc-ture
pun-gent
pu-pa
pu-pil
pu-pil-la
pu-pil-lar-y
pu-pil-lom-e-ter
pur-ga-tion
pur-ga-tive
purge
purg-ing

pu-ri-fied
pu-rine
Purkinje fi-bers
pur-pu-ra
purr
pu-ru-lence
pu-ru-lent
pus
pus—tube
pus-tu-lant
pus-tu-lar
pus-tu-la-tion
pus-tule
pus-tu-lo-sis
pu-ta-men
pu-tre-fac-tion
pu-tre-fac-tive
pu-tre-fy
pu-tres-cent
pu-trid
py-ar-thro-sis
pyc-nom-e-ter
pyc-no-sis
pyc-not-ic
py-e-li-tis
py-e-lo-cys-ti-tis
py-e-lo-gram
py-e-log-ra-phy
py-e-lo-li-thot-o-my
py-e-lo-ne-phrit-ic
py-e-lo-ne-phri-tis
py-e-los-to-my
py-e-mi-a
py-en-ceph-a-lus
pyg-my
pyk-nic
pyk-no-lep-sy
py-le-phle-bi-tis
py-le-throm-bo-sis
py-lor-i-ste-no-sis
py-lor-o-gas-trec-to-my
py-lor-o-my-ot-o-my

py-lor-o-plas-ty
py-lor-o-spasm
py-lor-o-ste-no-sis
py-lor-ot-o-my
py-lo-rus
py-o-col-pos
py-o-cy-an-ic
py-o-der-ma
py-o-der-ma-ti-tis
py-og-e-nes
py-o-gen-ic
py-o-he-mo-tho-rax
py-o-me-tra
py-o-ne-phri-tis
py-o-ne-phro-sis
py-o-per-i-car-di-um
py-o-per-i-to-ni-tis
py-o-pneu-mo-tho-rax
py-or-rhe-a
py-o-sal-pinx
py-o-sis
py-o-stat-ic
pyr-a-mid
py-ram-i-da-lis
py-ra-mid-ot-o-my
py-ra-nose
pyr-a-zine
pyr-a-zole
py-rec-tic
py-re-thrum
py-ret-ic
pyr-e-to-gen-ic
pyr-e-tol-y-sis
pyr-e-to-ther-a-py
py-rex-i-a
pyr-i-dine
pyr-i-dox-ine
py-ril-a-mine
py-rim-i-dine
py-ro-din
py-ro-gal-lol
py-ro-gen

py-ro-gen-ic
py-ro-glob-u-li-ne-mi-a
py-ro-ma-ni-a
py-rom-e-ter
py-ro-pho-bi-a
py-ro-phos-pha-tase
py-ro-phos-phate
py-ro-phos-phor-ic ac-id
py-ro-scope
py-ro-sis
py-rox-y-lin
pyr-role
py-ru-vate
py-ru-vic ac-id
py-u-ri-a

Q

Q fe-ver
quack-er-y
quad-ran-gu-lar
quad-rant
quad-rate
quad-ra-tus
quad-ri-ceps
quad-ri-gem-i-nal
quad-ri-ple-gi-a
quad-ri-va-lent
quad-ru-ped
quad-ru-plet
qual-i-ta-tive
qual-i-ty
quan-ta
quan-ti-ta-tive
quan-tum
quar-an-tine
quar-tan
quar-ter
quartz
qua-ter-na-ry

Queckenstedt's sign
Quervain's dis-ease
Quick meth-od
quick-en-ing
quick-lime
quick-sil-ver
quin-a-crine
quin-a-liz-a-rin
quin-hy-drone
quin-i-dine
qui-nine
qui-nin-ism
qui-none
quin-ox-a-line
quin-sy
quin-tu-plet
quo-tid-i-an
quo-tient

R

rab-bit fe-ver
rab-id
ra-bies
race
ra-ce-mic
ra-ce-mic ac-id
rac-e-mor-phan hy-dro-
    bro-mide
rac-e-mose
ra-chi-cele
ra-chi-o-camp-sis
ra-chi-om-e-ter
ra-chi-ot-o-my
ra-chi-re-sis-tance
ra-chis
ra-chit-ic
ra-chit-ic ro-sa-ry
rach-i-to-gen-ic
ra-cial

ra-clage
ra-dec-to-my
ra-di-al
ra-di-a-lis
ra-di-an
ra-di-ant
ra-di-a-tion
rad-i-cal
ra-dic-u-lar
ra-dic-u-lec-to-my
ra-dic-u-li-tis
ra-dic-u-lo-neu-ri-tis
ra-dic-u-lo-neu-rop-a-thy
ra-di-o-ac-tin-i-um
ra-di-o-ac-tive
ra-di-o-ac-tiv-i-ty
ra-di-o-au-to-graph
ra-di-o-bi-ol-o-gy
ra-di-o-chem-is-try
ra-di-o-co-balt
ra-di-o-cur-a-bil-i-ty
ra-di-o-cys-ti-tis
ra-di-o-der-ma-ti-tis
ra-di-o-don-ti-a
ra-di-o-gold
ra-di-o-graph
ra-di-og-ra-pher
ra-di-og-ra-phy
ra-di-o-hu-mer-al
ra-di-o-i-o-dine
ra-di-o-i-ron
ra-di-o-i-so-tope
ra-di-ol-o-gist
ra-di-ol-o-gy
ra-di-o-lu-cent
ra-di-o-lu-mi-nes-cence
ra-di-om-e-ter
ra-di-o-ne-cro-sis
ra-di-o-paque
ra-di-o-pel-vim-e-try
ra-di-o-phos-pho-rus
ra-di-o-po-tas-si-um

ra-di-o-re-sist-ance
ra-di-os-co-py
ra-di-o-sen-si-tiv-i-ty
ra-di-o-sil-i-con
ra-di-o-so-di-um
ra-di-o-ster-e-os-co-py
ra-di-o-stron-ti-um
ra-di-o-sul-fur
ra-di-o-ther-a-peu-tic
ra-di-o-ther-a-py
ra-di-o-tox-e-mi-a
ra-di-o-trans-par-ent
ra-di-o-ul-nar
ra-di-um
ra-di-um can-non
ra-di-um—F
ra-di-us
ra-dix
ra-don
ra-don seed
rag-weed
Rail-li-e-ti-na
rale
ra-mi
ram-i-fi-ca-tion
ram-i-fy
ra-mose
Ramstedt's op-er-a-tion
ram-u-lus
ra-mus
ran-cid
range
Rankin's op-er-a-tion
ran-u-la
Ranvier's nodes
rape oil
ra-phe
rar-e-fac-tion
rar-e-fy
rar-i-tas
rash
Ra-so-ri-an

rasp-ber-ry
rat—bite fe-ver
Rathke's pouch
ra-tio
ra-tion
ra-tion-al
ra-tion-al-i-za-tion
rats-bane
rat-tle
rat-tle-snake
Rau-wol-fi-a
Raynaud's syn-drome
re-ac-quired
re-ac-tion
re-ac-ti-vate
re-ac-ti-va-tion
re-a-gent
re-a-gin
ream-er
re-am-pu-ta-tion
re-an-i-mate
re-bound
re-cal-ci-fi-ca-tion
re-cal-ci-fied
re-ca-pit-u-la-tion
re-ceiv-er
re-cep-tive
re-cep-tor
re-cess
re-ces-sion
re-ces-sive
re-cid-i-va-tion
re-cid-i-vism
re-cid-i-vist
rec-i-div-i-ty
rec-i-pe
rec-li-na-tion
re-com-bi-na-tion
re-com-po-si-tion
re-com-pres-sion
re-con-sti-tu-tion
re-con-struc-tion

re-cov-er-y
re-cru-des-cence
re-cruit-ment
rec-tal shelf
rec-ti-fi-ca-tion
rec-to-ab-dom-i-nal
rec-to-cele
rec-toc-ly-sis
rec-to-coc-cyg-e-al
rec-to-fis-tu-la
rec-to-gen-i-tal
rec-to-la-bi-al
rec-to-scope
rec-to-sig-moid
rec-to-sig-moid-ec-to-
    my
rec-to-sig-moid-os-co-
    py
rec-to-ste-no-sis
rec-to-u-ter-ine
rec-to-vag-i-nal
rec-to-vag-i-no-ab-dom-
    i-nal
rec-to-ves-i-cal
rec-tum
rec-tus
re-cum-ben-cv
re-cum-bent
re-cu-per-ate
re-cu-per-a-tion
re-cu-per-a-tive
re-cur-rence
re-cur-rent
re-cur-va-tion
Red Cross
re-dif-fer-en-ti-a-
    tion
red-out
re-dox
re-dox po-ten-tial
re-duce
re-duced

re-du-ci-ble
re-duc-tant
re-duc-tase
re-duc-tion
re-du-pli-ca-ted
re-du-pli-ca-tion
Red-u-vi-i-dae
Re-du-vi-us per-son-a-
   tus
Reed—Sternberg cells
re-ed-u-ca-tion
reef-ing
re-ex-ci-ta-tion
re-fine
re-flect-ed
re-flec-tion
re-flec-tor
re-flex
re-flex-o-gen-ic
re-flux
re-fract
re-frac-tion
re-frac-tive
re-frac-tiv-i-ty
re-frac-tom-e-ter
re-frac-to-ry
re-frac-ture
re-fresh
re-frig-er-ant
re-frig-er-a-tion
ref-use
re-fu-sion
re-gen-er-ate
re-gen-er-a-tion
reg-i-men
re-gion
reg-is-ter
reg-is-trar
reg-is-tra-tion
reg-is-try
reg-le-men-ta-tion
re-gres-sion

re-gres-sive
reg-u-lar
reg-u-la-tion
reg-u-la-tive
re-gur-gi-tant
re-gur-gi-ta-tion
re-ha-bil-i-ta-tion
re-ha-la-tion
Rehfuss tube
re-im-plan-ta-tion
re-in-fec-tion
re-in-force-ment
re-in-fu-sion
re-in-ner-va-tion
re-in-oc-u-la-tion
re-in-te-gra-tion
re-in-ver-sion
Reiter's syn-drome
re-ju-ve-na-tion
re-lapse
re-la-tion
re-lax
re-lax-a-tion
re-lax-in
rel-e-vant
re-lief
re-lieve
re-me-di-al
rem-e-dy
re-min-er-al-i-za-tion
re-mis-sion
re-mit-tence
re-nal
ren-i-form
re-nin
ren-i-punc-ture
ren-nin
Rènon—Delille syn-
   drome
ren-o-va-tion
re-or-gan-i-za-tion
re-pair

re-pel-lent
re-pel-ler
re-per-cus-sion
re-pet-i-tive
re-place-ment
re-plan-ta-tion
re-plete
re-pli-ca-tion
re-po-lar-i-za-tion
re-po-si-tion
re-pous-soir
re-pres-sion
re-pro-duc-tion
re-pro-duc-tive
re-pul-sion
re-sect
re-sec-tion
re-sec-to-scope
re-ser-pine
re-serve
res-i-dent
re-sid-u-al
res-i-due
re-sil-i-ence
re-sil-i-ent
res-in
res-in-oid
re-sist-ance
res-o-lu-tion
re-solve
re-sol-vent
re-solv-ing pow-er
res-o-nance
res-o-nant
res-o-na-tor
re-sorb-ent
re-sor-cin-ol
re-sorp-tion
res-pi-ra-tion
res-pi-ra-tor
re-spire
res-pi-rom-e-ter

res-pi-rom-e-try
re-sponse
re-spon-si-bil-i-ty
res-ti-form
rest-ing
res-ti-tu-tion
res-to-ra-tion
re-stor-a-tive
re-straint
re-stric-tion
re-sub-li-ma-tion
re-sul-tant
res-ur-rec-tion
re-sus-ci-tate
re-sus-ci-ta-tion
re-sus-ci-ta-tor
re-su-ture
re-tain-er
re-tard-ed
retch-ing
re-te peg
re-ten-tion
re-tic-u-lar
re-tic-u-la-ted
re-tic-u-lo-cyte
re-tic-u-lo-cy-to-sis
re-tic-u-lo-en-do-the-
li-al
re-tic-u-lo-en-do-the-
li-o-ma
re-tic-u-lo-en-do-the-
li-o-sis
re-tic-u-lo-sar-co-ma
re-tic-u-lum
re-ti-form
ret-i-na
ret-i-nac-u-lum
ret-i-nene
ret-i-ni-tis cir-cum-
pap-il-lar-is
ret-i-ni-tis ex-u-da-ti-
va

ret-i-ni-tis hem-or-
rhag-i-ca
ret-i-ni-tis pig-men-to-
sa
ret-i-ni-tis pro-lif-
er-ans
ret-i-ni-tis sym-pa-
the-ti-ca
ret-i-no-blas-to-ma
ret-i-no-cho-roid-i-tis
ret-i-no-pap-il-li-tis
ret-i-nop-a-thy
ret-i-nos-co-py
re-tir-ing
re-tort
re-tract
re-trac-tile
re-trac-tion
re-trac-tor
ret-ro-ac-tion
ret-ro-an-ter-o-grade
ret-ro-bul-bar
ret-ro-car-di-ac
ret-ro-ce-cal
ret-ro-cele
ret-ro-dis-place-ment
ret-ro-flexed
ret-ro-flex-ion
ret-ro-grade
ret-ro-gres-sion
ret-ro-len-tal
ret-ro-lin-gual
ret-ro-na-sal
ret-ro-per-i-to-ne-al
ret-ro-pha-ryn-ge-al
ret-ro-posed
ret-ro-po-si-tion
ret-ro-pul-sion
ret-ro-tar-sal
ret-ro-ver-sion
ret-ro-vert-ed
re-tru-sion

re-un-ion
re-vac-ci-na-tion
re-ver-ber-a-tion
rev-er-ie
re-ver-sal
re-verse
re-ver-sion
re-vi-tal-i-za-tion
re-vive
re-vul-sive
rhab-do-my-o-blas-to-ma
rhab-do-my-o-ma
rhab-do-my-o-sar-co-ma
rhag-a-des
rham-ni-nose
rham-nose
rhe
rhe-ni-um
rhe-o-base
rhe-om-e-ter
rhe-o-scope
rhe-o-stat
rhe-o-tax-is
rhe-o-tome
rheu-mat-ic
rheu-ma-tism
rheu-ma-toid
rheu-ma-tol-o-gy
rhex-is
rhic-no-sis
rhi-nal
rhi-nal-gi-a
rhi-nel-cos
rhi-nen-ceph-a-lon
rhi-nism
rhi-ni-tis
rhi-no-chei-lo-plas-ty
rhi-no-der-ma
rhi-no-ky-pho-sis
rhi-no-lar-yn-gol-o-gy
rhi-nol-o-gist
rhi-nol-o-gy

rhi-no-mi-o-sis
rhi-no-phar-yn-gi-tis
rhi-no-pho-ni-a
rhi-no-phy-ma
rhi-no-plas-ty
rhi-no-pol-yp
rhi-nop-si-a
rhi-nor-rhe-a
rhi-no-scle-ro-ma
rhi-nos-co-py
Rhi-no-spo-rid-i-um
Rhi-pi-ceph-a-lus
   san-guine-us
rhi-zoid
rhi-zome
Rhi-zop-o-da
rhi-zot-o-my
rho-di-um
rho-do-gen-e-sis
rho-dop-sin
rhom-ben-ceph-a-lon
rhom-boid
rhom-boi-de-us
rhon-chi-al
rhon-chus
Rh fac-tors
rhu-barb
Rhus tox-i-co-den-dron
rhythm
rhyth-mic
rhyth-mic-i-ty
rhyt-i-do-plas-ty
ri-bon-fla-vin
ri-bo-nu-cle-ase
ri-bo-nu-cle-ic ac-id
ri-bose
ri-bo-side
ric-i-nine
ric-in-o-le-in
rick-ets
Rick-ett-si-a moo-
   ser-i

Rick-ett-si-a prow-a-
   zek-i
Rick-ett-si-a rick-
   ett-si-i
rick-ett-si-al-pox
rid-er's bone
Riedel's stru-ma
rig-id
ri-gid-i-ty
rig-or mor-tis
ri-mose
rin-der-pest
ring com-pound
Ringer's so-lu-tion
ring-worm
Rinne's test
ri-sus sar-don-i-cus
ri-val-ry
riz-i-form
roar-ing
Rochelle salt
rock-ing meth-od
Rock-y Moun-tain spot-
   ted fe-ver
ro-den-ti-cide
ro-dent ul-cer
roent-gen
roent-gen-o-gram
roent-gen-ol-o-gist
roent-gen-ol-o-gy
roent-gen-os-co-py
Rolando's a-re-a
rol-ler
Romberg's sign
ron-geur
root ca-nal
Rorschach test
ro-sa-ce-a
ro-sa-ce-i-form
ros-an-i-line
rose ben-gal
rose fe-ver

rose hips
rose-mar-y oil
Rosenheim's so-lu-tion
rose oil
ro-se-o-la
ro-se-o-lous
ro-sette
rose wa-ter
ros-in
ros-tel-lum
ros-tra
ros-tral
ros-trum
ro-tate
ro-ta-ting
ro-ta-tion
ro-ta-to-res
ro-te-none
rough-age
rou-leau for-ma-tion
round-worm
roup
Rous sar-co-ma
row-ing meth-od
rub-ber
ru-be-do
ru-be-fa-cient
ru-be-fac-tion
ru-bel-la
ru-be-o-la
ru-be-o-sis i-rid-is
ru-bes-cence
ru-bi-a
ru-bid-i-um
ru-big-i-nous
Rubin test
ru-bor
ru-bri-cyte
ruc-ta-tion
ruc-tus
ru-di-ment
ru-di-men-ta-ry

Ruffini's cor-pus-cle
ru-fous
ru-gae
ru-gose
ru-gos-i-ty
rum-bling
ru-men
ru-mi-nant
ru-mi-na-tion
rump
run—a-round
ru-pi-a
rup-ti-o
rup-ture
rup-tured
rust
rut
ru-the-ni-um
ruth-er-ford
ru-tin
ry-an-o-dine
rye smut

S

sab-a-dil-la
Sabouraud's a-gar
sab-u-lous
sac
sac-cha-rase
sac-cha-ra-ted
sac-cha-ride
sac-char-i-fy
sac-cha-rim-e-ter
sac-cha-rin
sac-cha-roids
sac-cha-rose
sac-cu-lar
sac-cu-la-ted
sac-cu-la-tion

sac-cule
sac-cu-lus
sa-cral-i-za-tion
sa-cro-an-te-ri-or
sa-cro-coc-cyg-e-al
sa-cro-coc-cyg-e-us
sa-cro-dyn-i-a
sa-cro-il-i-ac
sa-cro-lum-bar
sa-cro-pos-te-ri-or
sa-cro-spi-na-lis
sa-crum
sad-ism
sad-ist
sad-o-mas-o-chism
Saemisch's ul-cer
Saenger's op-er-a-tion
saf-fron
saf-ra-nine
saf-ra-no-phile
saf-role
sage-brush
sag-it-tal
sa-go
Saint Agatha's dis-ease
Saint Anthony's fire
Saint Martin's dis-ease
Saint Vitus' dance
sal a-er-a-tus
sal so-da
sa-la-cious
sal-e-ra-tus
sal-i-cin
sal-i-cyl al-co-hol
sal-i-cyl-al-de-hyde
sal-i-cyl-am-ide
sal-i-cyl-an-i-lide
sal-i-cyl-ate
sal-i-cyl-a-zo-sul-fa-
    pyr-i-dine
sal-i-cyl-ic ac-id
sal-i-cyl-ism

sa-lim-e-ter
sa-line
sa-li-va
sal-i-vate
sal-i-va-tion
Salk vac-cine
Sal-mo-nel-la a-bor-tus
Sal-mo-nel-la en-ter-
    i-ti-dis
Sal-mo-nel-la par-a-
    ty-pho-sa
Sal-mo-nel-la schott-
    mul-ler-i
Sal-mo-nel-la ty-phi
Sal-mo-nel-la ty-phi-
    mu-ri-um
Sal-mo-nel-la ty-pho-
    sa
sal-mo-nel-lo-sis
sal-pin-gec-to-my
sal-pin-gi-tis
sal-pin-gol-y-sis
sal-pin-go—o-o-pho-
    rec-to-my
sal-pin-go—o-o-pho-
    ri-tis
sal-pin-go-per-i-to-
    ni-tis
sal-pin-go-plas-ty
sal-pin-gos-to-my
sal-pin-gys-ter-o-cy-
    e-sis
sal-pinx
sal-ta-to-ry
salt-ing out
salt pe-ter
sa-lu-bri-ous
sal-u-tar-y
salve
sa-ma-ri-um
sam-ple
san-a-to-ri-um

san-dal-wood
san-da-rac var-nish
sand flea
sand-fly
sane
san-guic-o-lous
san-guine
san-guin-e-ous
san-gui-suc-tion
san-i-ta-ri-an
san-i-tar-y
san-i-ta-tion
san-i-tize
san-i-ty
san-to-nin
Santorini's duct
sa-phe-na
sa-phe-nous
sa-po
sap-o-na-ceous
sa-pon-i-fi-ca-tion
sa-pon-i-form
sap-o-nin
sa-pre-mic
sap-ro-gen-ic
sa-proph-a-gous
sap-ro-phyt-ic
sar-co-en-do-the-li-o-ma
sar-co-gen-ic
sar-coid
sar-coid-o-sis
sar-co-lem-ma
sar-co-ma
sar-co-ma-to-sis
sar-co-ma-tous
sar-co-mere
sar-co-mes-o-the-li-o-ma
Sar-cop-tes sca-bi-ei
sar-co-spo-rid-i-o-sis
sar-don-ic grin
sar-sa-pa-ril-la

sar-to-ri-us
sas-sa-fras
sas-sy bark
sat-el-lite
sat-el-li-to-sis
sa-ti-e-ty
sat-u-ra-ted
sat-u-ra-tion
sat-ur-nine
sat-ur-nism
sat-y-ri-a-sis
sat-yr tu-ber-cle
sau-cer-ize
sau-ri-a-sis
sa-vo-ry
Sayre's ap-pa-ra-tus
scab
scab-bard
scabbed
sca-bi-cide
sca-bi-es
sca-bi-ous
sca-bri-ti-es
sca-la
scald
scald-ing
scale
sca-lene
sca-le-nec-to-my
sca-le-not-o-my
sca-le-nus
sca-ler
sca-ling
scalp
scal-pel
sca-ly
scan-di-um
Scanzoni's ma-neu-ver
scaph-o-ceph-al-ic
scaph-oid
scap-u-la
scap-u-lo-hu-mer-al

scar-i-fi-ca-tion
scar-la-ti-na
scar-la-ti-ni-form
scar-let fe-ver
scar-let red
Scarpa's tri-an-gle
sca-to-ma
sca-toph-a-gous
scat-ter
scat-ter-ing
scav-en-ger
scav-en-ging
scent
Schaffer's re-flex
Schamberg's dis-ease
sche-ma
sche-mat-ic
Scheuermann's dis-ease
Schick test
Schilder's dis-ease
Schiller test
Schilling's meth-od
schis-to-cy-to-sis
schis-tor-rha-chis
Schis-to-so-ma haem-a-
 to-bi-um
Schis-to-so-ma ja-pon-
 i-cum
Schis-to-so-ma man-so-
 ni
schis-to-so-mi-a-sis
schiz-o-gen-e-sis
schiz-oid
schiz-o-ma-ni-a
schiz-ont
schi-zon-ti-cide
schiz-o-phre-ni-a
schiz-o-thy-mic
Schlemm's ca-nal
Schmincke's tu-mor
Schmorl's nod-ules
Schneider's in-dex

207

Schuffner's dots
Schultze's meth-od
schwan-no-ma
schwan-no-sar-co-ma
Schweizer—Foley Y—
    plasty
sci-age
sci-at-ic
sci-at-i-ca
scil-lism
scin-ti-gram
scin-til-la-scope
scin-til-la-tion
scin-til-la-tion
    coun-ter
scin-ti-scan-ner
scir-rhoid
scir-rhous
scis-sors
scis-su-ra
scle-ra
scle-ra-ti-tis
scler-ec-ta-si-a
scle-rec-to-ir-i-dec-
    to-my
scle-rec-to-my
scler-e-de-ma
scle-re-ma
scle-rit-ic
scle-ri-tis
scle-ro-cho-roid-i-tis
scle-ro-con-junc-ti-
    val
scle-ro-con-junc-ti-vi-
    tis
scle-ro-cor-ne-al
scle-ro-dac-ty-ly
scle-ro-der-ma
scle-ro-der-ma-ti-tis
scle-rog-e-nous
scle-roid
scle-ro-ker-a-ti-tis

scle-ro-ker-a-to-i-ri-
    tis
scle-ro-ma
scle-ro-ma-la-ci-a
scle-ro-nych-i-a
scle-ro-plas-ty
scle-ro-sant
scle-rosed
scle-ro-sis
scle-ro-ste-no-sis
scle-ros-to-my
scle-rot-ic
scle-rot-o-my
scle-rous
sco-lex
sco-li-o-lor-do-sis
sco-li-o-sis
scoop
sco-pol-a-mine
sco-pom-e-ter
scor-bu-ti-gen-ic
scor-pi-on
scot-o-din-ia
sco-to-ma
sco-tom-e-ter
sco-top-ic
scours
scrap-ie
scra-pings
scrof-u-lous
scrof-u-lo-der-ma
scro-tal
scro-tum
scrub ty-phus
scru-ple
scru-pu-lous
scurf
scur-vy
scul-te-tus band-age
scu-tate
scute
scu-tu-lum

scyb-a-lous
scy-phi-form
sea-sick-ness
seat-worm
se-ba-ceous
seb-or-rhe-a
se-bum
se-clu-sion of pu-pil
sec-o-dont
sec-ond-ar-y
se-cre-ta
se-cre-ta-gogue
se-crete
se-cre-tin
se-cret-ing
se-cre-tion
se-cre-to-ry
sec-ta-ri-an
sec-tion
sec-to-ri-al
se-cun-di-grav-i-da
sec-un-dines
se-da-tion
sed-a-tive
sed-en-tar-y
sed-i-ment
sed-i-men-ta-tion
seg-ment
seg-men-tal
seg-men-ta-tion
seg-re-ga-tion
Seidel's sign
Seitz fil-ter
sei-zure
se-junc-tion
se-lec-tion
se-lec-tor
se-le-ni-ate
se-le-ni-um
self—a-buse
self—fer-ti-li-za-tion
self—in-duc-tance

self—lim-it-ed
sel-la tur-ci-ca
se-man-tics
se-men
sem-i-car-ba-zide
sem-i-car-ba-zone
sem-i-car-ti-lag-i-nous
sem-i-com-a-tose
sem-i-lu-nar
sem-i-mem-bra-no-sus
sem-i-mem-bra-nous
sem-i-nal
sem-i-na-tion
sem-i-nif-er-ous
sem-i-no-ma
sem-i-nor-mal
sem-i-spi-na-lis
sem-i-ten-di-no-sus
sem-i-ten-di-nous
se-nes-cence
se-nes-cent
se-nile
se-nil-i-ty
sen-na
se-no-pi-a
sen-sa-tion
sense or-gan
sen-si-bil-i-ty
sen-si-ble
sen-si-tiv-i-ty
sen-si-ti-za-tion
sen-si-tized
sen-so-ri-mo-tor
sen-so-ri-um
sen-so-ry
sen-su-al-ism
sen-tient
sen-ti-ment
sep-a-ra-tor
sep-sis
sep-tal
sep-tic

sep-ti-ce-mi-a
sep-to-mar-gi-nal
sep-tum
se-quel-ae
se-quence
se-quen-ti-al
se-ques-ter
se-ques-tra-tion
se-ques-trec-to-my
se-ques-trum
se-ral-bu-min
se-ries
ser-ine
se-ro-der-ma-ti-tis
se-ro-di-ag-no-sis
se-ro-fi-brin-ous
se-ro-log-ic
se-rol-o-gist
se-rol-o-gy
se-ro-mem-bra-nous
se-ro-mu-cous
se-ro-pu-ru-lent
se-ro-re-sis-tant
se-ro-sa
se-ro-san-guin-e-ous
se-ro-si-tis
se-ro-syn-o-vi-tis
ser-o-to-nin
se-rous
ser-pen-tine
ser-pig-i-nous
ser-ra-tion
ser-ra-tus
Sertoli cells
se-rum
shad-ow
sha-king
sham rage
shank
shears
sheath
shed-ding

shell
shel-lac
shell-shock
shel-tered
Shepherd's frac-ture
Sherman plates
shield
shift
Shi-gel-la
shi-gel-lo-sis
shin
shin-gles
shiv-er
shock
short cir-cuit
shoul-der
show
Shrapnell's mem-brane
shreds
shriv-el
shud-der
shunt
si-a-li-thot-o-my
si-a-lo-ad-e-ni-tis
si-a-lo-do-chi-tis
si-a-log-e-nous
si-a-log-ra-phy
si-a-loid
si-al-o-lith
si-a-lo-li-thot-o-my
si-a-lor-rhe-a
sib-i-lant
sib-ling
sic-cant
sic-cus
sick-le—form
sick-le-mi-a
sick-ness
sid-er-ite
sid-er-o-fi-bro-sis
sid-er-o-pe-ni-a
sid-er-o-phil ·

sid-er-o-sis
sid-er-ot-ic
Siegle's o-to-scope
sigh
sight
sig-moid
sig-moid-ec-to-my
sig-moid-i-tis
sig-moi-do-scope
sig-moid-os-co-py
sig-moid-os-to-my
sig-na-ture
sig-nif-i-cant dif-fer-ence
si-lent
sil-i-ca
sil-i-cate
si-li-ceous
sil-i-con
si-li-co-si-der-o-sis
sil-i-co-sis
sil-i-co-tu-ber-cu-lo-sis
sil-lo-neur
sil-ver
Silvester's meth-od
sim-i-an
Simmonds' dis-ease
sim-ple
Simpson's for-ceps
Sims' spec-u-lum
sim-u-la-tion
si-na-pis
sin-ci-put
sin-ew
sin-gul-tus
sin-is-ter
sin-is-tral
sin-is-tra-tion
sin-is-tro-car-di-al
sin-is-tro-cer-e-bral
sin-is-tro-gy-ra-tion
sin-is-tro-tor-sion

sin-is-trous
si-no-a-tri-al
si-no-au-ric-u-lar
sin-u-ous
si-nus
si-nus-i-tis
si-nus-oid
si-nus-oi-dal
si-nus-ot-o-my
si-phon
Sippy di-et
si-ren
site
si-tol-o-gy
si-tos-ter-ol
sit-ting height
si-tus in-ver-sus
skat-ole
skel-e-tal trac-tion
skel-e-ti-za-tion
skel-e-ton
Skene's glands
ske-nei-tis
skew de-vi-a-tion
ski-ag-ra-phy
ski-as-co-py
skin graft-ing
skin-ny
skin trac-tion
skull-cap
skunk cab-bage
slake
slap-ping
slav-er
sleep-ing sick-ness
sleep-less-ness
sli-cer
slide
sling
slit
slough
Sluder's snare

sludge
slum-ber
small-pox
smear
smeg-ma
Smellie's for-ceps
smell-ing salts
Smith's in-ci-sion
Smith—Petersen's nail
Smithwick's op-er-a-tion
smudg-ing
smut
snail
snake-root
snap
snare
sneeze
Snellen chart
snore
snow-blind-ness
snuff-box
so-cial
so-ci-ol-o-gy
so-ci-o-med-i-cal
sock-et
so-da lime
so-di-um
so-do-ku
sod-om-ist
sod-om-y
sof-ten-ing
sol
sol-a-na-ce-ous
so-lar-i-za-tion
so-lar plex-us
sole
so-le-us
sol-id
so-lid-i-fi-ca-tion
sol-ip-sism
sol-i-tar-y
sol—lu-nar

sol-u-bil-i-ty
sol-u-ble
so-lum tym-pa-ni
sol-ute
so-lu-tion
sol-vate
sol-vent
so-ma
so-mat-ic
so-ma-tist
so-ma-ti-za-tion
so-ma-to-gen-ic
so-ma-tol-o-gy
so-ma-to-plasm
so-ma-to-psy-chic
so-ma-to-tro-pin
so-ma-to-type
so-mes-thet-ic
so-mite
som-nam-bu-la-tion
som-nam-bu-lism
som-nam-bu-list
som-ni-fa-cient
som-nif-er-ous
som-nif-ic
som-nil-o-quism
som-nil-o-quy
som-no-lence
som-no-les-cent
som-nus
so-phis-ti-ca-tion
so-po-rif-ic
sor-bic ac-id
sor-bi-tan
sor-des
sor-did
sore
sor-ghum
so-ro-ri-a-tion
sor-rel
souf-fle
sound

Sourdille's op-er-a-tion
soy-bean
spa
space med-i-cine
spal-la-tion
Span-ish wind-lass
Spar-ga-num
spar-go-sis
spasm
spas-mod-ic
spas-mo-lyt-ic
spas-mus
spas-tic
spas-tic-i-ty
spa-tial
spat-u-la
spav-in
spay
spear-mint
spe-cial-ist
spe-cial-ty
spe-cies
spe-cif-ic
spec-i-fic-i-ty
spec-ta-cles
spec-tro-col-or-im-e-ter
spec-tro-gram
spec-tro-graph
spec-trom-e-ter
spec-tro-pho-te-lom-e-
    ter
spec-tro-pho-tom-e-ter
spec-tro-po-lar-im-e-
    ter
spec-tro-scope
spec-tros-co-py
spec-trum
spec-u-lum
speech
sperm
sper-ma-cet-i
sper-ma-ta-cra-si-a

sper-mat-ic
sper-ma-tid
sper-ma-to-cele
sper-ma-to-ci-dal
sper-ma-to-cide
sper-ma-to-cyst
sper-ma-to-cys-ti-tis
sper-ma-to-cy-te
sper-ma-to-gen-e-sis
sper-ma-to-gen-ic
sper-ma-to-go-ni-um
sper-ma-toid
sper-ma-tol-y-sis
sper-ma-to-phore
sper-ma-tor-rhe-a
sper-ma-tu-ri-a
sper-mi-cide
sphac-e-la-tion
sphac-e-lo-der-ma
sphac-e-lus
sphe-ni-on
sphe-no-eth-moid
sphe-noid
sphe-noid-i-tis
sphe-no-man-dib-u-lar
sphe-no-max-il-lar-y
sphe-no—oc-cip-i-tal
sphe-no-pal-a-tine
sphe-no-pa-ri-e-tal
sphe-no-pe-tro-sal
sphe-no-sis
sphe-no-tribe
sphe-no-trip-sy
sphe-ro-cyl-in-der
sphe-ro-cyte
sphe-ro-cy-tic
sphe-ro-cy-to-sis
sphe-roid
sphe-rom-e-ter
sphinc-ter
sphinc-ter-ec-to-my
sphinc-ter-ol-y-sis

sphinc-ter-ot-o-my
sphin-go-my-e-lin
sphin-go-sine
sphyg-mo-chron-o-graph
sphyg-mod-ic
sphyg-mo-gram
sphyg-mo-graph
sphyg-moid
sphyg-mo-ma-nom-e-ter
sphyg-mo—os-cil-lom-e-ter
sphyg-mo-phone
sphyg-mus
spi-ca
spic-ule
spi-der
spike—and—wave
spi-lo-ma
spi-na
spi-nal cord
spi-na-lis
spin-dle
spine
spi-no-cel-lu-lar
spi-no-tec-tal
spi-ral
spi-reme
spir-il-lo-sis
Spi-ril-lum
spir-it
Spi-ro-chae-ta
Spi-ro-chae-ta-ce-ae
Spi-ro-chae-ta-les
spi-ro-chete
spi-ro-che-ti-cide
spi-ro-che-to-sis
spi-ro-gram
spi-ro-graph
spi-rom-e-ter
splanch-nic
splanch-ni-cot-o-my
spleen

sple-nal-gi-a
sple-nec-to-my
splen-ic
splen-i-co-pan-cre-at-ic
splen-i-form
sple-ni-tis
sple-ni-us
splen-i-za-tion
sple-no-dyn-i-a
sple-no-gran-u-lo-ma-to-sis sid-er-ot-i-ca
sple-no-hep-a-to-meg-a-ly
sple-noid
sple-no-ma-la-ci-a
sple-no-meg-a-ly
sple-no-pex-y
sple-nop-to-sis
sple-not-o-my
splice
splint
splin-ter
splint-ing
split-ting
spoke-shave
spon-dy-li-tis
spon-dy-lo-ar-thri-tis
spon-dy-lo-dyn-i-a
spon-dy-lo-lis-the-sis
spon-dyl-ol-y-sis
spon-dy-lo-sis
spon-dy-lo-syn-de-sis
spon-dy-lot-o-my
sponge
spon-gi-o-blast
spon-gi-o-blas-to-ma
spon-gi-o-cyte
spon-gi-o-cy-to-ma
spon-gi-oid
spon-gi-ose
spon-gy
spon-ta-ne-ous

spoon
spoon-er-ism
spo-rad-ic
spo-ran-gi-o-phore
spo-ran-gi-o-spore
spo-ran-gi-um
spore
spo-ri-cide
spo-ro-cyst
spo-ro-cyte
spo-ro-gen-e-sis
spo-ro-phyte
spo-rot-ri-chin
spo-ro-tri-cho-sis
Spo-ro-trich-um
Spo-ro-zo-a
spo-ro-zo-an
spo-ro-zo-ite
sport
spor-u-late
spot-ting
sprain
spray
spread-ing
sprue
spud
spur
spu-tum
squa-ma
squa-mo-sa
squa-mous
squill
squint
stab
sta-bile
sta-bi-li-zer
sta-ble
stac-ca-to
sta-di-um
staff
stage
stag-gers

stag-na-tion
stain
stalk
sta-men
stam-i-na
stam-mer-ing
stand-ard
stand-ard-i-za-tion
stand-still
Stanford—Binet test
stan-nic
stan-nous
sta-pe-dec-to-my
sta-pe-di-al
sta-pe-di-us
sta-pes
staph-y-lec-to-my
staph-yl-e-de-ma
staph-y-li-tis
staph-y-lo-coc-cal
staph-y-lo-coc-cic
staph-y-lo-coc-cus
staph-y-lo-der-ma-ti-tis
staph-y-lo-ki-nase
staph-y-lol-y-sin
staph-y-lo-ma
staph-y-lo-plas-ty
staph-y-lot-o-my
staph-y-lo-tox-in
starch
Starling's law
start-er
star-va-tion
sta-sis
state-ment
stat-ic
stat-ics
stat-im
sta-tion
sta-tis-ti-cal
sta-tis-tics
stat-ure

sta-tus
sta-tus asth-ma-ti-cus
sta-tus ep-i-lep-ti-cus
sta-tus lym-pha-tic-us
stead-y state
steap-sin
stear-ate
ste-ar-ic ac-id
stear-in
ste-a-ti-tis
ste-a-to-ma
ste-a-to-py-gi-a
ste-a-tor-rhe-a
Steinmann's pin
stel-late
sten-o-pe-ic
ste-nosed
ste-no-sis
ste-nos-to-my
Stensen's du-et
stent
step-page gait
ster-co-ro-ma
ster-cus
ster-e-o-chem-is-try
ster-e-og-no-sis
ster-e-o-gram
ster-e-og-ra-phy
ster-e-o-i-so-mer
ster-e-op-sis
ster-e-op-ter
ster-e-o-ra-di-og-ra-phy
ster-e-o-scop-ic
ster-e-o-tax-is
ster-e-ot-ro-pism
ster-ic hin-drance
ster-ile
ste-ril-i-ty
ster-i-li-za-tion
ster-i-lize
ster-i-li-zer
ster-na-lis

ster-no-cla-vic-u-lar
ster-no-clei-do-mas-toid
ster-no-hy-oid
ster-no-mas-toid
ster-no-thy-roid
ster-num
ster-nu-ta-tor
ster-oid
ster-ol
ster-tor-ous
steth-o-phone
steth-o-scope
sthen-ic
stib-i-um
stic-tac-ne
sti-fle
stig-ma
stig-ma-tism
stil-bam-i-dine
stil-bes-trol
still-birth
still-born
Still's dis-ease
stim-u-lant
stim-u-late
stim-u-la-tion
stim-u-lus
stip-pling
stir-rup
stock-i-net
stock-ing
Stokes—Adams syn-
    drome
sto-ma
stom-ach
sto-mach-ic
sto-mat-ic
sto-ma-ti-tis
sto-ma-tol-o-gy
sto-ma-tot-o-my
sto-mo-de-um
stool

stop-cock
stop-page
storm
stra-bis-mus
strain
strait-jack-et
stra-mo-ni-um
stran-gle
stran-gu-la-tion
stran-gu-ry
strat-i-fi-ca-tion
strat-i-fied
strat-o-sphere
strat-um
straw-ber-ry mark
streak
stream
strep-i-tus
strep-ti-ce-mi-a
strep-to-an-gi-na
strep-to-ba-cil-lus
strep-to-coc-cal
strep-to-coc-ce-mi-a
strep-to-coc-ci
Strep-to-coc-cus
strep-to-dor-nase
strep-to-ki-nase
strep-to-ly-sin
Strep-to-my-ces
strep-to-my-cin
Strep-to-thrix
stress in-con-ti-nence
stretch
stretch-er
stri-a
stri-ae grav-i-dar-um
stri-a-ted
stri-a-tum
stric-ture
stri-dor
strid-u-lous
strin-gent

string—gal-va-nom-e-ter
strip-ping
strob-ic
stro-bi-la
strob-i-la-tion
strob-ile
stro-bi-lus
stro-bo-scope
Stroganoff's meth-od
stro-ma
stro-ma-tin
Stromeyer's splint
Stron-gy-loi-des
stron-gy-loi-di-a-sis
stron-ti-um
stro-phan-thin
stroph-u-lus
struc-ture
stru-ma
stru-mi-tis
Strumpell—Marie dis-
    ease
strych-nine
stump
stunt-ing
stupe
stu-pe-fa-cient
stu-pe-fac-tion
stu-pid-i-ty
stu-por
stur-dy
Sturge—Weber—Dimitri
    dis-ease
stut-ter-er
stut-ter-ing
sty
sty-let
sty-lo-glos-sus
sty-lo-hy-oid
sty-lo-man-dib-u-lar
sty-lo-mas-toid
sty-lo-pha-ryn-ge-us

sty-lus
styp-tic
sty-rol
sub-ab-dom-i-nal
sub-ac-e-tate
sub-a-cro-mi-al
sub-a-cute
sub-ap-i-cal
sub-ap-o-neu-rot-ic
sub-a-rach-noid
sub-a-re-o-lar
sub-a-tom-ic
sub-au-ric-u-lar
sub-cal-ca-rine
sub-cal-lo-sal
sub-cap-su-lar
sub-car-bon-ate
sub-chron-ic
sub-cla-vi-an
sub-clin-i-cal
sub-con-junc-ti-val
sub-con-scious
sub-con-scious-ness
sub-cor-a-coid
sub-cor-ti-cal
sub-cos-tal
sub-cul-ture
sub-cu-ta-ne-ous
sub-cu-tic-u-lar
sub-del-toid
sub-di-a-phrag-mat-ic
sub-di-vi-ded
sub-duc-tion
sub-du-ral
sub-e-pen-dy-mo-ma
sub-fam-i-ly
sub-gle-noid
sub-in-vo-lu-tion
sub-ja-cent
sub-jec-tive
sub-la-tion
sub-le-thal

sub-li-mate
sub-li-ma-tion
sub-lim-i-nal
sub-li-mis
sub-lin-gual
sub-lux-a-tion
sub-mal-le-o-lar
sub-man-dib-u-lar
sub-ma-rine
sub-max-il-lar-y
sub-men-tal
sub-mi-cro-scop-ic
sub-mu-co-sa
sub-ni-trate
sub-nor-mal
sub-nu-cle-us
sub-oc-cip-i-tal
sub-or-di-na-tion
sub-per-i-os-te-al
sub-per-i-to-ne-al
sub-phren-ic
sub-pla-cen-tal
sub-pu-bic
sub-scap-u-lar
sub-scrip-tion
sub-se-rous
sub-si-dence
sub-sist-ence
sub-spi-nous
sub-stage
sub-stance
sub-stan-ti-a
sub-ster-nal
sub-sti-tu-tion
sub-strate
sub-sul-tus
sub-ten-to-ri-al
sub-thal-a-mus
sub-to-tal
sub-tro-chan-ter-ic
sub-trop-i-cal
sub-un-gual

sub-vo-lu-tion
suc-ce-da-ne-ous
suc-cif-er-ous
suc-cin-ic ac-id
suc-cin-yl-cho-line
suc-cu-lent
suc-cus-sion
suck-ing
suck-le
suck-ling
su-crose
su-cro-su-ri-a
suc-tion
Su-dan
su-da-tion
su-da-to-ri-um
Sudeck's at-ro-phy
su-dor-if-er-ous
su-dor-if-ic
su-dor-ip-a-rous
su-et
suf-fo-cate
suf-fo-ca-tion
suf-fu-sion
sug-ar
sug-ar-ine
sug-gest-i-bil-i-ty
sug-gest-i-ble
sug-ges-tion
sug-gil-la-tion
su-i-cide
sul-cus
sul-fa-di-a-zine
sul-fa-guan-i-dine
sul-fa-mer-a-zine
sul-fa-meth-a-zine
sul-fa-nil-a-mide
sul-fa-nil-ic ac-id
sul-fa-pyr-a-zine
sul-fa-pyr-i-dine
sulf-ars-phen-a-mine
sul-fate

sul-fa-thi-a-zole
sulf-he-mo-glo-bin
sulf-he-mo-glo-bi-ne-
    mi-a
sulf-hy-dryl
sul-fide
sul-fite
sul-fon-a-mide
sul-fo-na-tion
sul-fo-sal-i-cyl-ic
    ac-id
sul-fur
sul-fu-ra-ted
sul-fu-ric ac-id
sul-fu-rous
Sulkowitch re-a-gent
su-mac
sum-ma-tion
sun-burn
sun-stroke
su-per-ab-duc-tion
su-per-a-cute
su-per-al-i-men-ta-tion
su-per-cil-i-ar-y
su-per-e-go
su-per-ex-ci-ta-tion
su-per-ex-ten-sion
su-per-fe-cun-da-tion
su-per-fe-cun-di-ty
su-per-fe-ta-tion
su-per-fi-cial
su-per-in-fec-tion
su-per-in-vo-lu-tion
su-pe-ri-or
su-per-lac-ta-tion
su-per-na-tant
su-per-nor-mal
su-per-nu-mer-ar-y
su-per-sat-u-rate
su-per-scrip-tion
su-per-sen-si-tive
su-per-sen-si-ti-za-tion

su-per-son-ic
su-per-spi-na-tus
su-per-ven-tion
su-per-vi-sor
su-pi-na-tion
su-pi-na-tor
su-pine
sup-ple-men-tal
sup-port
sup-pos-i-to-ry
sup-pres-sion
sup-pu-rant
sup-pu-ra-tion
sup-pu-ra-tive
su-pra-cla-vic-u-lar
su-pra-con-dy-lar
su-pra-gle-noid
su-pra-hy-oid
su-pra-or-bit-al
su-pra-pa-tel-lar
su-pra-pu-bic
su-pra-re-nal
su-pra-scap-u-lar
su-pra-sel-lar
su-pra-spi-na-tus
su-pra-spi-nous
su-pra-ster-nal
su-pra-ton-sil-lar
su-pra-troch-le-ar
su-pra-vi-tal stain-ing
surd-i-ty
sur-face
sur-geon
sur-ger-y
sur-ro-gate
sur-sum-duc-tion
sur-sum-ver-gence
sur-sum-ver-sion
sur-vi-vor
sus-cep-ti-bil-i-ty
sus-cep-ti-ble
sus-ci-tate

sus-pend-ed
sus-pen-sion
sus-pen-so-ri-um
sus-pen-so-ry
sus-ten-tac-u-lum
su-sur-ra-tion
su-tu-ra
su-ture
swab stick
swag-ing
swal-low-ing
sway—back
sweat
swel-ling
swiv-el stir-rup
sy-co-sis
Sydenham's cho-re-a
syl-la-ble
syl-la-bus
syl-vat-ic plague
sym-bi-o-sis
sym-bleph-a-ron
sym-bleph-a-ro-sis
sym-bol
sym-bol-ism
sym-bol-i-za-tion
sym-me-try
sym-pa-thec-to-my
sym-pa-thet-ic
sym-pa-thet-i-co-mi-
   met-ic
sym-path-i-co-blas-to-ma
sym-path-i-co-to-ni-a
sym-path-i-co-trop-ic
sym-pa-thin
sym-pa-thism
sym-pa-thi-zer
sym-path-o-lyt-ic
sym-path-o-mi-met-ic
sym-pa-thy
sym-phys-i-on
sym-phy-si-ot-o-my

sym-phy-sis
symp-tom
symp-to-mat-ic
symp-tom-a-tol-o-gy
syn-an-the-ma
syn-apse
syn-ar-thro-sis
syn-chon-dro-sis
syn-chro-nous
syn-chro-tron
syn-chy-sis scin-til-lans
syn-cli-tism
syn-clo-nus
syn-co-pe
syn-cyt-i-um
syn-dac-tyl
syn-dac-ty-ly
syn-des-mi-tis
syn-des-mo-cho-ri-al
syn-des-mo-sis
syn-drome
syn-ech-i-a
syn-ech-ot-o-my
syn-er-e-sis
syn-er-get-ic
syn-er-gism
syn-er-gis-tic
syn-er-gy
syn-ga-my
syn-os-tosed
syn-os-to-sis
syn-o-vec-to-my
syn-o-vi-al
syn-o-vi-o-ma
syn-o-vi-tis
syn-the-sis
syn-thet-ic
syn-ton-ic
syn-troph-o-blast
syph-i-lid
syph-i-lis
syph-i-lit-ic

syph-i-lo-derm
syph-i-loid
syph-i-lol-o-gist
syph-i-lo-ma
syph-i-lo-ther-a-py
syr-inge
syr-in-go-ma
sy-rin-go-my-e-li-a
sy-rin-go-my-e-lo-cele
syr-inx
syr-up
sys-tem
sys-to-le
sys-tol-ic
syz-y-gy

T

tab-a-co-sis
tab-a-nid
ta-bel-la
ta-bes
ta-bet-ic
ta-ble
ta-ble-spoon
tab-let
ta-bo-pa-re-sis
tab-u-lar
tache
ta-chet-ic
ta-chis-to-scope
ta-chog-ra-phy
ta-chom-e-ter
tach-y-car-di-a
tach-y-graph
ta-chym-e-ter
tach-yp-ne-a
ta-chys-ter-ol
tac-tile
Tae-ni-a sag-i-na-ta

Tae-ni-a so-li-um
tae-ni-a cho-roi-de-a
tae-ni-form
tail
taint
talc
tal-cum
tal-i-pes
tal-low
Tallqvist's meth-od
ta-lus
tam-bour
tam-pon
tam-pon-ade
tan-nic ac-id
tan-nin
tan-ta-lum
tan-trum
tape-worm
tap-i-o-ca
ta-pote-ment
tap-ping
tap-root
ta-ran-tu-la
ta-rax-is
tard-ive
tared
tar-get
ta-ro
tars-ad-e-ni-tis
tars-al-gi-a
tars-ec-to-my
tar-si-tis
tar-so-met-a-tar-sal
tar-so-plas-ty
tar-sot-o-my
tar-sus
tar-tar
tar-tar-ic ac-id
tat-too-ing
tau-tom-er-al
tau-tom-er-ism

tax-is
tax-on-o-my
Tay—Sachs dis-ease
Taylor brace
tears
tease
tea-spoon
teat
tech-ne-ti-um
tech-ni-cian
tech-nique
tec-ti-form
tec-to-ri-al
tec-to-spi-nal
tec-tum
te-di-ous
teeth-ing
teg-men
teg-men-tum
te-la cho-roi-de-a
tel-al-gi-a
tel-an-gi-ec-ta-sis
tel-an-gi-i-tis
tel-an-gi-o-ma
tel-e-cep-tor
tel-e-ki-ne-sis
tel-en-ceph-a-lon
tel-e-o-log-ic
te-lep-a-thy
tel-es-the-si-a
tel-lu-ri-um
tel-o-den-dron
tel-o-lec-i-thal
tel-om-er-i-za-tion
tel-o-phase
tem-per
tem-per-a-ment
tem-per-ance
tem-per-ate
tem-per-a-ture
tem-ple
tem-po-ral

tem-po-rar-y
tem-po-ri-za-tion
tem-po-ro-man-dib-u-lar
tem-po-ro—oc-cip-i-tal
tem-po-ro-pa-ri-e-tal
tem-po-ro-pon-tile
te-na-cious
te-nac-i-ty
te-nac-u-lum
ten-der-ness
ten-din-o-plas-ty
ten-di-nous
ten-do
ten-dol-y-sis
ten-don
te-nec-to-my
te-nes-mus
ten-nis el-bow
ten-o-de-sis
ten-o-dyn-i-a
ten-o-my-ot-o-my
Tenon's cap-sule
ten-on-i-tis
ten-o-nom-e-ter
ten-o-plas-ty
ten-or-rha-phy
ten-os-to-sis
ten-o-syn-o-vec-to-my
ten-o-syn-o-vi-tis
te-not-o-my
ten-o-vag-i-ni-tis
ten-si-om-e-ter
ten-sion
ten-si-ty
ten-sive
ten-sor
ten-sure
ten-ta-tive
ten-tig-i-nous
ten-to-ri-um
ten-u-ate
ten-u-ous

tep-id
te-rat-ic
ter-a-tism
ter-a-to-car-ci-no-ma
ter-a-tog-e-ny
ter-a-toid
ter-a-tol-o-gy
ter-a-to-ma
ter-a-to-sis
ter-bi-um
te-re
te-res
ter-mi-nal
ter-mi-na-tion
ter-mi-nol-o-gy
ter-na-ry
ter-pene
ter-pin hy-drate
ter-ra
ter-tian
ter-ti-ar-y
tes-ta-ceous
tes-ti-cle
tes-tic-u-lar
tes-tis
tes-tos-te-rone
te-tan-ic
te-tan-i-form
tet-a-nism
tet-a-ni-za-tion
tet-a-no-can-na-bin
tet-a-noid
tet-a-no-ly-sin
tet-a-nus
tet-a-ny
tet-ra-ba-sic
tet-ra-bro-mo-phthal-
ein
tet-ra-caine hy-dro-
chlo-ride
tet-ra-chlo-ro-eth-
ane

tet-ra-chlo-ro-eth-yl-
ene
tet-rad
tet-ra-eth-yl-am-mo-
ni-um
tet-ra-eth-yl-lead
tet-ra-eth-yl-py-ro-
phos-phate
tet-ra-gen-ic
te-trag-e-nous
tet-ra-hy-dro-can-nab-
in-ol
tetralogy of Fallot
tet-ra-nu-cle-o-tide
tet-ra-pep-tide
tet-ra-ple-gi-a
tet-ra-ploid
tet-ra-thi-o-nate
tet-ra-vac-cine
tet-ra-va-lent
tet-ra-zole
tet-rose
te-trox-ide
tex-ti-form
tex-ture
tha-lam-ic
thal-a-mo-cor-ti-cal
thal-a-mo-len-tic-u-
lar
thal-a-mo-mam-mil-lar-y
thal-a-mo-teg-men-tal
thal-a-mot-o-my
thal-a-mus
tha-las-se-mi-a
Tha-lic-trum
thal-li-um
Thal-loph-y-ta
thal-lus
than-a-to-gno-mon-ic
than-a-toid
than-a-to-pho-bi-a
than-a-top-sy

than-a-tos
Thebesian veins
the-ca
the-ci-tis
the-co-dont
the-co-ma
the-e-lin
the-ine
The-la-zi-a
the-le-plas-ty
the-li-tis
the-li-um
the-nar
then-yl-pyr-a-mine
The-o-bro-ma
the-o-bro-mine
the-o-ma-ni-a
the-o-phyl-line
the-o-ret-i-cal
the-o-ry
ther-a-peu-tic
ther-a-peu-tist
ther-a-pist
ther-a-py
therm
ther-mal
therm-es-the-si-a
ther-mic
ther-mite
ther-mo-an-al-ge-si-a
ther-mo-an-es-the-si-a
ther-mo-cau-ter-y
ther-mo-chem-is-try
ther-mo-cou-ple
ther-mo-dy-nam-ics
ther-mo-gen-ic
ther-mo-hy-per-al-ge-si-a
ther-mo-in-hib-i-to-ry
ther-mo-la-bile
ther-mol-y-sis
ther-mo-lyt-ic

ther-mo-mas-sage
ther-mom-e-ter
ther-mo-met-ric
ther-mom-e-try
ther-mo-phile
ther-mo-phil-ic
ther-mo-pho-bi-a
ther-mo-phyl-ic
ther-mo-pile
ther-mo-ple-gi-a
ther-mo-reg-u-la-tion
ther-mo-reg-u-la-tor
ther-mo-sta-ble
ther-mo-stat
ther-mo-tac-tic
ther-mo-tax-is
ther-mo-ther-a-py
ther-mo-tox-in
ther-mot-ro-pism
the-sis
thi-a-min-ase
thi-a-mine
thi-a-zine
thi-a-zole
thigh
thi-mer-o-sal
thi-o-bac-te-ri-a
thi-o-bar-bi-tu-ric ac-id
thi-o-car-ban-i-lide
thi-o-chrome
thi-o-cy-a-nate
thi-ol
thi-o-nine
thi-o-pen-tal so-di-um
thi-o-phil-ic
thi-o-sul-fate
thi-o-u-ra-cil
thi-o-u-re-a
thirst
thix-ot-ro-py
Thomas splint

Thomsen's dis-ease
tho-ra-cec-to-my
tho-ra-cen-te-sis
tho-rac-ic
tho-ra-ci-co-lum-bar
tho-ra-co-a-cro-mi-al
tho-ra-co-lum-bar
tho-ra-cop-a-gus
tho-ra-co-plas-ty
tho-ra-cos-to-my
tho-ra-cot-o-my
tho-rax
tho-ri-um
thorn—ap-ple
tho-ron
thought
thread
thread-worm
three-o-nine
thresh-old
thrill
throat
throb
throe
throm-bec-to-my
throm-bin
throm-bo-an-gi-i-tis ob-lit-er-ans
throm-bo-ar-te-ri-tis
throm-bo-clas-tic
throm-bo-cyte
throm-bo-cyt-ic
throm-bo-cyt-ic se-ries
throm-bo-cy-to-crit
throm-bo-cy-to-pe-ni-a
throm-bo-cy-to-pe-nic pur-pu-ra
throm-bo-cy-to-sis
throm-bo-em-bo-lism
throm-bo-gen-ic
throm-bo-kin-ase
throm-bo-lyt-ic

throm-bo-pe-ni-a
throm-bo-phle-bi-tis
throm-bo-plas-tin
throm-bo-plas-tin-o-gen
throm-bose
throm-bosed
throm-bo-sis
throm-bo-sta-sis
throm-bot-ic
throm-bus
throt-tle
throw-back
thrush
thu-li-um
thyme oil
thy-mec-to-my
thy-mic
thy-mi-co-lym-phat-ic
thy-mi-tis
thy-mol
thy-mo-ma
thy-mus
thy-re-o-gen-ic
thy-ro-ad-e-ni-tis
thy-ro-ar-y-te-noid
thy-ro-ep-i-glot-tic
thy-ro-glob-u-lin
thy-ro-glos-sal
thy-ro-hy-al
thy-ro-hy-oid
thy-roid
thy-roid-ec-to-my
thy-roid-ism
thy-roid-i-tis
thy-ro-par-a-thy-roid-
  ec-to-my
thy-ro-phar-yn-ge-us
thy-ro-pri-val
thy-ro-pro-te-in
thy-ro-ther-a-py
thy-ro-tox-ic
thy-ro-tox-i-co-sis

thy-rot-ro-pin
thy-rox-in
tib-i-a
tib-i-a-lis
tib-i-o-fib-u-lar
tic
tic dou-lou-reux
tick-ling
ti-dal drain-age
ti-groid
tim-bre
tim-o-thy
tinc-tu-ra
tinc-ture
tin-e-a bar-bae
tin-e-a cap-i-tis
tin-e-a cor-po-ris
tin-e-a cru-ris
tin-e-a fa-vo-sa
tin-e-a pe-dis
tin-e-a un-gui-um
tin-e-a ver-si-col-or
tin-gle
tin-ni-tus
Tiselius ap-pa-ra-tus
Tissot gas-om-e-ter
tis-sue
ti-ta-ni-um
ti-ter
tit-il-la-tion
ti-trate
ti-tra-tion
toad-skin
to-bac-co
to-coph-er-ol
to-kog-ra-phy
tok-o-pho-bi-a
tol-er-ance
tol-er-ant
to-lu bal-sam
tol-u-ene
to-lu-i-dine blue

tol-u-ol
to-mo-gram
to-mog-ra-phy
tongue
ton-ic
to-nic-i-ty
ton-i-co-clon-ic
to-no-fi-brils
to-nom-e-ter
ton-sil
ton-sil-lec-to-my
ton-sil-li-tis
ton-sil-lo-lith
ton-sure
to-nus
tooth-ache
toothed
tooth-paste
Topfer's re-a-gent
to-pha-ceous
to-phus
top-i-cal
top-o-an-es-the-si-a
top-o-graph-ic
to-pog-ra-phy
top-ol-o-gy
tor-pid
tor-pid-i-ty
tor-por
torque
tor-sion
tor-so
tor-ti-col-lis
tor-tu-ous
Tor-u-la his-to-lyt-i-ca
tor-u-lo-sis
tor-u-lus
to-rus
tour-ni-quet
tox-a-phene
tox-e-mi-a
tox-e-mic

220

tox-i-cant
tox-ic-i-ty
Tox-i-co-den-dron
tox-i-co-der-ma-ti-tis
tox-i-col-o-gist
tox-i-col-o-gy
tox-i-co-sis
tox-if-er-ous
tox-ig-e-nous
tox-in
tox-in—an-ti-tox-in
tox-oid
tox-o-plas-min
tox-o-plas-mo-sis
tra-bec-u-la
tra-cer
tra-che-a
tra-che-i-tis
tra-che-o-bron-chi-al
tra-che-o-bron-chi-tis
tra-che-o-la-ryn-ge-al
tra-che-o-lar-yn-got-
o-my
tra-che-oph-o-ny
tra-che-os-co-py
tra-che-os-to-my
tra-che-ot-o-mize
tra-che-ot-o-my
tra-cho-ma
trac-ing
tract
trac-tion
trac-tor
trac-tot-o-my
trac-tus
trade-mark
trag-a-canth
tra-gus
trail-er
train-ing
trait
trance

trans-am-i-nase
trans-am-i-na-tion
trans-duc-tion
tran-sec-tion
trans-fer-ence
trans-fix-ion
trans-for-ma-tion
trans-form-er
trans-fuse
trans-fu-sion
tran-sient
trans-il-lu-mi·na-tion
tran-sis-tor
tran-si-tion-al
trans-lu-cent
trans-meth-yl-a-tion
trans-mi-gra-tion
trans-mis-si-ble
trans-mis-sion
trans-mit-tance
trans-mu-ta-tion
trans-par-ent
trans-phos-phor-yl-ase
tran-spi-ra-tion
trans-plant
trans-plan-ta-tion
trans-pose
trans-po-si-tion
tran-su-date
tran-su-da-tion
trans-u-re-thral
trans-vag-i-nal
trans-ver-sa-lis
trans-verse
trans-ver-sus
trans-ves-ti-tism
tra-pe-zi-um
tra-pe-zi-us
trap-e-zoid
Traube's sign
trau-ma
trau-mat-ic

trau-ma-tize
trav-ail
treat-ment
Treitz's lig-a-ment
trem-a-tode
trem-bles
trem-bling
trem-o-lo
trem-or
trem-u-lous
trench foot
trench mouth
Trendelenburg's po-si-
tion
trep-a-nize
tre-phine
tre-phin-ing
trep-i-da-tion
Trep-o-ne-ma pal-li-dum
trep-o-ne-mi-cid-al
tri-ad
tri-age
tri-al
tri-an-gle
tri-an-gu-la-ris
tri-ax-i-al
tri-bro-mo-eth-a-nol
tri-cal-ci-um phos-
phate
tri-ceps
trich-i-a-sis
Trich-i-nel-la
trich-i-no-sis
tri-chlo-ro-a-ce-tic
ac-id
tri-chlo-ro-eth-yl-ene
trich-o-be-zoar
Trich-o-ceph-a-lus
trich-o-cyst
Trich-o-der-ma
trich-o-ep-i-the-li-o-ma
trich-o-glos-si-a

221

trich-o-ma-ni-a
trich-o-ma-to-sis
trich-o-mo-na-cide
Trich-o-mo-nas vag-i-nal-is
Trich-o-my-ce-tes
trich-o-my-co-sis
trich-o-no-sis
trich-oph-a-gy
trich-o-phy-to-be-zoar
Trich-o-phy-ton
trich-o-phy-to-sis
Trich-o-spo-ron
trich-o-til-lo-ma-ni-a
tri-chro-mat-ic
tri-chro-mic
Trich-u-ris trich-i-u-ra
tri-cre-sol
tri-crot-ic
tri-cus-pid
tri-dent
tri-den-tate
tri-eth-a-nol-am-ine
tri-eth-yl-ene gly-col
tri-eth-yl-ene mel-a-mine
tri-fid
tri-gas-tric
tri-gem-i-nal
tri-gem-i-nus
tri-gem-i-ny
tri-glyc-er-ide
tri-gone
tri-go-ni-tis
tri-go-num
tri-i-o-do-thy-ro-nine
tri-lam-i-nar
tri-lo-bate
tri-loc-u-lar
tri-mes-ter
tri-meth-a-di-one
tri-mor-phism

tri-ni-tro-phe-nol
tri-ni-tro-tol-u-ene
tri-ose
tri-pep-tide
tri-pha-sic
tri-phos-pho-pyr-i-dine nu-cle-o-tide
trip-le point
trip-le re-sponse
trip-let
trip-sis
tri-que-trum
tri-sac-cha-ride
tris-mus
tri-so-mic
tris-tis
trit-i-a-tion
trit-i-um
trit-u-rate
trit-u-ra-tion
tri-va-lent
tri-valv-u-lar
tro-car
tro-chan-ter
tro-che
troch-le-a
troch-le-ar
troch-o-gin-gly-mus
tro-choid
Trom-bic-u-la
Trom-bid-i-um
tro-pane
tro-phe-de-ma
troph-ic
troph-ism
tro-pho-blast
tro-pho-derm
tro-pho-zo-ite
trop-i-cal
trop-in
tro-pism
tro-po-sphere

Trousseau's sign
trun-cat-ed
trun-cus
truss
try-pan-o-ci-dal
Tryp-a-no-so-ma cru-zi
Tryp-a-no-so-ma gam-bi-en-se
Tryp-a-no-so-ma rho-de-si-en-se
tryp-a-no-so-mi-a-sis
tryp-ars-a-mide
tryp-sin
tryp-sin-o-gen
tryp-to-phan
tset-se fly
tsut-su-ga-mush-i dis-ease
tu-bage
tu-bal
tu-bec-to-my
tu-ber
tu-ber-cle
tu-ber-cu-lar
tu-ber-cu-lid
tu-ber-cu-lin
tu-ber-cu-loid
tu-ber-cu-lo-ma
tu-ber-cu-lo-pro-te-in
tu-ber-cu-lo-sis
tu-ber-cu-lous
tu-ber-cu-lum
tu-ber-os-i-ty
tu-bo-cu-ra-rine
tu-bo—o-va-ri-an
tu-bo-u-ter-ine
tu-bu-lar
tu-bule
tu-bu-lo-al-ve-o-lar
tu-bu-lo-rac-e-mose
tu-bu-lus
tu-bus

tug-ging
tu-la-re-mia
tum-bu fly
tu-me-fa-cient
tu-me-fac-tion
tu-mes-cence
tu-mes-cent
tu-mid
tu-mid-i-ty
tu-mor
tu-mor-ous
tu-mul-tus
Tun-ga
tun-gi-a-sis
tung-sten
tu-nic
tu-ni-ca
tu-ning fork
tun-nel
tur-bid
tur-bi-dim-e-ter
tur-bi-nate
tur-bi-nec-to-my
tur-ges-cence
tur-ges-cent
tur-gid
tur-gor
turn-ing
tur-pen-tine
tur-tle
tus-sal
tus-sis
tus-sive
tweez-ers
twi-light sleep
twinge
twin-ning
twitch-ing
ty-lo-ma
ty-lo-sis
tym-pan-ic nerve
tym-pa-ni-tes

tym-pa-nit-ic
tym-pa-ni-tis
tym-pa-ny
Tyndall ef-fect
typh-li-tis
ty-phoid
ty-phus
typ-i-cal
ty-ping
ty-ra-mine
ty-rant
tyr-an-ny
ty-rem-e-sis
ty-rog-e-nous
ty-ro-sin-ase
ty-ro-sine
ty-ro-thri-cin
Tyrrell's hook

U

u-cam-bin
ud-der
ul-cer
ul-cer-ate
ul-cer-a-tion
ul-cer-a-tive
ul-cer-o-mem-bra-nous
ul-cus
u-li-tis
ul-na
ul-nar
u-loid
u-lo-sis
u-lot-ic
ul-ti-mo-bran-chi-al
ul-tra-cen-tri-fuge
ul-tra-fil-ter
ul-tra-fil-tra-tion
ul-tra-mi-cro-scope

ul-tra-mi-cros-cop-y
ul-tra-red
ul-tra-son-ic
ul-tra-son-o-scope
ul-tra-struc-ture
ul-tra-vi-rus
um-ber
um-bi-lec-to-my
um-bil-i-cal
um-bil-i-cate
um-bil-i-ca-tion
um-bil-i-cus
um-bo
un-ci-form
Un-ci-na-ri-a
un-ci-na-ri-a-sis
un-ci-nate
un-con-scious
un-con-scious-ness
unc-tion
unc-tu-ous
un-cus
un-dec-y-len-ic ac-id
un-der-weight
un-do-ing
un-du-lant fe-ver
un-du-la-tion
un-du-la-to-ry
un-guen-tum
un-guis
un-gual
un-gu-late
un-health-y
u-ni-ar-tic-u-lar
u-ni-cam-er-al
u-ni-cel-lu-lar
u-ni-cen-tral
u-ni-cus-pid
u-ni-fi-lar
u-ni-lat-er-al
u-ni-loc-u-lar
u-ni-oc-u-lar

un-ion
u-ni-ov-u-lar
u-nip-a-rous
u-ni-po-lar
u-ni-po-ten-tial
u-ni-sex-u-al
u-nit
u-ni-tar-y
u-ni-va-lent
u-ni-ver-sal do-nor
Un-na's paste boot
un-of-fi-cial
un-or-gan-ized
un-rest
un-sat-u-ra-ted
un-sound
un-stri-a-ted
un-u-ni-ted
un-well
u-ra-chus
u-ra-cil
u-ra-gogue
u-ran-i-nite
u-ra-ni-um
u-ra-no-plas-ty
u-ra-no-ple-gi-a
u-ra-nor-rha-phy
u-ra-nos-chi-sis
u-ra-no-staph-y-lor-
  rha-phy
u-ra-nyl
u-rate
u-ra-te-mi-a
u-ra-tu-ri-a
ur-ban-i-za-tion
u-re-a
u-re-ase
u-re-mi-a
u-re-sis
u-re-ter
u-re-ter-ec-to-my
u-re-ter-i-tis

u-re-ter-o-cele
u-re-ter-o-co-los-to-
  my
u-re-ter-o-cys-tic
u-re-ter-o-cys-tos-
  to-my
u-re-ter-o-en-ter-os-
  to-my
u-re-ter-og-ra-phy
u-re-ter-o-hy-dro-ne-
  phro-sis
u-re-ter-o—in-tes-ti-
  nal a-nas-to-mo-sis
u-re-ter-o-li-thi-a-
  sis
u-re-ter-o-li-thot-o-my
u-re-ter-o-ne-phrec-to-
  my
u-re-ter-o-pel-vic
u-re-ter-o-plas-ty
u-re-ter-o-py-e-li-tis
u-re-ter-o-py-e-log-
  ra-phy
u-re-ter-o-py-e-lo-ne-.
  phri-tis
u-re-ter-o-py-e-lo-plas-
  ty
u-re-ter-os-to-my
u-re-ter-ot-o-my
u-re-ter-o-u-ter-ine
u-re-ter-o-vag-i-nal
u-re-thra
u-re-threc-to-my
u-re-thri-tis
u-re-thro-bulb-ar
u-re-thro-cele
u-re-thro-cys-ti-tis
u-re-thro-gram
u-re-throg-ra-phy
u-re-thro-plas-ty
u-re-thro-pro-stat-ic
u-re-thro-scope

u-re-thros-co-py
u-re-thro-spasm
u-re-thro-ste-no-sis
u-re-thro-tome
u-re-throt-o-my
u-re-thro-tri-go-ni-tis
u-re-thro-vag-i-nal
ur-gen-cy
u-ric ac-id
u-ric-ac-i-du-ri-a
u-ri-ce-mi-a
u-ri-cos-u-ri-a
u-ri-cos-u-ric
u-ri-nal
u-ri-nal-y-sis
u-ri-nate
u-ri-na-tion
u-rine
u-ri-nif-er-ous
u-ri-nip-a-rous
u-ri-nom-e-ter
u-ri-nous
u-ro-bi-lin
u-ro-bi-li-ne-mi-a
u-ro-bi-lin-o-gen
u-ro-bi-li-noi-din
u-ro-bi-li-nu-ri-a
u-ro-chrome
u-ro-cy-an-o-gen
u-ro-cy-a-no-sis
u-ro-fla-vin
u-ro-fus-cin
u-ro-gen-i-tal
u-rog-e-nous
u-ro-gram
u-rog-ra-phy
u-ro-lith
u-ro-li-thi-a-sis
u-ro-lith-ot-o-my
u-rol-o-gist
u-rol-o-gy
u-ron-ic ac-id

u-rop-a-thy
u-ro-por-phy-rin
u-ros-co-pist
u-ros-co-py
u-ro-tox-ic
u-ro-xan-thin
ur-ti-ca-ri-a
ur-ti-ca-ri-al
ur-ti-cate
ur-ti-ca-tion
us-ti-lag-i-nism
u-ter-al-gi-a
u-ter-ine
u-ter-is-mus
u-ter-i-tis
u-ter-o-ab-dom-i-nal
u-ter-o-cer-vi-cal
u-ter-o-col-ic
u-ter-og-ra-phy
u-ter-o-in-tes-ti-nal
u-ter-o—o-va-ri-an
u-ter-o-pel-vic
u-ter-o-pex-y
u-ter-o-pla-cen-tal
u-ter-o-plas-ty
u-ter-o-rec-tal
u-ter-o-sa-cral
u-ter-o-sal-pin-gog-ra-phy
u-ter-o-ton-ic
u-ter-o-tu-bal
u-ter-o-vag-i-nal
u-ter-o-ves-i-cal
u-ter-us
Uthoff's sign
u-tri-cle
u-tric-u-li-tis
u-tric-u-lus
u-ve-a
u-ve-al
u-ve-i-tis
u-ve-o-par-o-ti-tis

u-vu-la
u-vu-lec-to-my
u-vu-li-tis
u-vu-lot-o-my

V

vac-ci-nal
vac-ci-nate
vac-ci-na-tion
vac-cine
vac-cin-i-a
vac-cin-i-form
vac-cin-i-o-la
vac-ci-noid
vac-ci-no-ther-a-py
vac-u-o-lar
vac-u-o-la-ted
vac-u-o-la-tion
vac-u-ole
vac-u-um
va-gal
va-gal es-cape
va-gi-na
vag-i-nal
vag-i-nec-to-my
vag-i-nis-mus
vag-i-ni-tis
vag-i-no-my-co-sis
vag-i-no-plas-ty
vag-i-not-o-my
va-gi-tus u-ter-in-us
va-got-o-mized
va-got-o-my
va-go-ton-ic
va-go-trop-ic
va-grant
va-gus
va-lence

va-le-ri-an
va-ler-ic ac-id
val-gus
val-ine
val-late
val-lec-u-la
Valsalva's test
valve
val-vot-o-my
val-vu-la
val-vu-lar
val-vu-li-tis
val-vu-lo-tome
val-vu-lot-o-my
vam-pire
va-na-di-um
Van Allen belt
Van de Graaff gen-er-a-tor
van den Bergh's test
va-nil-la
van-il-lin
Van Slyke's meth-od
va-por
va-por-i-za-tion
va-por-i-zer
va-ri-a-bil-i-ty
va-ri-a-ble
va-ri-ance
va-ri-ant
va-ri-a-tion
var-i-ca-tion
var-i-cec-to-my
var-i-cel-la
var-i-cel-li-form
var-i-ces
va-ric-i-form
var-i-co-cele
var-i-co-ce-lec-to-my
var-i-cog-ra-phy
var-i-coid
var-i-co-phle-bi-tis

var-i-cose
var-i-cos-i-ty
var-i-cot-o-my
va-ri-e-ty
va-ri-form
va-ri-o-la
va-ri-o-lar
var-i-o-late
var-i-o-li-form
var-i-o-loid
va-ri-o-lo-vac-cine
var-ix
va-rus
va-sa va-sor-um
va-sa def-er-ens
vas-cu-lar
vas-cu-lar-i-ty
vas-cu-lar-i-za-tion
vas-ec-to-my
vas-i-tis
vas-o-con-stric-tion
vas-o-con-stric-tive
vas-o-con-stric-tor
vas-o-de-pres-sor
vas-o-dil-a-ta-tion
vas-o-di-la-tor
va-sog-ra-phy
vas-o-in-hib-i-tor
vas-o-li-ga-tion
vas-o-mo-tor
vas-o-pa-ral-y-sis
vas-o-pres-sin
vas-o-re-lax-a-tion
vas-or-rha-phy
vas-o-sec-tion
vas-o-spasm
vas-o-stim-u-lant
vas-ot-o-my
vas-o-ton-ic
vas-o-to-nin
vas-o-va-gal
vas-tus

vault
vec-tor
vec-tor-car-di-o-gram
vec-tor-car-di-o-graph
veg-e-tal
veg-e-ta-tion
ve-hi-cle
veil
vein
vel-a-men-tous
vel-a-men-tum
vel-li-ca-tion
Vel-peau's band-age
ve-lum
ve-na ca-va
ve-na-tion
ven-ec-to-my
ven-e-nif-er-ous
ve-ne-re-al
ve-ne-re-ol-o-gy
ven-e-sec-tion
ven-i-punc-ture
ve-noc-ly-sis
ve-no-gram
ven-og-ra-phy
ven-om
ven-om-ous
ve-no-per-i-to-ne-os-to-my
ve-no-scle-ro-sis
ve-nos-i-ty
ve-no-sta-sis
ve-not-o-my
ve-nous
ve-no-ve-nos-to-my
vent
ven-ti-late
ven-ti-la-tion
ven-ti-lom-e-ter
ven-tral
ven-tri-cle
ven-tric-u-lar

ven-tric-u-li-tis
ven-tric-u-lo-gram
ven-tric-u-log-ra-phy
ven-tric-u-lom-e-try
ven-tric-u-lo-punc-
ture
ven-tric-u-los-to-my
ven-tric-u-lus
ven-tri-duc-tion
ven-tril-o-quism
ven-tri-me-sal
ven-tro-lat-er-al
ven-tro-me-di-an
ven-tu-ri tube
ven-ule
ve-nus
ve-ra-trum vi-ri-de
ver-big-er-a-tion
ver-di-gris
ver-do-he-min
ver-gen-ces
ver-gens
ver-ger prism
Verhoeff's op-er-a-tion
ver-mi-ci-dal
ver-mi-cide
ver-mic-u-lar
ver-mic-u-late
ver-mic-u-la-tion
ver-mic-u-lose
ver-mic-u-lus
ver-mi-form
ver-mi-fuge
ver-min
ver-min-ous
ver-mis
ver-ni-er
ver-nix ca-se-o-sa
ver-ru-ca a-cu-mi-na-ta
ver-ru-ca plan-tar-is
ver-ru-ca se-nil-is
ver-ru-ca vul-gar-is

226

ver-ru-ci-form
ver-ru-cous
ver-si-col-or
ver-sion
ver-te-bra
Ver-te-bra-ta
ver-te-brate
ver-te-brec-to-my
ver-tex
ver-ti-cal
ver-tig-i-nous
ver-ti-go
ver-u-mon-ta-num
ver-i-ca
ves-i-cal
ves-i-cant
ves-i-ca-tion
ves-i-ca-to-ry
ves-i-cle
ves-i-co-pro-stat-ic
ves-i-cot-o-my
ves-i-co-u-ter-ine
ve-sic-u-la
ve-sic-u-lar
ve-sic-u-la-tion
ve-sic-u-li-tis
ve-sic-u-lo-bul-lous
ve-sic-u-lo-pap-u-lar
ve-sic-u-lo-pus-tu-lar
ves-sel
ves-tib-u-lar
ves-ti-bule
ves-tige
ves-tig-i-al
ves-tig-i-um
vet-er-i-na-ri-an
vet-er-i-nar-y
vi-a-ble
vi-al
vi-brate
vi-bra-tion
vi-bra-tor

vi-bra-to-ry
Vib-ri-o com-ma
vi-bris-sa
vi-car-i-ous
vi-cious
vid-e-og-no-sis
Vidian ar-ter-y
vig-il
vig-i-lance
vil-lous
vil-lus
Vincent's an-gi-na
vin-e-gar
vi-nyl
vi-o-la-tion
vi-o-let
vi-o-my-cin
vi-per
Vi-per-i-dae
Virchow's node
vi-re-mi-a
vir-gin
vir-gin-al
vir-gin-i-um
vir-ile
vir-i-lism
vi-ril-i-ty
vi-rol-o-gist
vi-rol-o-gy
vir-u-lence
vir-u-lent
vi-rus
vis
vis-ce-ra
vis-cer-op-to-sis
vis-cer-o-sen-so-ry
vis-cid
vis-co-sim-e-ter
vis-cos-i-ty
vis-cous
vis-cus
vis-i-bil-i-ty

vis-i-ble
vi-sion
vis-u-al
vis-u-al-i-za-tion
vis-u-o-psy-chic
vis-u-o-sen-so-ry
vi-tal
vi-tal-ism
vi-tal-i-ty
vi-tal-ize
vi-tals
vi-ta-mer
vi-ta-min
vi-tel-lin
vi-tel-lus
vi-ti-a-tion
vit-i-lig-i-nes
vit-i-li-go
vit-re-ous
vi-tres-cence
vit-re-um
vit-ric
vit-ri-ol-ic
vit-ri-tis
vit-rum
viv-i-dif-fu-sion
viv-i-fi-ca-tion
vi-vip-a-rous
viv-i-sec-tion
viv-i-sec-tion-ist
viv-i-sec-tor
Vleminckx's so-lu-tion
vo-cal
vo-ca-lis
voice
void
vo-lar
vol-a-tile
vo-le-mic
vo-li-tion
Volkmann's pa-ral-y-sis
vol-ley

227

vol-age
vol-ta-ic
volt-am-me-ter
volt-me-ter
vol-ume
vol-u-met-ric
vol-un-tar-y
vol-vu-lus
vo-mer
vom-it
vom-it-ing
vom-i-tive
vom-i-to-ry
vom-i-tus
von Economo's dis-ease
Voorhees bag
vo-ra-cious
vor-tex
vor-ti-cose
vo-yeur
vo-yeur-ism
vu-e-rom-e-ter
vul-can-ize
vul-ner-a-ble
vul-va
vul-vec-to-my
vul-vi-tis
vul-vo-vag-i-ni-tis

wad-ding
wad-dle
wa-fer
waist-line
wake-ful-ness
Waldeyer's ring
walk-ing i-ron
Wallerian de-gen-er-a-
    tion

wall-eye
wan-der-ing
Wangensteen's tube
war-bles
war-far-in
wart
Wasserman test
wa-ter
Waterhouse—
    Friderichsen
    syn-drome
wa-ter moc-ca-sin
wa-ters
watt
watt-me-ter
wave-length
weav-ers' bot-tom
Weber's test
Wechsler—Bellevue in-
    tel-li-gence scale
weep-ing
Weidel re-ac-tion
weight
Weil's dis-ease
Weil—Felix test
wen
Wenckebach's phe-
    nom-e-non
Werdnig—Hoffmann
    syn-drome
Wernicke's sign
Wertheim's op-er-a-tion
Westergren meth-od
wet-ting a-gent
Wetzel's grid
Wharton's duct
wheal
Wheat-stone bridge
wheeze
whey
whiff
Whipple's dis-ease

Whipple's op-er-a-tion
whip-worm
whis-per
Whitfield's oint-ment
whit-low
whoop-ing cough
wick-ing
Widal test
Wigand's ma-neu-ver
Wilms's tu-mor
Wilson's dis-ease
wind-lass
win-dow
wind-pipe
wine spot
win-ter-green
Wintrobe meth-od
wir-ing
Wirsung's duct
wir-y
wis-dom teeth
witch ha-zel
witch's milk
with-draw-al
Wolff—Parkinson—White
    syn-drome
wolfs-bane
womb
Wood's light
wood al-co-hol
wool fat
word blind-ness
word sal-ad
Wormian bones
wound
Wright's stain
wrin-kles
wrist
wry-neck
Wuch-er-er-i-a ban-
    crof-ti
wuch-er-e-ri-a-sis

X

xan-tha-line
xan-the-las-ma
xan-thene
xan-thine
xan-tho-chro-mat-ic
xan-tho-chro-mic
xan-tho-der-ma
xan-tho-gran-u-lo-ma-to-sis
xan-tho-ma
xan-tho-ma-to-sis
xan-thom-a-tous
xan-tho-pro-te-in
xan-thop-si-a
xan-thop-ter-in
xan-thor-rhe-a
xan-tho-sis
xe-nol-o-gy
xe-non
xen-oph-thal-mi-a
xe-no-plas-ty
xe-ran-tic
xe-ro-der-ma
xe-roph-thal-mi-a
xe-ro-sis
xe-ro-sto-mi-a
xe-rot-ic
xiph-i-ster-nal
xiph-o-cos-tal
xiph-oid
xiph-o-ster-nal crunch

x—ray
xy-lan
xy-lene
xy-len-ol
xy-lol
xy-lose

Y

yawn-ing
yaws
yeast
yel-low
yo-him-bine
yolk sac
Young's op-er-a-tion
y-per-ite
Y—plas-ty
yt-ter-bi-um
yt-tri-um

Z

ze-in
Zenker's fix-ing flu-id
ze-o-lite
ze-ro
Ziehl—Neelsen stain
zinc ox-ide oint-ment
Zinn's lig-a-ment
Zinsser's a-gar slant

zir-co-ni-um
zo-na
zone
zon-es-the-si-a
zon-ule
zon-u-li-tis
zo-o-ge-og-ra-phy
zo-ol-o-gist
zo-ol-o-gy
zo-o-no-sis
zo-o-par-a-site
zo-o-phyte
zo-o-plas-ty
zos-ter
zos-ter-i-form
Z—plas-ty
zwit-ter-i-on
Zy-ga-de-nus ve-nen-o-sus
zy-ga-poph-y-sis
zy-go-ma
zy-go-mat-ic
zy-go-mat-i-co-fa-cial
zy-go-mat-i-co-tem-po-ral
zy-go-mat-i-cus
zy-go-my-ce-tes
zy-gote
zy-mase
zy-mo-gen
zy-mo-gen-ic
zy-mo-hy-drol-y-sis
zy-mol-o-gy
zy-mo-phor-ic
zy-mo-pro-te-in
zy-mo-sis